NURSING
SUPERVISION

Lee Hand

NURSING
SUPERVISION

Reston Publishing Company, Inc.
A Prentice-Hall Company
Reston, Virginia

Library of Congress Cataloging in Publication Data

Hand, Lee
  Nursing supervision.

  Includes index.
  1. Nursing service administration.   2. Supervision
of employees.   I. Title.   [DNLM: 1. Nursing,
Supervisory.   WY105 H236n]
RT89.H36   362.1'7   80–18509
ISBN 0–8359–5044–1
ISBN 0–8359–5043–3 pbk.

© 1981 by Reston Publishing Company, Inc.
A Prentice-Hall Company
Reston, Virginia 22090

10   9   8   7   6   5   4   3   2   1

PRINTED IN THE UNITED STATES OF AMERICA

To Bruce,
who knew I could do it

Contents

Contents

Contents

ix

Preface

Because the public forms an opinion of health care by those administering direct patient care, the obligation of every supervisor is to have all the skills necessary to lead others to perform to their maximum efficiency. This goal can be accomplished only through sound knowledge of management and supervision. Yet the problem with learning supervision is trying to limit the subject to a manageable size. There is so much to learn for good supervision that the supervisor feels overwhelmed. New information appears every day, and it seems impossible to keep up. Although those in industry have studied the principles of management and applied them to train new supervisors, nurses have not always studied management as a science. Only now are they beginning to apply the industrial principles of management to their profession. For this reason, the text not only gives you a basis of the principles of management, but it also uses these principles to enable you to integrate this information with your own experience. In fact, the primary emphasis is on applying this newly gained knowledge to your own experience. You are asked to learn in an active, rather than in a passive way.

The entire text is action-oriented. Students generate their own data through the use of discussion questions, problem-solving situations, role playing, questionnaires, programmed learning lessons, and thought-provoking questions. Students are encouraged to think in terms of their own experience and to relate this experience to learning leadership behaviors that can improve their own leadership style. The use of questionnaires helps students share and record personal problems, as well as to find solutions to these problems through sound problem-solving techniques. Some of the applications are perfect for a classroom setting, but most can be done independently.

In many texts on supervision, you are the passive learner, simply reading material that may or may not apply to you. In this text, you can take an active part. Your participation in the exercises puts you in the role of an active learner. Your initial response to this type of situation may be one of confusion or anxiety because an entirely new role is asked of you. With some application, however, your feelings will change to excitement, challenge, and confidence. The best supervisors are aware of the major responsibility of their role, and they feel confident of their ability to handle it.

The study of supervision cannot provide rules, formulas, or methods to solve all problems or to handle all situations. Yet the study of supervision can provide you with the tools necessary to apply managerial and supervisory principles to a specific situation and to deal with it in an intelligent and rational way. Although the study of leadership behavior is sometimes presented in black and white terms, supervisors know that they live and work in a "gray" world. Serious students learn, apply, and practice those skills necessary to function in that world. Students who are willing to participate in the learning experience and to transform principles into techniques that work for a given circumstance become supervisors who are assets to health care.

The goal of this text is to teach the student *foresight*. In other words, the students learn to anticipate the results of their behavior and then behave in a way to achieve the desired results. Supervisors manipulate subordinates' behavior to reach the goal of the organization through the use of administrative principles. Sneaky? Yes, but effective.

ACKNOWLEDGMENTS

The writing of a textbook is never accomplished alone, and I owe thanks to many individuals for their help and encouragement.

This book would not be a reality without the input of the hundreds of nurses who shared their accomplishments and problems with me in the many supervisory classes and seminars held throughout the country. I always maintain that I learn more at each class than the students, and it is this knowledge that I share. Merced Community Medical Center must be singled out as a real training ground for my management theories.

I owe a real debt of gratitude to the University of LaVerne and especially to Jerry Ford for letting me "try my wings." My thanks go to Peggy Bivens for the many hours of typing and retyping, and to Brian Shepard for his art work. The major push to write, and my biggest encouragement, came from my husband Bruce. I thank him and my boys for believing in me and for putting up with my work hours.

LEE HAND

1

Introduction to nursing supervision

Good supervision is one of the cornerstones of successful nursing operations. No health agency, regardless of the size or scope of its operations, can function at maximum efficiency without a high quality of supervisory control and coordination among all personnel.

Professionalization of nursing services is one of the most pressing problems facing our modern, highly complex society today. Only a highly professional body of nurses can cope with the complicated problems and pressures imposed by society and by the various groups concerned with health care. The specialization of health care services and multiplicity of personnel have presented a whole new series of problems to the nurse practitioner and nurse administrator. Solutions to these problems will not be simple, and seeking solutions is a primary responsibility of nursing management. Proper implementation of policy and procedure rests with the supervisors, and thus the supervisory role takes on added significance and importance.

The public view of health care is largely determined by the way the average person sees nurses, usually the most visible persons in health care. We are all familiar with the "horror stories" of patients and families concerning their care in a particular institution. Most of these stories deal directly with the role of nurses. A major responsibility of supervisors is to see that the actions of nursing personnel create a favorable impression of our profession. Supervisors have the task of realizing the importance of public relations and of impressing upon staffs their vital role as "public relations experts."

Due to the emotional state of patients, their families, and friends, we do not ordinarily deal with people who are functioning at their emotional and intellectual best. Illness is frightening—a threat to the well-being of both the patient and the family. This threat impairs the patient's ability to function rationally, and the individual is generally unable to cope with the myriad problems associated with illness. As supervisors, we must deal with people on this level, meeting their psychological as well as their physical needs.

Another major problem facing the nursing supervisor today is a lack of training and education. Due to the rapidly expanding population, the increased number of health care agencies, the rapid turnover rate in hospitals, and the numerous educational preparation programs, the supervisor is sometimes "caught in the middle." Most training institutions are so pressed by tight finances and tight schedules that leadership or supervisory training is either ignored or skimmed over. In nurse's training, learning leadership behavior usually means learning the functional tasks involved in leadership roles, not the attitudes and attributes necessary to lead others. Simply "playing the role" of team leader, head nurse, or supervisor, even with the guidance and support of an instructor, is not adequate instruction to take over these responsibilities in health care upon graduation. With the majority of health care agencies relying heavily on auxiliary personnel, the registered nurse is usually placed in a position of authority within months of graduation. Also, because of the rapidly expanding population, new health care agencies are springing up almost overnight. Each of these agencies needs supervisors, and more and more nurses are being asked to function in this role.

Yet expertise in nursing does not necessarily mean expertise in supervision. These new leaders are still learning the skills necessary to be proficient nurses, much less leaders. Many nurses are promoted to a level of authority *because* they are already proficient nurses. (It is well known that the best nurses are usually the ones that are promoted, so we see many skilled practitioners elevated to management roles.) These nurses, although skilled, do not always possess the leadership behaviors necessary to guide others.

The turnover rate in hospitals and in other health care agencies is very rapid, and many supervisors are promoted just because they have seniority. Although experience is one of the qualities of a good leader, it does not automatically mean success. As supervisors, persons must develop an entirely new concept of the work process. They must see the responsibility of the job as accomplishing work through others instead of doing it personally.

We are therefore faced with an army of nurses in supervisory roles who lack the specific education and training for the functions they are performing. Leadership is a learned function—one that requires practice to achieve excellence.

Even experienced supervisors face their own set of problems in today's health care setting. With specialization the rule rather than the exception, they are called upon to supervise others in tasks for which they may not be skilled. This requirement makes managerial skills even more important, for nurses trained in management and supervision can guide and direct others no matter which function they are performing. "Managerial skills" does not mean that supervisors need know only how to lead and forget all the principles of nursing; rather, it means that they must learn the management function in addition to their basic nursing knowledge.

Supervisors become the "rag dolls" in the health care industry. They are the links between the nursing staff and the management of the hospital. These two factions pull in opposite directions, and supervisors feel allegiance to each group. They feel as though they are being "pulled apart." Supervisors—new or experienced—must learn to deal with these feelings of being in the middle in order to accomplish the goals of the health care agency. Many nurses, forced into positions of authority without proper training, feel left out. They no longer belong to the comfortable group of the nursing staff, and they don't really belong to management. Old friendships are lost, and new ones are difficult to develop because of the tremendous responsibility of leading others.

All these problems point up the need to teach leadership as a science. Supervisors must know themselves, their goals, their interests, their emotions, their personalities. They must feel comfortable with themselves as persons in order to move into the role of supervisor.

THE RESPONSIBILITIES
OF THE SUPERVISOR

Supervision is an exacting job that includes many duties and responsibilities. Some of these are:

1. understanding the role of supervision, specifically the many behaviors that are lumped together under the title of "leader";
2. making sure that all subordinates are qualified for the tasks they are performing, and training subordinates to carry out these tasks;
3. knowing their place in the organization, how to enforce the lines of authority and make them work;
4. developing an appreciation of modern methods of handling people;
5. enforcing the rules of the organization and making sure that all subordinates strive to achieve the organizational objectives.

These concepts, as well as others that complete the role of supervisor, are discussed in depth in subsequent chapters. In this text, the phrase *health care* includes all persons who are actively engaged in nursing, preventative health care, and the care and treatment of illness. The term *supervisor* is used to apply to all persons who guide and direct the activities of others. Since all nurses are placed in such a role in many ways every day, leadership principles apply to every nurse in every health care setting. The specific tasks necessary to function in positions of authority vary according to the level of authority, the size of the agency, the specialization of the nursing function, and the policies of the specific health care agency. For this reason, leadership attitudes and behaviors are taught, rather than specific tasks.

DISCUSSION QUESTIONS

1. Why is good supervision essential to health care?
2. What are some of the major problems facing supervisors today?
3. Why is "professional expertise" not a good basis for promotion?
4. What is a supervisor, and what is his or her role in health care?

APPLICATION: ORGANIZATIONAL SOCIALIZATION

Objectives

- To introduce the concept of the psychological contract.
- To articulate and share your expectations of the learning experience provided in this text book.
- To identify problem areas based on conflicting expectations of your role in management, and the expectations of your health care agency.
- To resolve any of these conflict areas.

Introduction

When you join a specific agency, the terms of employment do not always spell out the expected behaviors in terms of psychological commitment. A psychological contract is a contract formed between the individual and the organization of which he or she is a member. Not always written in terms of goals and expectations, this contract deals with your expectations of the organization, and the organization's expectations of you as a supervisor. It is a written record of the goals and expectations, that define the dynamic, changing relationship necessary for mutually shared goals. This contract should be one that is always in a state of flux, continually being renegotiated as your needs, and the needs of the organization, change.

This exercise deals with such areas. If an individual expects too much of the health care agency, which is unable to meet these needs, he or she feels cheated. On the other hand, a person who refuses to meet the organization's standards is a stumbling block, and no growth can take place. The writing of a psychological contract leaves room for growth and increased creativity. The goals of the individual and those of the health care agency mutually influence each other. High expectations on the agency's part can produce increased individual contribution, and this increases your personal growth and learning.[1]

Activity—Part I

Students will evaluate and list their expectations for this educational experience. They will analyze what they hope to learn, and how this learning can be put to use in their health care agencies.

1. What are your goals for this learning experience (to learn theories, to practice new behaviors, to achieve a promotion, and so on)?

2. In what ways do you feel you can achieve these goals?

3. What are your personal resources for this study?

Activity—Part II

Students will assess the needs of the organization, as well as how they can best meet these needs.

1. What does your health care agency expect in a supervisor?

[1] David Kolb, Irwin Rubin, and James M. McIntyre, *Organizational Psychology: An Experiential Approach* (Englewood Cliffs, N.J.: Prentice-Hall, Inc., 1971), pp. 7–17. Reprinted by permission of Prentice-Hall, Inc.

2. What skills do you need to learn in order to meet the needs of your health care agency?

3. How can the study of management and supervision help your organization?

Activity—Part III

Student will identify any conflict areas and try to resolve them.

1. In which areas do your goals and those of the organization differ?

2. What steps must be taken to resolve these conflicts?

3. In what way can this learning experience help you to resolve these conflicts?

REFERENCES

DRUCKER, PETER F., *Management: Tasks, Responsibilities, Practices.* New York: Harper & Row, Publishers, Inc., 1973.

GULICK, LUTHER, "Management Is a Science," *Journal of the Academy of Management* (March 1965).

KOONTZ, HAROLD AND O'DONNELL, CYRIL, *Principles of Management,* 5th ed. New York: McGraw-Hill Book Company, 1972.

MELNICOE, WILLIAM B., AND JOHN P. PEPER, *Supervisory Personnel Development.* Sacramento, Cal.: California State Department of Education, 1965.

MINER, JOHN, *The Management Process.* New York: Macmillan, Inc., 1973.

PFIFFNER, JOHN M. AND MARSHALL FELS, *The Supervision of Personnel,* 3rd ed. Englewood Cliffs, N.J.: Prentice-Hall, Inc., 1964.

2

Health delivery organizations

THE NEED FOR MANAGER/TECHNICIANS

The American health care system has entered a "crisis" period. Some of the symptoms of its illness are the rising cost of health care, shortages in and the poor distribution of many kinds of personnel, and the lack of consumer participation in the decisions that control health care. A particularly ironic symptom is the ineffective use of health care delivery systems. Although the United States has the best trained health care professionals, our health care delivery by no means measures up. At a time when research and technology are at an all-time high, consumer dissatisfaction is also at a peak.

Answers to the health care problem come from everywhere. These solutions run the gamut from a "do-nothing-because-nothing-is-wrong" attitude to total government regulation. Since the solution probably lies in the middle ground between these extremes, we must realize that there is indeed a problem; ignoring it will not make it go away. The health care crisis will not disappear because nurses complain, rebel, and perhaps leave the profession because they feel "unfulfilled." The only solution is to use the health care systems in existence—and learn to "manage" them.

All health care facilities are staffed by highly skilled and professional workers. The administration of health care has always required great knowledgeability and proficiency of its practitioners. The problem is that the health care industry is managed by skilled technicians, not by professional managers. Because a skilled manager must be trained specifically in the tasks and behaviors necessary in management, a person who is a good physician, nurse, or technologist is not necessarily an effective manager. The effective physician, nurse, or technologist, however, who trains to be a skilled manager not only has the best of both worlds, but is also a real asset to health care.

Persons with management responsibility see the danger in failing to manage effectively, and they also see the opportunity that such know-how gives them. The responsibility of any nurses in a management role is to know as much about that function as they know about the patient care role. One of the comments often made by nurses in a supervisory role is that they miss "nursing" and wish they could stop pushing papers and go back to patient care. This desire is fine, if it is really what the nurse wants, but it is usually not the problem at all. Too many nurses lose sight of the fact that the supervision and management of nursing services is "nursing" too. Just as bathing or medicating patients is essential to their well-being, so are the myriad functions of management necessary to the care and well-being of recovering patients. We are all parts of a whole. Each of us does a task so that the common goal can be reached.

Pushing papers? Perhaps, but without those papers, there would be no quality nursing care. As a supervisor, your responsibility is to your employer, to the health care agency. The organization that hired you and that pays your salary expects you to work toward meeting its goals and objectives.

THE BASIC PURPOSE OF HEALTH CARE AGENCIES

The purpose of most health care agencies is to serve the health care needs of the public. An agency may meet these needs in a variety of ways: administering patient care, patient education, education of future health care workers, research into better care and treatment, and protection of the general public from further illness. The emphasis is determined by the type of agency. No matter which type of health care agency employs you and no matter what its emphasis, you must know its goals and work with all your effort to meet those goals. All organizations are slightly different, but they all share four common elements:

1. *equipment*—those instruments and machines necessary to accomplish the work of the organization;
2. *methods*—the policies and procedures set by the organization for smooth and coordinated goal achievement;
3. *materials*—the supplies necessary for continued operation, from paperclips to mops (as well as the personnel necessary to do the job, the "raw material"); and

4. *finances*—as unpleasant as it may be, every organization is ruled by a budget, and its final results are sometimes limited by finances.

No matter how your organization uses these four common elements, its basic goal is the same: to satisfy the health needs of the public.

ORGANIZATION OF HEALTH CARE AGENCIES

You cannot meet the goals and objectives of your particular health care agency, unless you know its organizational structure. The type of structure determines how much authority you possess as a supervisor and enables you to function in your role more effectively.

Types of Agencies

The organizational structures in health care are of three basic types:

1. official,
2. voluntary, and
3. proprietary.

Each type serves a specific segment of the population, and each performs a function necessary to the maintenance of health.

OFFICIAL HEALTH CARE AGENCIES   Set up by the federal, state, county, or city government by law or statute, official health care agencies are tax-supported and serve a specific group of people within the community. Examples of federal health care agencies are military hospitals, clinics, and welfare health care agencies. The state, county, or city may set up a tax-supported health care agency to meet the needs of, say, low-income individuals who need health care but who are unable to pay the cost. Since these agencies are run by the government, all decisions are made by the official agency set up by the governing body.

VOLUNTARY HEALTH CARE AGENCIES   Voluntary health care agencies are defined as nonprofit agencies set up to serve the general public. The operating capital to run these agencies comes partially from fees paid by the clients and, largely, from private gifts made to the agency by interested individuals. The authority for running the agency and all decision-making power come from the Board of Trustees, who are the elected or appointed officials responsible for the management of the hospital. In some cases, the trustees may all be from a certain ethnic or religious group, and the general thrust or tone of the agency reflects their views.

PROPRIETARY HEALTH CARE AGENCIES   A proprietary health care agency is privately owned and operated for profit by either an individual or a group of people. The decision-making power rests with the owners of the agency, but many times their authority is shared with the actual providers of the care. Often nurses working in a proprietary health care agency feel as though they have more authority over decisions concerning the goals and objectives of the organization than a nurse working in a voluntary agency. Proprietary health care agencies may receive public funds if they are performing a service to a specific group of people, such as military personnel unable to reach a military hospital for hemodyalisis and indigent patients receiving welfare.

Departmentalization

Obviously, as the health care agency grows, the management of the agency must also change. When expansion has reached a point that one person or one group of people is no longer able to manage the day-to-day activities of the agency, activities must be grouped—or "departmentalized."

Departmentalization may be accomplished according to three divisions:

1. territory,
2. function, and
3. diagnosis.

BY TERRITORY   If a health care agency is grouped by territory, the agency serves a group of clients who are geographically united. For example, visiting nurses might see patients in a certain geographical area, or a traveling clinic might be driven out to a rural community.

BY FUNCTION   Departmentalization by function is seen in major cities, which have clinics set up to perform one specific function, such as well-baby clinics. The Red Cross is a functional department, set up to provide, among other things, blood.

DIAGNOSIS   The most common division is diagnosis—what we see most often in hospitals. The areas of the hospital are divided according to the patients' diagnoses: pediatrics, medical, surgical, cardiac care, and so on.

Basic Structures

Each type of health care agency has its peculiar type of basic structure. The official agency is structured as shown by Figure 2–1: Authority descends from the governing body to the director of the agency and then to the various directors of departments. As the agency grows, the number of departments increases, and the structure expands vertically and horizontally. A sample organizational structure for a voluntary health care agency is seen in Figure 2–2; the agency is not responsible to the federal, state, or local government. Proprietary hospitals may be set up as seen in Figure 2–3; the owners are directly responsible for the management.

Delegation of Authority

In a large agency, delegating authority to subordinates is necessary to get the work done. This delegation can be either centralized or decentralized.

CENTRALIZED DELEGATION   In this setup, all planning is done by managers. Nursing assignments come from the nursing office, and the staff has little to say over decision making. This type of delegation tends to be task-oriented and ignores the human element. The organization is set up to accomplish work and cares only secondarily about the creativity and concerns of its employees. In centralized delegations, supervision must be close, and control must remain with those on the highest levels.

DECENTRALIZED DELEGATION   In this sort of agency, decisions are made by those closest to the situation. The rationale is that the people who work in any given area know more about its day-to-day activities, and that they are better equipped to make decisions pertinent to the area. In a very large agency, this type of delegation is absolutely necessary because of the wide scope of the agency. No one manager, or even a group of managers, could know everything necessary to control the many departments operating at once. This type of agency uses the chain of command or pyramid organization.

HOSPITALS

Qualifications

The health care agency that most nurses are familiar with is the hospital, whose basic goal, as in any health care agency, is to perform a service to the public. The American Hospital Association says that a

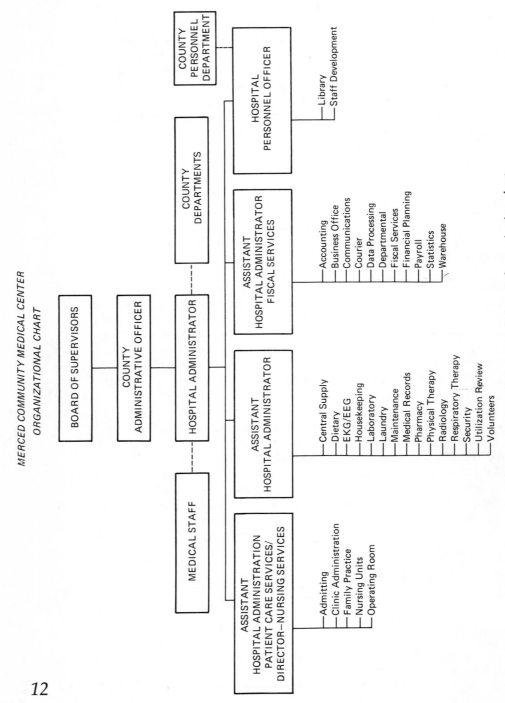

MERCED COMMUNITY MEDICAL CENTER
ORGANIZATIONAL CHART

BOARD OF SUPERVISORS

COUNTY ADMINISTRATIVE OFFICER

MEDICAL STAFF

HOSPITAL ADMINISTRATOR

COUNTY DEPARTMENTS

COUNTY PERSONNEL DEPARTMENT

ASSISTANT HOSPITAL ADMINISTRATION PATIENT CARE SERVICES/ DIRECTOR—NURSING SERVICES
- Admitting
- Clinic Administration
- Family Practice
- Nursing Units
- Operating Room

ASSISTANT HOSPITAL ADMINISTRATOR
- Central Supply
- Dietary
- EKG/EEG
- Housekeeping
- Laboratory
- Laundry
- Maintenance
- Medical Records
- Pharmacy
- Physical Therapy
- Radiology
- Respiratory Therapy
- Security
- Utilization Review
- Volunteers

ASSISTANT HOSPITAL ADMINISTRATOR FISCAL SERVICES
- Accounting
- Business Office
- Communications
- Courier
- Data Processing
- Departmental
- Fiscal Services
- Financial Planning
- Payroll
- Statistics
- Warehouse

HOSPITAL PERSONNEL OFFICER
- Library
- Staff Development

Figure 2–1. A typical nonprofit hospital organization chart.

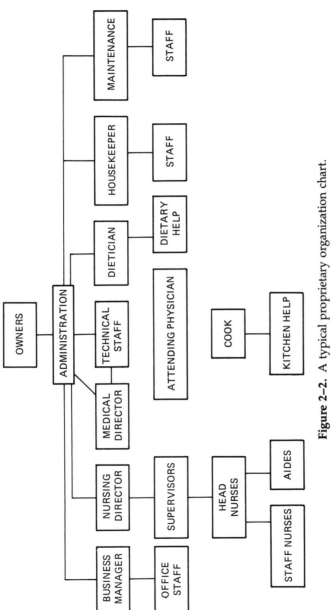

Figure 2–2. A typical proprietary organization chart.

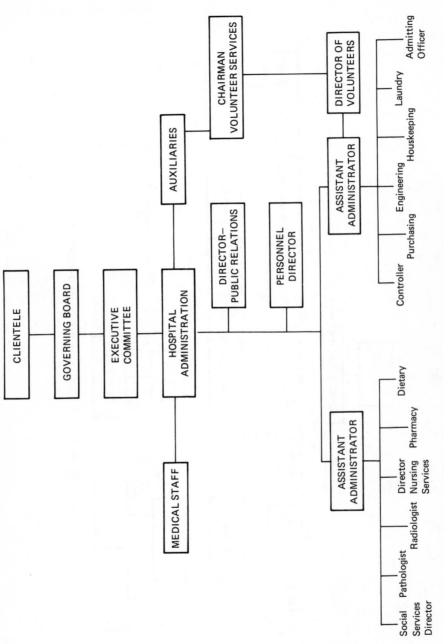

Figure 2–3. A typical voluntary hospital organization chart.

hospital is an institution with the primary function of providing patient services, both diagnostic and therapeutic, for a variety of medical conditions, both surgical and nonsurgical. To qualify as a hospital, an agency must meet other requirements:

1. It must maintain at least six inpatient beds, which shall be continuously available for the care of patients who are nonrelated and who stay on the average in excess of twenty-four hours per admission.
2. It must be constructed, equipped, and maintained to insure the health and safety of patients and to provide uncrowded, sanitary facilities for the treatment of patients.
3. It must be under the direction of an identifiable governing authority that is legally and morally responsible for the conduct of the hospital.
4. There must be a chief executive to whom the governing authority delegates the continuous responsibility for the operation of the hospital in accordance with established policy.
5. The agency must have an organized medical staff of physicians that may include, but need not be limited to, dentists. The medical staff should be accountable to the governing authority for maintaining proper standards of medical care, and it should be governed by by-laws adopted by the staff and approved by the governing authority.
6. Each patient must be admitted on the authority of a member of the medical staff who is directly responsible for the patient's diagnosis and treatment. Any graduate of a foreign medical school who is permitted to assume responsibilities for patient care must possess a valid license to practice medicine, be certified by the Educational Council for Foreign Medical Graduates, or have successfully completed an academic year of supervised clinical training under the direction of a medical school approved by the Liaison Committee on Medical Education of the American Medical Association and the Association of American Medical Colleges.
7. Registered nurse supervision and other nursing services must be continuous.
8. The institution must maintain a current and complete medical record for each patient and make it available for reference.
9. Pharmacy service must be maintained in the institution and supervised by a registered pharmacist.
10. The institution must provide patients with food service that meets their nutritional and therapeutic requirements; special diets must also be available.
11. The institution must maintain diagnostic X-rays service, with facilities and staff for a variety of procedures.

12. The institution must also maintain a clinical laboratory service, with facilities and staff for a variety of procedures. Anatomical pathology services must be regularly and conveniently available.

13. The institution must, finally, offer operating room service with facilities and staff.[1]

Hospital Organization

Due to the many different functions and operations going on in a hospital, the activities of all individuals must be coordinated so that the work of the institution can be accomplished. In many large industries, this organization is usually the pyramid structure, which has proven so successful in most large bureaucratic organizations. The problem is that hospitals do not easily fit into this mold. Health care would be better off if they did!

The health care industry presents the unique situation of having two distinct groups present in the hierarchy. One is represented by the administrative authority they possess (the Governing Board) and the other by the professional authority they have (the Medical Staff). The only individuals who fit the classic pyramid structure mold are those whose salaries are paid by the hospital. The Medical Staff, however, is an independent group; they are financially responsible to their patients, not to the hospital. This difference sets up the unusual situation of a "bi-pyramid" or dual pyramid structure, as seen in Figure 2–4. Harvey L. Smith, who has described the basic duality of hospitals, maintains

Figure 2–4. The dual pyramid (bi-pyramid) structure.

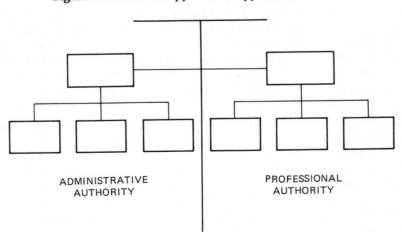

ADMINISTRATIVE
AUTHORITY

PROFESSIONAL
AUTHORITY

[1] Adapted from *Guide to the Health Care Field* (American Hospital Association, 1974), pp. 15–16.

that two lines of authority, lay and professional, exist in the hospital. One is the hierarchy that extends from the Trustees through the administrator and the department heads to the various categories of hospital workers. The second is composed of the various roles held by professional persons in the organization, especially the physicians. While physicians may have very little formal authority in the organization, their actual authority is very great indeed.[2]

Often ignored in the complex structure of hospital organization is the basic principle of organization that a person should have only one immediate supervisor. The nature of the bi-pyramid makes each person responsible to more than one supervisor. As the organization grows and becomes more departmentalized, more and more areas need coordination. Although all departments have the same goal of patient care, each one brings its own needs and desires into the plan and colors the basic goals of the organization. Trying to meet the goals of the organization through the coordinated efforts of these departments often leads to conflict.

As a result of these dual lines of authority and despite the fact that each hospital differs its chart's setup, all hospitals have in common the organizational triad shown in Figure 2–5. The triad consists of the Governing Board, the Administrative Staff, and the Medical Staff. These three divisions share the same goals, but they differ in individual motivation.

THE GOVERNING BODY   Legally constituted to maintain and operate the hospital, by law the Governing Body has the power to make decisions and is responsible for the care and treatment of patients in the hospital.

THE ADMINISTRATOR   As the chief executive in the hospital, the administrator, with his or her assistants, is responsible for managing the hospital to achieve the desired results. The Administrator is responsible for setting and meeting the objectives of the hospital, using the available

Figure 2–5. The organizational triad.

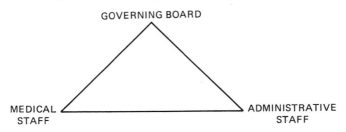

GOVERNING BOARD

MEDICAL STAFF

ADMINISTRATIVE STAFF

[2] Harvey L. Smith, "Two Lines of Authority Are One Too Many," *Modern Hospital* (March 1955), pp. 59–64.

resources to achieve these goals, dealing with the people responsible for carrying out the tasks of goal-attainment, and being the one person to institute change in the hospital.

THE MEDICAL STAFF   The physicians and dentists allowed by charter to care for the patients in the hospital constitute the Medical Staff. Their administration of the hospital is done chiefly through committees. To simplify the enormous job of administering medical care, most hospitals are organized by departments, with a medical staff member in charge of each area, such as obstetrics, pediatrics, gerontology, and so on.

CATEGORIES OF NURSING PERSONNEL

Within each health care agency there are many categories of nursing personnel. The training and functions of each category vary from state to state, but basically they are as follows:

1. nurses' aides or practical nurses,
2. licensed vocational nurses or licensed practical nurses, and
3. registered nurses.

Nurses' Aides or Practical Nurses

The main function of a nursing aide is to perform unskilled or basic nursing tasks under the direct supervision of a licensed nurse. The training varies from a few weeks of on-the-job education to a formal course of study leading to employment in the health care field. Although some hospitals are still training their own nurses' aides, most training is done by private educational organizations, correspondence training, and state junior colleges. In California, for example, a state-funded occupational program prepares nurses' aides.

Since the training for this job is minimal, these assistants are very limited in the scope of their functions. Without a license or special training, they are unable to do the more complicated procedures or to administer medication. Although the salary for nurses' aides is usually low, they are still not cost-effective to the hospital, because they are so limited in the tasks they may perform. As more and more hospitals are changing to more efficient systems of administering patient care, such as primary care, the nurses' aide job is being phased out.

Licensed Vocational Nurses or Licensed Practical Nurses

The licensed vocational nurse (LVN) or the licensed practical nurse (LPN) is another member of the nursing team. The functions of these nurses are greater than aides' because they are licensed by the state in which they work. The duties of LVNs or LPNs are similar to those of nurses' aides, with the addition of treatments and medications. Licensed vocational nurses function as members of the nursing team; they care for patients, they work with the patients' families, and they have an expanded role in the community health care field. In the hospital setting, LVNs are often asked to supervise nurses' aides, thus increasing their responsibilities.

The State Board sets the criteria for licensure, and it is the basis for the authority granted to an LVN or LPN. The scope of the licensed vocational nurse's or the licensed practical nurse's legally described duties is set by the policies and procedures of the hospital and by the Board of Nursing of the particular state.

Vocational or practical nurses may or may not have had formal training for the job. Many LVNs and LPNs receive their licenses by waiver from the state. In some states, nurses' aides who are skilled on the job and who function at a high degree of proficiency for a prescribed period are eligible to apply for the licensure that enables them to function in an expanded role of LVN or LPN.

The formal training course for LVNs or LPNs is offered in many educational settings, and it usually consists of a year of study leading to a licensing examination. At the end of the training, and after successfully completing the examination, the nurse is able to function in the health care setting as a licensed vocational nurse.

Registered Nurses

The highest category of nursing personnel in health care is that of the registered nurse. The state sets the criteria for educational preparation for the registered nurse and is responsible for licensure, testing, and definition of authority.

One of the major issues facing nursing today is the actual definition of duties for each registered nurse. As they are defined today, they do not differ by law from the duties performed by nurses from any type of educational preparation. Many agencies are looking for stricter guidelines to limit the scope of activities of nurses from various academic programs. The idea of "technical" vs. "professional" preparation is a debate that goes on daily in health care. In 1967, the Western Council on Higher Education in Nursing came out with proposed guidelines delineating the duties for registered nurses. Their recommendations are that the nurses be limited by their academic preparation to only specific tasks and that, in order to progress in nursing, their educational preparation must increase. The Curriculum Content Commission of the Associate Degree Seminar of the Western Council on Higher Education in Nursing made the following distinctions:

a. associate degree registered nurse,
b. diploma graduate,
c. baccalaureate degree nurse, and
d. nurse practitioner.

ASSOCIATE DEGREE REGISTERED NURSE   This nurse receives his or her nursing training in conjunction with a two-year college degree at a community college. The Council feels that such experience and training are adequate for quality nursing care, patient teaching, family counseling, and primary care. Yet the Associate Degree nurse is not prepared to work in administration without further educational preparation and experience.

DIPLOMA GRADUATE   These nurses function as generalists in health care. They are skilled in administering the patient care functions, in giving quality nursing care with a broad background of knowledge, and in administering therapeutic, rehabilitative, educational, and preventative medical care. The recommendation of the Council on Higher Education is that these nurses not be allowed to function in roles of authority without additional educational preparation. In essence, they are considered "technical" nurses.

BACCALAUREATE DEGREE NURSE (BSN)   Nurses prepared in baccalaureate degree programs are trained in and perform all the functions of patient care described so far. In addition, their college degree is geared specifically to preparing them to take over positions of authority in health care. The training concentrates on leadership and management skills to prepare "professional" nurses to function in the expanded roles of leaders and supervisors of the nursing team.

NURSE PRACTITIONERS   The American Nurses' Association defines the nurse practitioner as a nurse "with specific preparation to take over a much expanded role. His or her duties include: taking histories and doing physicals, admitting patients, assisting the patient during recovery, managing the patient care independently with standing orders, teaching, counseling, supervising and managing the care of healthy pregnant women, and doing well-child care and education."

Defining Duties

The problems inherent in categorizing nurses is that no clear-cut line of demarcation has been established. Although many agencies concerned with health care have made recommendations, no one plan has been established. Also, each state follows its own directives, with no continuity from state to state. Finally, the nursing associations themselves disagree with the Council on Higher Education in Nursing concerning their position of "technical" vs. "professional" preparation.

Understandably, many nurses feel threatened by these proposed guidelines. Functions traditionally performed by RNs are no longer included in their job descriptions, due to their educational preparation. Diploma graduates are the most verbal in their disagreement with these limitations on their functions: They feel that they are well enough prepared to function in any nursing role, including administration, and they do not wish to be referred to as "technical" nurses.

In actuality, most hospitals expect not only baccalaureate degree registered nurses, but diploma and associate degree nurses to function in leadership roles. The general feeling in the nursing community is that nurses should be allowed to perform tasks for which they are adequately prepared. All registered nurses should receive the additional training and education necessary to assume the supervision roles. They should not be distinguished by their general educational preparation programs, but by their specific education. If nurses are educationally prepared to lead, then they have the right to do so.

Nurses today demand a higher degree of autonomy and power. As hospital administrators feel this pressure from nurse leaders, they begin to comply and give nurses positions of authority. Nurses must be prepared for this and not fail in the task, because of a lack of preparation. The Surgeon General of the United States has become interested in the role of nursing in health care. The findings of his report indicate a need for increased research into both the practice of nursing and the role of educational preparation. The educational systems and curricula should be standardized and enhanced. Career opportunities in nursing are increasing, and financial support should be increased to attract the type of people necessary to meet these needs.

The Commission on Nursing Practice and Education recommends a change in professional institutional patterns and an end to the professional controversy. These aims could be accomplished through the formulation of new ideas for the development of nurses, allowance for career mobility among various educational programs, and the preparation of all nurses to assume the responsibilities of leadership. Due to the development of new health occupations, nurses are taking over some of the functions that were previously assigned only to physicians. These new duties serve to point out even more vividly the need for an expansion of the health team in all settings.

DELIVERY OF NURSING CARE

No one system of health care delivery is best for all situations; each has merit in its own setting. One of the ways that the health team could be more effective in its present setting is to improve the delivery systems presently in use. Many nurses are unaware of the many types of health delivery and patient care organization methods. Patient care can be accomplished by means of four basic methods:

1. functional,
2. team nursing,
3. case method, and
4. primary care.

FUNCTIONAL NURSING   This method can be called task-oriented nursing because the emphasis is on task behavior. All nursing care for a specific group of patients is divided into the tasks necessary for good patient care. These tasks are then assigned according to each nursing team member's individual skills and ability. Each person is responsible for one or more tasks for a given number of patients; for example, each team might have a medication nurse, a treatment nurse, an "A.M.-Care" aide, and so on. The cost of functional nursing is very low because fewer staff members are necessary to carry out the tasks, and each staff member is utilized to the fullest extent.

Some of the disadvantages of functional nursing are that the patient gets fragmented care. Many people are responsible for many functions, and patients feel that no one person is aware of all of their needs. Another problem is that it becomes repetitious and boring, and this factor can lead to mistakes. A routine task becomes automatic, and the staff member does not give full attention to detail. This causes mistakes.

If time and cost are major factors in the administration of nursing care, then functional nursing is a good method to use. It gets the work done well, at the lowest possible cost. (See Figure 2–6.)

CASE METHOD   In this method, also called "one-to-one nursing," one staff member is responsible for all the needs of one or more patients. The patient feels very secure, and usually the care is better than that provided by functional nursing, because one person is aware of all as-

Figure 2–6. Functional nursing.

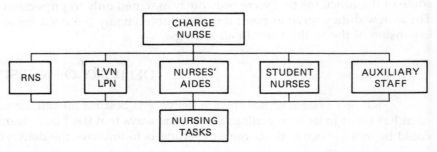

22

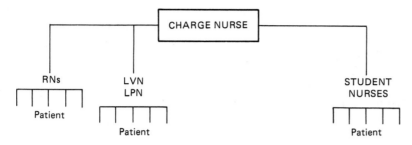

Figure 2–7. Case method of nursing.

pects of a patient's program of care. This method takes a larger, more skilled staff to administer, and, for this reason, it is more expensive to use. Examples of this technique are intensive care and private duty nursing (Figure 2–7).

TEAM NURSING   This way of organizing patient care was developed in the 1950s. The idea of team nursing is that a team of staff members is jointly responsible for the care of a group of patients. Each staff member cares for certain patients on the team, but responsibility is shared. A leader coordinates the activities of the team and serves as resource person. Each member's contribution to the patient care is important, and members are considered equal. Team nursing is cost-effective and one of the most common ways of organizing patient care (Figure 2–8).

PRIMARY CARE NURSING   Developed in 1968, primary care nursing is one of the newest methods of organizing patient care. By definition, it is a nursing organization in which the nurse is able to form a meaningful relationship with a patient, make decisions about that patient's care, assume responsibility for the patient and his or her health care needs, interview and assess the patient, evaluate data received, and plan and

Figure 2–8. Team nursing.

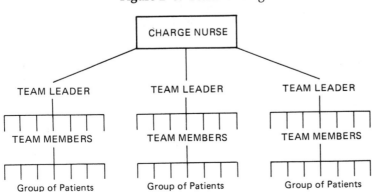

23

direct that care for a 24-hour period. The primary care nurse works with two associate nurses, who care for the patient during the 16 hours that the primary care nurse is off duty. The associate nurses, directly responsible to the primary care nurse, use that nurse's care plan as a basis for their activities. Primary care nursing gives greater responsibility to the nurse, who is placed in the position of planning, coordinating, directing, and administering patient care. The primary care nurse works with the doctor and the patient as a team to obtain the best possible results.

Many hospitals are using primary care as a basis for organizing patient care, and they find it very effective. Since one person is the sole provider of patient care, primary care requires that only licensed personnel administer the care. Even with all licensed personnel, hospitals find the approach to be cost-effective because of the high degree of utilization of all existing personnel. Patients are very satisfied with this method of care because there is real continuity of care, and patients are involved in their own care plan (Figure 2–9).

Figure 2–9. Primary care nursing.

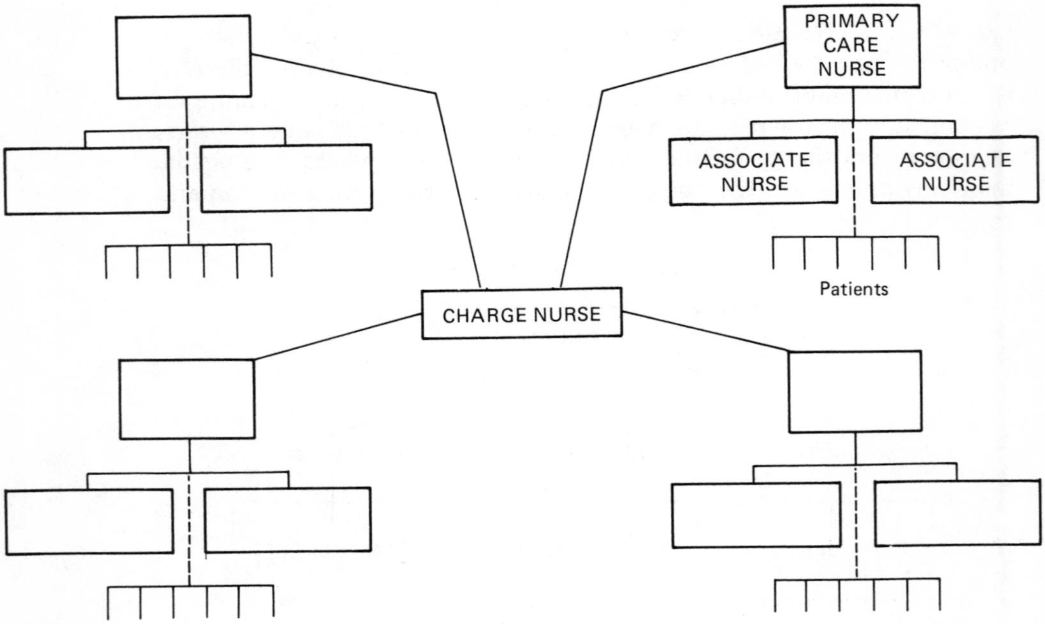

DISCUSSION QUESTIONS

1. Is there a difference between professional and technical preparation for nurses?
2. Must nurses who want more responsibility, such as physicians' assistants, divorce themselves from nursing?
3. What is the expanded role of nurses? Where is the legal limitation?
4. Should all educational programs teach leadership? If not, which programs should teach leadership?
5. How much responsibility should each group labeled "nurse" be given? (e.g. BSN, RN, LVN, Nurse's Aide)
6. Do employers have the right to expect all licensed nurses to possess leadership skills?

APPLICATION: BASIC PRINCIPLES OF NURSING ORGANIZATION

Objectives

- To list five methods of organizing and dividing the work of patient care.
- To list and define the four basic principles in the philosophy of team nursing.

Directions

Refer to the page numbers in the top right corner. Start at page 1, Segment 1, and read the information presented. Turn to subsequent pages as instructed in the program. Answer the questions asked by drawing a circle around T for true or F for false, and proceed as directed, according to your answer. When you have completed the program, answer the questions on the last page.

SEGMENT 1 Every hospital, whether large or small, performs approximately the same functions. The major difference is the degree of specialization found in the larger agency.

    These nursing functions, or tasks, should be organized and delegated according to recognized management principles which take into account the size of the hospital, the relative importance of each function, and the objectives of the health care system.

Turn to page 2, Segment 1.

SEGMENT 2 You seem to be having some difficulty with this organizational principle because you chose the wrong answer.

Turn back to page 5, Segment 1, and reread the statement.

SEGMENT 3 With the thrust toward "liberation" of nurses and the move toward extending the scope of nursing practice, another type of patient care specialist has emerged. The independent nurse practitioner functions independently to provide nursing care.

Turn to page 2, Segment 3.

SEGMENT 4 False is the right answer.

A nursing team, whenever possible, includes each and every member in the development and implementation of nursing care.

Turn to page 4, Segment 4.

SEGMENT 5 You were right in answering false.

There must be only one coordinator who is aware of all assignments.

Turn to page 6, Segment 4.

Supervisors have the final responsibility for the efficiency and effectiveness of their departments. Because they can never relinquish their responsibility for seeing that all tasks are properly carried out, they may organize their departments as they think best without having to follow specific management principles.

SEGMENT 1

T   If you answered true, turn to page 4, Segment 1.
F   If you answered false, turn to page 3, Segment 1.

Organizing and assigning patients by giving responsibility for total patient care to one nurse is called the"case method."

SEGMENT 2

T   If you answered true, turn to page 4, Segment 2.
F   If you answered false, turn to page 1, Segment 2.

The independent nurse practitioner functions in a traditional role as a special duty nurse.

SEGMENT 3

T   If you answered true, turn to page 4, Segment 3.
F   If you answered false, turn to page 3, Segment 3.

The team member, although important to the finished outcome, is only a means to an end. His or her contributions and ideas are not important.

SEGMENT 4

T   If you answered true, turn to page 3, Segment 4.
F   If you answered false, turn to page 1, Segment 4.

According to the principle of members as equals, the team leader should be aware of the common goal of the team and function cooperatively with the members to provide care.

SEGMENT 5

T   If you answered true, turn to page 7, Segment 4.
F   If you answered false, turn to page 6, Segment 5.

SEGMENT 1   Very Good. False is the correct answer. *All* administrators and supervisors must follow certain recognized management principles that have been proven successful over the years.
Turn to page 5, Segment 1, and continue.

SEGMENT 2   Another technique of dividing patient care is by function. This method involves a division of care that is job-centered or task-oriented. Personnel are fitted into fixed slots; one person passes medications, another does treatments, and others make beds or give baths.
Turn to page 5, Segment 2.

SEGMENT 3   You were right in marking this one false. Hopefully you didn't get it by guessing or miss it on your first try. The more independent nurse practitioner bridges the gap from health practitioners to the patient and family.
You are doing fine. For a fifth method of organizing nursing care, turn to page 5, Segment 3.

SEGMENT 4   Wrong. The team method uses each and every team member as an individual and as a contributing member of the nursing care plan.
Review these points on page 8, Segment 3, and try the question again.

SEGMENT 5   A nursing team is changeable and adaptable, and it undergoes never-ending reorganization. This is the philosophy of adaptability and change.
Turn to page 5, Segment 5.

Sorry, your answer is incorrect. While you were correct in your conclusion that department heads have final responsibility for the efficiency of their departments, they must follow recognized management principles in organizing their departments and in assigning tasks to be carried out by subordinates.

Please return to page 1, Segment 1, and try again.

SEGMENT 1

Right you are! Case method is used most often in the acute setting, such as intensive care, or when the patient requires isolation. If this was your first choice, you are progressing nicely. If this is your second choice, you are back on the right track.

Turn to page 3, Segment 2.

SEGMENT 2

You guessed wrong on this item, but it was a tough question. Nurse practitioners are able to function more independently and with greater initiative than ever before. They are breaking away from traditional roles.

Please return to page 1, Segment 3, and give it another try.

SEGMENT 3

The nursing team recognizes the need for a prepared person to be the overall coordinator and interpreter of plans of care.

Turn to page 5, Segment 4.

SEGMENT 4

You are right. Being rigid in the team situation causes nothing but confusion.

You have now completed the nine principles of effective nursing care organization presented in this booklet.

Please turn to page 9, and complete the summary.

SEGMENT 5

SEGMENT 1   There are at least five basic methods of organizing nursing care. Sometimes two or more of these methods may be applied at the same time.

 The first method of nursing care is the one-to-one, or case, method. The practitioner has responsibility for providing complete nursing care to one or more patients. Case assignment requires that the designated nurse be capable of fulfilling all requirements of the assignment.

Turn to page 2, Segment 2.

SEGMENT 2   Assigning personnel to fixed tasks is the organizational method called "functional."

T   If you answered true, turn to page 6, Segment 1.
F   If you answered false, turn to page 8, Segment 5.

SEGMENT 3   We have now considered case, functional, clinical nurse specialist, and independent nurse practitioner as methods of organizing nursing care. The last is the team method.

Turn to page 8, Segment 2.

SEGMENT 4   It would be an acceptable procedure for a supervisor to give a general list of assignments and allow each head nurse to choose which he or she would accept without consulting the supervisor.

T   If your answer is true, turn to page 8, Segment 4.
F   If your answer is false, turn to page 1, Segment 5.

SEGMENT 5   The team members must be aware of the constant change of a patient's condition and be ready to change the nursing care plan whenever necessary.

T   If you answered true, turn to page 4, Segment 5.
F   If you answered false, turn to page 7, Segment 5.

Right again! Agencies using a task-centered approach. They have borrowed this concept from industry, in which the assembly line approach has proved to be the most effective one when mass production is desired.

Turn to page 7, Segment 1.

SEGMENT 1

Absolutely correct! This new approach is being used in combination with other methods in large medical centers.

Turn to page 1, Segment 3.

SEGMENT 2

No, but you are partly right. The team does function cooperatively, but the major thrust in team nursing is considering the individual, not the task.

Turn to page 5, Segment 3, and come back through again.

SEGMENT 3

Next, we will consider the philosophy of team members functioning as equals. In the team method there should be minimal emphasis on *hierarchical lines of demarcation between the leader and the led.*

Turn to page 2, Segment 5.

SEGMENT 4

Somehow you missed the key point. "Equal" means that all members, including the team leader, work together as partners in patient care.

Please return to page 6, Segment 4.

SEGMENT 5

SEGMENT
1

Due to the increasing complexity of hospital services, a new method of patient care has been established. This is the clinical nurse specialist who has had specialized preparation in a clinical area, usually at the masters level.

Turn to page 8, Segment 1.

SEGMENT
2

Wrong! Those are all examples of areas in which a clinical nurse specialist functions. Others are rehabilitation, family health, and maternal–child.

Review the statement on page 7, Segment 1, and continue.

SEGMENT
3

You're right, the answer is false.

As we said before, team nursing is a cooperative effort, but all activities are based on a concern for the *individuals* served, not for the task.

You've done quite well to this point. Please turn to page 8, Segment 3.

SEGMENT
4

Right! You have taken into account the fact that all members work together to provide the best possible care for the patient.

Turn to page 3, Segment 5.

SEGMENT
5

Wrong! Think only of the word *change*, and remember that the nursing team must always be adaptable.

Return to page 3, Segment 5, and try once more.

Providing significant nursing skills to patients in selected specialty areas SEGMENT
such as medical–surgical, mental health, and community health is the 1
function of the clinical nurse specialist.

T   If you answered true, turn to page 6, Segment 2.
F   If you answered false, turn to page 7, Segment 2.

In team nursing a group of people, led by a qualified nurse, provide for SEGMENT
the health needs of an individual or a group of people through a collab- 2
orative and cooperative effort. The major thrust is task-oriented.

T   If you answered true, turn to page 6, Segment 3.
F   If you answered false, turn to page 7, Segment 3.

Team nursing is a system of providing care in which a professional nurse SEGMENT
facilitates the efforts of a group of diversified health care personnel to 3
provide for the health needs of an individual. The first principle in the
philosophy of team nursing is realizing the worth of the individual, both
patient and team member.
        Turn to page 2, Segment 4.

Sorry, back to the drawing board. While some supervisors are not directly SEGMENT
aware of what goes on in their departments, correct team method phi- 4
losophy says that one coordinator should be aware of all assignments.
If everyone chose what they would do independently of the others, there
would be chaos.
        Turn to page 4, Segment 4, and review this principle.

Wrong! A common example of dividing work by functional method is SEGMENT
assigning TPRs to one person which is common to most hospitals. 5
        Return to page 3, Segment 2, and try again.

Please copy your answers from the programmed instruction booklet to this page as follows:

PAGE	SEGMENT	ANSWER
2	1	T F
2	2	T F
2	3	T F
2	4	T F
2	5	T F
5	2	T F
5	4	T F
5	5	T F
8	1	T F
8	2	T F

List the five methods of organizing patient care as discussed in this booklet.

1.

2.

3.

4.

5.

List the four principles of the philosophy of team nursing.

1.

2.

3.

34   **4.**

REFERENCES

DIEKELMANN, NANCY L. AND MARTIN M. BROADWELL, *The New Hospital Supervisor.* (Boston, Mass.: Addison–Wesley Publishing Company, 1977).

DOUGLASS, LAURA MAE AND EM OLIVIA BEVIS, *Nursing Leadership in Action.* St. Louis: The C. V. Mosby Company, 1974.

MAHLER, WALTER R. *Diagnostic Studies.* Boston, Mass.: Addison–Wesley Publishing Company, 1974.

RUBIN, IRWIN M., RONALD E. FRY, AND MARK S. PLOVNICK, *Managing Resources in Health Care Organizations.* Reston, Va.: Reston Publishing Co., 1978.

3

Personal qualifications of the nurse/leader

THE SUPERVISOR'S PERSPECTIVE

As a nurse, you enter a whole new world when you accept a position of supervision. Everything that was secure and comfortable in your old position is changed into a new, strange feeling. You enter the area of supervision filled with conflicting emotions: fear, excitement, anxiety, regret, and loneliness. All these feelings seem to be present at once, and you feel as though you will never be able to cope with it all.

Before actually taking charge, you may feel very sure of your ability to supervise; perhaps you received special training for the job. Yet the day you start that new position, everything seems to change. What seemed so simple is now very complex. Problems that you glibly solved for everyone else now seem very different—when you are the one who must make the final decision. Every doubt you ever felt now seems magnified in your mind. Part of the reason for this reaction is your realization that everyone is looking to you for solutions to their problems, answers to their questions, and organization for their confusion. The job that you awaited so eagerly does not seem quite so desirable now.

A Case in Point

In one hospital a nurse found out the hard way how different it is to be inside, looking out. This particular nurse was very skilled in her day-to-day tasks. She loved nursing and found joy in doing every

36

nursing activity. She was very popular with her co-workers, partly because of her high degree of skill, but more because of her bright disposition and cheerful attitude. Her fellow workers enjoyed working with her because she was so organized and seemed to be able to get everything done without much hassle. Frequently other nurses would make comments to her about her leadership ability and how much they would enjoy working for someone like her.

Eventually a promotion was offered, and our nurse was the logical choice for the position. She was delighted, as were her co-workers. The first few weeks went by in a flash of learning all there was to learn about the new tasks. Then, after a few weeks of the new job, she realized that she was not as optimistic as before. The sunny disposition was replaced by a serious, thoughtful self. The staff noticed the change and commented on it. Her defense was that she no longer had time to be friendly and cheerful; there was too much to do. She found herself snapping at the staff and becoming very impatient with even the smallest slip-up.

Everything seemed different. It was so much easier to do the jobs herself, rather than ask someone else to do them. After all, she had the final responsibility, and if she did the job, she knew that it was being done correctly. Now, instead of delegating authority to others so that she could go about the job of supervision, she was trying to do everything herself. The tasks that she had done so well as a staff nurse were done quickly, almost carelessly, with much less care and patience. Her supervision was minimal, and what supervision she did offer seemed to be mainly criticism. She was trying to be everything to everyone, and failing in the attempt.

This nurse was learning the hard way that supervision requires a completely new set of standards and behaviors. Luckily, this nurse was smart enough to realize quickly the dangers of her behavior and was able to relieve the problem before it became serious. She learned to accomplish work through others. She learned the importance of positive reinforcement, rather than criticism. Most importantly, she learned

Figure 3–1. The supervisor takes on a new perspective.

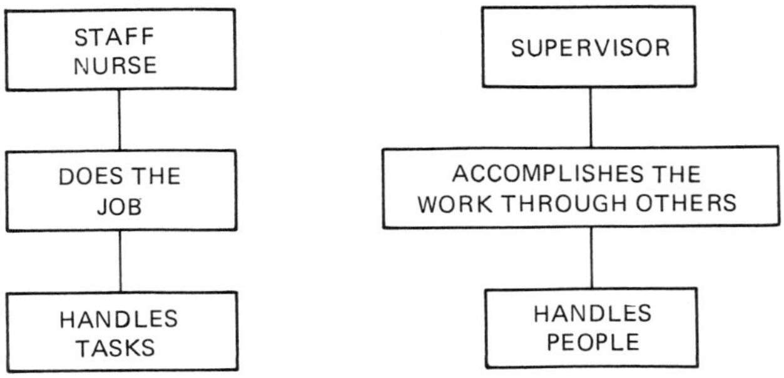

37

to back off and let others do their work. She learned to *supervise*. The smile came back, and, with the smile, came the joy of work again. She now felt the same satisfaction from supervising others that she had felt by giving the care herself. She was a fine staff nurse, and now she is a fine supervisor, one that everyone likes to work for and with.

When you become the supervisor, you will miss the companionship of your fellow workers at times. The times spent over a cup of coffee were precious and hard to give up. Even harder to accept is the fact that *you* are now the subject of conversation at coffee break time.

Supervision is satisfying, very satisfying, but it is a job that must be worked at and practiced just like any other. Every minute of every day, you are faced with new situations that must be faced. Although every situation is different, all the dealings you have as a supervisor have one thing in common: You deal with the human element. If you can remember that one factor, you will succeed. Just as no one answer is best for every question, no one style of supervision is perfect for every situation. Wise supervisors know themselves, know their staff, and feel comfortable in the role of leader.

The term "supervise" means literally to "look over." As a supervisor you are not only expected to look over your staff's work, you must take final responsibility for the work. This is a major responsibility and one that does not come easily. Doing a job well is one thing; teaching someone else to do the job well is an entirely different thing. The best supervisor knows when to work, and when to watch.

PERSONAL QUALITIES

A supervisor must have "leadership," which implies direction and guidance. Leadership ability may be inherited by a few lucky people, but most of us need to develop it, like any talent. Just as a talent for music does not necessarily mean that a person is able to play an instrument without practice, a leadership talent is nonproductive unless it is developed and practiced. The successful supervisor knows the tools of leadership and knows how to develop and maintain them. To develop your leadership potential to its fullest, you must know your strengths and weaknesses. Everyone is different and everyone uses his or her own personality to set a style of supervision, but some elements are common to all good leaders. See Figure 3–2.

Appearance

The jokes about the supervisor's being "a vision in white with clipboard in hand" may have hidden meanings. Your staff judges you on the first impression you present, part of which is based on your appearance. Too many nurses feel that what they do is more important

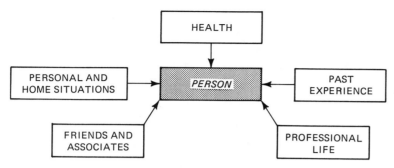

Figure 3–2. People are different due to the factors affecting their lives. We change as those factors change.

than how they look. The impression that you impart to the public and to your staff is colored by how you look. A neat, efficient-looking supervisor creates a picture of efficiency to a distraught family. A well-groomed supervisor sets an example for the staff and generates a feeling of organization. Whether you wear a uniform or street clothes in your area, your appearance should make a favorable statement about your ability. You are the example for your staff, and your appearance may not deviate from acceptable standards.

Punctuality

As in all areas of supervision, "Do as I say, not as I do" is *not* the rule. No one respects the supervisor who is consistently late. Being punctual is not just getting somewhere on time, though. Punctuality also implies that tasks are done when they are due, reports turned in on time, promises kept. All these factors combine to build your staff's confidence in you.

Integrity

It goes without saying that the supervisor must be honest. The profession has no place for anything less. Yet, integrity means even more: Honesty is obeying the letter of the law; integrity is obeying the spirit of the law. Integrity means adhering to your personal and professional obligations and responsibilities. Supervisors may be subject to criticism if any of the aspects of their personal lives are not maintained in the expected manner. This is not to say that supervisors must be paragons of virtue, but they must be discreet in their personal lives. A supervisor must also be totally discreet about confidential matters, whether they concern patients or staff.

Total loyalty to the health care agency is essential. There is no place for idle conversation or information that reflects unfavorably on your organization. If you are asked a question about your health care agency by a lay or professional person, answer only if you can give a positive image. Real integrity means upholding the policies and procedures of your institution, no matter what your personal feelings may be. If you disagree with a policy, try to change it. But until that change is made, you must support your organization's stand.

Good Judgment

Listing this as a personality trait necessary to supervision puts some pressure on the new supervisor. Good judgment comes with experience, and novice leaders have no experience to guide them. Yet experience is not the only way to develop good judgment. A sound basis of common sense, a feeling for human nature, and an absolute knowledge of the policies and procedures of the hospital all take the supervisor through some difficult situations. Good judgment is often knowing when to act, and when to ask for assistance. A great deal of help is available to supervisors, if only they ask.

Empathy

The most effective nurse/leaders cultivate their leadership attitudes using empathy and objectivity. *Empathy,* or the ability to place one's self in the position of another, is necessary to gauge the tone of the group and respond in an appropriate fashion. *Objectivity,* or the ability to observe and evaluate the causes of events unemotionally, is necessary to maintain control and to guide and direct the group toward the established norms.

The staff looks to the supervisor for help in all things, both professional and personal. A kind, warm understanding of their needs as human beings helps you in all your dealings with the staff. Empathy, however, does not mean that you become emotionally involved with the personal problems of staff members, to the detriment of the organization. Supervisors must keep first and foremost in their minds the goals of the organization. It is helpful to be concerned and interested in the lives of the organization. It is helpful to be concerned and interested in the personal lives of your staff, but not so involved that the staff begins to manipulate you with their problems. It takes real discipline to stay interested but detached.

The successful supervisor is able to deal in the same way with patients and their families. Feeling pain with a patient or family shows love and caring. If you are dealing with a grieving family, you may feel moved to tears. There is nothing wrong with showing emotion as long as you are in control of yourself. The family will certainly know how deeply you care, and your staff will not see this sort of reaction as a sign of weakness.

Lack of Jealousy

If you are ambitious in your profession and seek to reach the highest levels, remaining free of jealousy is sometimes difficult. You must simply try to do the best job you can for the organization. This obligation might even entail watching someone else get the job or position you are seeking—an extremely difficult thing to do. No good comes from a show of jealousy, and a great deal of harm can occur. Everyone is working in the health care agency for the same goal, the good of the patient. If this is truly your motivation for work, it should not matter *who* does the tasks, as long as they are done.

A lack of jealousy does not mean meekness and modesty to the point of downgrading your abilities, but you must seek to elevate yourself on your own merit. Backbiting and petty jealousy do nothing to raise your esteem. Honest acceptance of the talents of others gains more than competition.

Tolerance

With tolerance goes patience, understanding, and fairness. All people are different, and each presents a uniquely individual set of behaviors and ideals. Dealing with these ideas as fairly as possible, without letting your personal opinion affect your treatment of staff members, is up to you. Not everyone is like you, not everyone behaves in the way you behave, and not everyone can do things the way you do them. Prejudices or preconceived ideas and methods have no place

Figure 3–3. The roles of supervision.

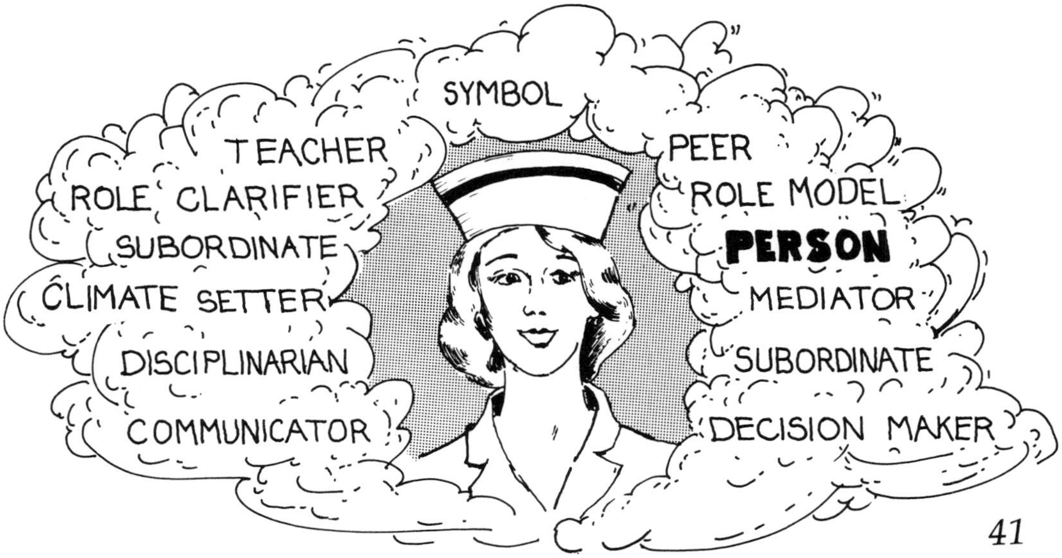

SYMBOL

TEACHER
ROLE CLARIFIER
SUBORDINATE
CLIMATE SETTER
DISCIPLINARIAN
COMMUNICATOR

PEER
ROLE MODEL
PERSON
MEDIATOR
SUBORDINATE
DECISION MAKER

41

in supervision. The wise supervisor allows staff members the freedom
to accomplish the goals of the agency in their own ways.

Responsibility

Being able to accept responsibility is a very difficult thing to
learn. The saying, "The buck stops here," is especially applicable to
supervisors. You are the one who takes the final responsibility for the
actions of others, and blaming *them* rather than yourself is very easy.
A supervisor must know that any task delegated to another is still his
or her responsibility. If the job is not done correctly, the fault might lie
in the supervision or in the training, not in the task accomplishment.
This is not to say that an error may go without punishment. Supervisors
learn from mistakes and take the responsibility for eliminating them.
They look into themselves and try to find the little extra that will eliminate the problem the next time.

Flexibility

The most important personal quality necessary in a leader is
flexibility—flexibility with fairness. The rigid person is never able to
succeed in the area of nursing, which demands quick, decisive action.
As an intelligent supervisor, you have a range of possible alternatives
in mind and can move from one choice to another with relative ease.
When you deal with the public and with the quirks of human nature,
you must be flexible and open to change. With flexibility comes innovation and creativity, qualities that are always desirable in health care.

Emotional Stability

To be an effective leader you must be free from undue insecurity, anxiety, overagressiveness, psychosomatic illness, and other neu-
rotic behaviors. You must try to adapt your emotional responses to the
needs of the situation. A person who is easily moved to fits of anger or
depression will have problems in a leadership role. One of the hardest
things to learn, but one of the most important, is to maintain your
composure in situations of stress or pressure.

Organization

No work can be done without planning and clear direction. A
supervisor must possess the ability to plan and organize work so that
it can be accomplished effectively, efficiently, and according to the
schedule. Much can be said about the benefits of list-making. Some

supervisors cannot begin the day without their lists. If this system helps you to remain organized, by all means, use it, but don't become compulsive about the accomplishment of your listed tasks.

Separation of Home and Profession

Male or female, the tie between home and professional life must be broken. The supervisor, when coming to work, must leave all home situations behind. The temptation is to blame mistakes made or errors in judgment on problems at home.

Unfortunately, women supervisors are considered more susceptible to this tendency than men. Women are frequently criticized as being poor leaders because they are "too emotional" and "too tied to the home situation." The comment has been made that women cannot lead other women because they lead with their hearts, not with their heads. Such statements should be false, but too often they prove to be true. Even though many women have worked for years and have supported their homes and families with little or no assistance, some are unable to fully commit themselves to their jobs because of the pressures of society.

As our society is becoming more aware of the blending of the male and female professional roles, the working women should become less of an issue. In many cases, the professional life of a woman is subject to, and secondary to, her family. If illness occurs in the household, the nurse becomes a mother and must take time off to care for her family. Until some equality in child care can be reached, women who have families and who continue to work outside the home will continue to feel this pull. The only solution to the problem is to make sure that provision is made for all but the most unusual emergencies and try to arrive on duty with your mind free to nurse.

Assuming you can do so, you must, as a supervisor, be aware of the same pressures on staff members, who might also be working mothers. If special arrangements must be made to accommodate an unusual problem, and if these arrangements fit into the hospital procedures, don't hesitate to be understanding and flexible. If your employees know that you understand the problems of raising a family and working at the same time, they will respect you and give you their best efforts.

Positive Attitude

As beauty is in the eye of the beholder, so too is success in leadership in the eye of the observer. Subordinates judge your success or your failure by their own standards and ideals. If you display confidence and a positive attitude, your staff feels secure and reacts positively to you.

The staff's perception of you depends partially, in turn, on your perception of yourself. You must therefore understand your own perception and your role in supervision. If that perception is positive, you will have fewer problems and greater harmony in your professional life. As a nurse, your total self goes into your perceptions. All your goals, desires, needs, experiences, feelings, ideals, and talents go into shaping the person who is uniquely you. You see yourself not necessarily by *what* you are but often by what you *think* you are. If you feel that you will be a failure in supervision, no amount of success is going to erase that feeling. If you program yourself for failure, you will fail. If you believe in yourself, in your skills, and in your talents, then you will succeed in whatever you attempt to accomplish.

Your perceptions involve more than what you see and hear; they also entail what you think and feel. Two people can witness the same occurrence—they see and hear the same thing—but their interpretation of that incident may be entirely different. The reason for the difference is that their personal feelings and thoughts influence their interpretations of the situation. Correspondingly, even more important than *getting* positive feedback from your staff is your ability to *interpret* that feedback, translating it into positive feelings about yourself. As an analogy, patients who are losing a great deal of weight often have difficulty "feeling" thin. The mirror tells them that they are slim, their friends see their "new" selves, the doctor encourages and compliments them—but until they interpret the data and change their own self-images, they continue to feel fat.

Personal Commitment

The leadership role is very personal. All the areas of your supervisory task involve your handling of people rather than things. In leadership, then, the most important tool you possess is your *self*. You are the instrument that gets results in your organization, and you cannot get those results by detached administration. You must be totally and personally committed to all areas of your role. Giving yourself so completely to your profession means successfully dealing with others. Leadership is not the blind leading the blind. Until you are aware of your own strengths and weaknesses, you cannot assist others in accomplishing their goals or the goals of the organization.

In a study at the University of Florida in 1974, perceptual psychologists studied persons in the helping professions. The purpose of the study was to determine the relationship of self-fulfillment to personal adequacy in leadership. The results of the study showed that effective leaders felt themselves to be:

1. identified with, rather than apart from, others;
2. basically adequate rather than inadequate;
3. trustworthy rather than untrustworthy;
4. wanted rather than unwanted or ignored; and,
5. worthy rather than overlooked or discounted.

Nurses with positive self-images, personal commitment, and positive feelings of adequacy project this image to their staffs. Members of the staff feel this personal confidence and develop their own positive support system.

THE ROLE OF SUPERVISION

The supervisor plays many roles when dealing with subordinates. Just as in your personal life you wear many hats, so too in your professional life you are many things to many people. As a leader, you must respond with the appropriate role for any situation. See Figure 3–3.

CLIMATE SETTER   You are responsible for the tone of your department. If you are anxious and tense, the staff pick up this feeling, and they feel unsure of themselves. If you try to accomplish work while remaining cheerful and optimistic, the staff imitate these behaviors, which are thus reflected in their attitudes.

SYMBOL   You, as the supervisor, stand for the entire organization. You *are* the organization. Think how many times patients or relatives of patients have demanded to "speak to the supervisor." Somehow, if they speak to you, they feel that more will be accomplished. A supervisor must resist the temptation to feel the effects of this power. Your responsibility is to your staff and to the organization, not to your public image.

ROLE MODEL   You are the embodiment of all the policies and procedures in the hospital. If you make an error, it is much more conspicuous and its consequences are more serious than errors by the staff. This does not mean that you are expected to be perfect. Far from it. Experienced supervisors know that sometimes mistakes will be made, problems will occur, and answers will not be available right at their fingertips. The successful role model knows how to find the answer, thus acknowledging a lack of omnipotence. The temptation is to try to bluff your way out of a situation. This tendency can only spell doom, because your tactic will be found out, and the staff will feel as though you have cheated them. If you make an error, the simplest and best way to deal with it is to admit it. "I made a mistake" is sometimes very difficult to say, but no words do more to raise the level of respect in the eyes of the staff.

MEDIATOR   You are expected to be the go-between for management and the staff—not a fence-walker, but a mediator. Trying to get these sometimes opposing factions together takes the patience of a saint, but the results are worthwhile. The trick to remember is that you must take a stand. You cannot vacillate between one group and the other. You cannot be on two sides at once, and, if you try to do so, you will lose both sides.

DECISION MAKER   Every day, almost every minute of every day, you are expected to make decisions. Many times, you have no one to go to for help, and you must make that final choice. The staff will respect you if you are able to make decisions based on sound judgment and experience, even if it is not the best decision. On the other hand, nothing is more frustrating for staff than asking for guidance or answers and then being put "on hold." At times, delaying a decision is best, but most of the time a well-thought-out and prompt decision is necessary. Too many supervisors are afraid to make decisions for fear of error, and their staff feel as though they have no leader.

COMMUNICATOR   Supervisors spend 50 percent of their time communicating. Whether you are using verbal or written communication, you must be sure that what you want to express is coming across. What seems very clear to you may not make any sense at all to your staff. So keep your verbal massages short and to-the-point, and your written communications clear and concise.

DISCIPLINARIAN   This is a role that most supervisors would rather not accept. There is little or no pleasure in disciplining a staff member. Yet you must always keep in mind that, with successful discipline, overall results are improved and the organization benefits. The rules of discipline are firmness, fairness, and consistency.

TEACHER   You are expected to convey many ideas, both by example and by formal instruction. Whether you are giving a lecture to many nurses or a one-to-one training explanation, you must explain carefully and wait with patience to make sure that you are understood. Allow time for the staff member's thought processes, and never become impatient.

SUBORDINATE   Within the hierarchy of authority in the health care setting, you report to your immediate superior. Tact, courtesy, and willingness all help you in these dealings. Sometimes it is very comforting to know that you have someone to go to, someone to guide you in your professional activities.

PEER   Relationships with other supervisors are very important to your feelings of satisfaction and success. Everyone leads differently and has a different set of perceptions, so you should not be quick to judge the style of your peers. Your fellow supervisors can be a source of friendship, guidance, support, resourcefulness, and assistance. Comfortable interdepartmental relationships without conflict or competition help everyone in reaching organizational goals. Never discuss your peers' professional or personal dealings with subordinates.

RÒLE CLARIFIER   Your staff are expected to function in many roles in their professional life, and they come to you for help in sorting out these sometimes conflicting roles. Before you can assist others to integrate the many facets of their lives, you must feel secure in the roles *you* play.

PERSON   You are you, with your own perceptions, emotions, and ideals. You as a person may be mother, father, friend, lover, among other things in your personal life. All these factors influence your thoughts and activities. Some of your personal skills enhance your supervision and enable you to deal more effectively in situations. All life's experiences that you have mold and shape you into a well-balanced, integrated person.

No matter how much you learn about supervision, you still bring to the job a special quality that is uniquely you. This is what makes the job of supervision so interesting and so rewarding.

DISCUSSION QUESTIONS

1. Discuss the "role theory" of supervision.
2. In addition to the roles discussed in the chapter, can you think of some other roles that the supervisor may be expected to play?
3. What is the role of "organizational climate" in supervision? How does the supervisor play a part in setting the climate?
4. Why is self-confidence so important to the supervisor?

47

APPLICATION: PERCEPTIONS
OF SELF AND OF OTHERS

Objectives

- To understand the factors that influence the perception of others.
- To understand how others' impressions of you influence relationships.
- To explore methods for giving and receiving feedback.
- To understand your own conceptual system.

Introduction

When we meet other persons, we do not judge them on the basis of their own personalities, but on the basis of their affect on us. At this first meeting, we tend to lump people into categories or concepts rather than distinguish them by their individual traits. This first impression is based on a multitude of factors related to our personal interpretations and understandings. So too do other people judge us by these first-impression interpretations. Understanding and analyzing these first-impression concepts can be very interesting and valuable pursuits. We can gain insight into the image we are projecting, and we can evaluate our impressions of others.

The categories we see in ourselves and in others do not stand alone. They tend to be tied together in a way that is unique to us, and they reflect our own images and stereotypes. In other words, when we see a warm, friendly, open, and pleasant smile, we may link this first impression with our own network of concepts and immediately like the person. Or we may see the same smile as suspicious, thus evoking distrust, fear, and caution. Our reactions can yield two totally different impressions to the first meeting. Right or wrong, these impressions may last and color our actions with that person. We must be aware of our perceptions of others and learn to deal with people on the basis of their personalities, not of our perception of them.

This exercise enables you to see the concepts you have of yourself and of others. By analyzing the findings, you will have a clearer picture of your interpersonal perceptions.[1]

Procedure

With your class, a group of associates, or some friends, form groups of four or five members each.

[1] David A. Kolb, Irwin M. Rubin, and James M. McIntyre, *Organizational Psychology: An Experiential Approach* (Englewood Cliffs, N.J.: Prentice-Hall, Inc., 1971), pp. 190–200. Reprinted by permission of Prentice-Hall, Inc.

STEP ONE Each individual fills out the perception matrix form, specifically the column entitled "How You See Yourself" (Table 3–1). It is important to work quickly; only first impressions are to be given.

   A. *Self-image:* As you think about the image you have of self, list:

      1. the first five or six words that come to your mind,
      2. an animal,
      3. a musical instrument,
      4. a food.

TABLE 3–1
Perception matrix (own perceptions)

MEMBER / CATEGORY	HOW YOU SEE:					
	YOURSELF	A	B	C	D	E
Five or Six Words		quiet	shy	smart	smile	honest
Animal		cat				
Musical Instrument		flute				
A Food		p+B s'nz				

   B. *Perception of others:* As you think about the image you have of each of the other members of your present group, list the same four categories. (Use columns A through E of Table 3–1.)

STEP TWO Share your impressions of yourself and of the other members of the group. List these shared impressions on the form provided in Table 3–2.

STEP THREE Analyze the data received, and try to make a pattern analysis of the major concepts expressed about you. See if there are any key concepts.

Major Concepts Expressed

  _____ _____ _____

  _____ _____ _____

  _____ _____ _____

STEP FOUR Discuss as a group any discrepancies between how you see yourself and how others see you.

TABLE 3–2
Perception matrix (others' perceptions)

MEMBER / CATEGORY	HOW I AM SEEN BY:				
	A	B	C	D	E
Five or Six Words					
An Animal					
A Musical Instrument					
A Food					

APPLICATION: JOHARI WINDOW

Objectives

- To understand how our self-perceptions affect our behavior.
- To understand how we shield ourselves from behaviors that we feel are undesirable.

Introduction

Sociologist Erving Goffman has described the tendency of people to preserve the "face" that others present to them. When people we know act in ways that we feel are "out of character," we tend to try to force them back into their accepted roles. In social situations, we try to protect our own self-image and the self-images of others. We feel that we would embarrass a person by mentioning a behavior that is contrary to the image they are trying to create—for example, telling a person that he has bad breath. This inclination can be graphically demonstrated by the use of a Johari Window, named after Joe Luft and Harry Ingraham.

Procedure

Fill out the Johari Window in Table 3–3. Try to decide for yourself which items should be moved from the hidden area to the open. With the use of feedback, move some items from the blind area into the open. It is only as we move from the hidden and blind areas into the open area that a true sharing of perceptions and understanding can develop.

APPLICATION: SELF-EVALUATION

Directions

What type of leader are you? Using the point system in Table 3–4, evaluate your personality assets and your nursing ability. If your total score is below 30, consider yourself below average.

TABLE 3–3
Johari window

	KNOWN TO SELF	UNKNOWN TO SELF
Known to Others	Free to Self and Others 1	Blind to Self and Seen by Others 2
UnKnown to Others	Hidden: Self Hidden from Others 3	Unknown: Self Unknown to Others and Self 4

OPEN AREA: This cell (1) includes all the factors on which the others and I have mutually shared perceptions.

UNKNOWN AREA: In this cell (4) are factors that I do not see in myself, nor do others see in me.

HIDDEN AREA: In this cell (3) are factors that I see in myself, but that I hide.

BLIND AREA: In this cell (2) are factors that other people perceive in me, but that I do not see in myself.

To move from a hidden area to an open one requires trust.
To move from a blind area to an open one requires feedback.

TABLE 3–4

	POINTS	ACTION TO BE TAKEN
Personal appearance	3	
Discretion in speech and manner	2	
Courtesy, manners, social sense	3	
Ability to work with others	2	
Acceptance of supervision	2	
Sense of responsibility	3	
Dependability	3	
Punctuality	2	
Tact	2	
Initiative	2	
Knowledge of procedures and treatments	2	
Recognition of total needs of patient	3	
Attention to comfort of patient	2	

TABLE 3–4 (*cont.*)

	POINTS	ACTION TO BE TAKEN
Ability to follow directions	2	
Ability to organize work well	2	
Ability to keep environment orderly	2	
Economy of time and material	2	
Total score		

If you consider yourself: then give yourself:
Above Average   3 points
Average   2 points
Below Average   1 point

REFERENCES

BASS, BERNARD M., *Leadership Psychology and Organizational Behavior.* New York: Harper & Row, Publishers, Inc., 1960.

CHRUDEN, HERBERT J. AND ARTHUR W. SHERMAN, JR., *Personnel Management*, 2nd ed. Cincinnati: South-Western Publishing Co., 1963.

DAVIS, KEITH, *Human Relations at Work.* New York: McGraw-Hill Book Company, 1962. Leon C. Meggison, *Personnel: A Behavioral Approach to Administration.* Homewood, Ill.: Richard D. Irwin, Inc., 1967.

GREENE, RICHARD M., JR., *The Management Game—How to Win with People.* Homewood, Ill., Dow Jones–Irwin, Inc., 1969.

GOFFMAN, ERVING, "On Face-work: An Analysis of Ritual Elements in Social Interaction," *Psychiatry*, 18 (1955), 213–31.

HECKMANN, I. L., JR. AND S. G. HUNERYAGER, *Human Relations in Management.* Chicago: South-Western Publishing Co., 1960.

INTERNATIONAL CITY MANAGERS' ASSOCIATION, *Municipal Personnel Administration*, 6th ed. Chicago: The International City Managers' Association, 1960.

KASSOFF, NORMAN C., *Organizational Concepts.* Washington, D.C.: International Association of Chiefs of Police, 1967.

MASSIE, JOSEPH L. AND HOHN DOUGLAS, *Managing: A Contemporary Introduction.* Englewood Cliffs, N.J.: Prentice-Hall, Inc., 1973.

SPRIEGEL, WILLIAM R., EDWARD SCHULZ, AND WILLIAM B. SPRIEGEL, *Elements of Supervision.* New York: John Wiley & Sons, Inc., 1967.

4

Leadership

WHAT IS LEADERSHIP?

Former President Eisenhower once stated, "Leadership is the art of getting somebody else to do something you want done because he wants to do it." True leadership is a positive rather than a negative force, based on cooperation and mutual trust, not coercion and fear. The essence of real leadership is the ability to obtain from subordinates the highest quality of service that they have the capacity to render. Good leadership does not involve the exercise of authority through commands and the threat of punishment for noncompliance, nor is it related to the strength with which commands are issued. No organization can function efficiently without competent leaders, but this maxim is particularly true in a health care agency.

Leadership consists of a set of actions that influence your group toward the attainment of the organizational goals. Expressed a different way, leadership is the accomplishment of organizational objectives as the result of interpersonal relationships between the leader and the led. As you can see by these definitions, leadership is a behavior, not a characteristic. Leadership is a role enactment of behaviors that guide others to reach goals. The behavior pattern of leadership is a learned behavior; anyone can learn the behaviors necessary to lead others.

Parts of this chapter have been adapted from *Supervision and Leadership*, Field Operations Management Series, Vol. 7 (Sacramento: Department of the California Highway Patrol, 1957), pp. 9–48.

There is a difference between managing and leading. A manager is responsible for the planning and organization necessary to achieve goals. A leader, by the simplest definition, must simply get others to follow those plans. To be a good leader, a nurse must learn the principles and behaviors of leadership, not the policies and operations. You must learn the behaviors of leadership, not just the rules and regulations of your health care agency.

Leadership is a *process* and must be thought of in terms of action orientation. The best leadership is obtained by using an organized system of problem solving, in other words, a type of information processing. The learning and experience that you possess, combined with your problem-solving techniques, give you the ability to predict the outcome of any given situation. This approach is called a predictive principle: Given a set of circumstances, the leader can decide on the desired outcome and use the type of leadership necessary to reach that goal.

No goal can be obtained without the total cooperation of the group. Cooperation is best accomplished by using feedback. By considering leadership as a process or as an active behavior, you see another definition of leadership. The best leadership is achieved by directing change toward an objective by using feedback.

To reach any goal you must understand the elements of goal attainment. There are three elements to consider:

1. *Purpose*—the reason for the movement toward an objective: To be really efficient, any goal-achievement activity must have a valid purpose, which is clear to all individuals involved in the process.
2. *Organization*—the way the activity is structured to reach a goal: This planning and directing stage is necessary for efficient operations.
3. *Predicted outcome*—the final result to which all your energy, and that of your staff, is directed.

THE DEVELOPMENT OF LEADERSHIP

The process of leadership involves three essential steps:

1. input,
2. operation, and
3. feedback.

Input

Input is the formulation and development of the principles of leadership through education. It is the process of *learning* the fundamental rules that leaders apply to influence, control, and guide their own actions and the actions of their subordinates.

Operation

In this process, leaders *utilize* the principles of leadership—put them to work. Skilled leaders are not persons armed with a lot of simple, fixed habits that they turn on with push-button directness. They are persons who possess general skills, based on a general understanding and insight, and who are able to apply these skills to any situation. No leader is effective unless he or she can *use* the skills of leadership.

Feedback

The most important part of the leadership process, the feedback stage is one in which leaders are able to evaluate their leadership techniques and strategies through the comments and criticisms of their groups. Understanding why an operation worked or did not work can be achieved only by listening to the opinions and feelings of the group. Leaders must be open to their communication and willing to learn from this feedback. Once the feedback is obtained, you must be willing to use this data base to improve your leadership.

In order to be a good leader, you must accept the entire role of leadership. The role of leadership includes the leader, the led, and the audience: The leader's purpose is to guide and direct, the led (or your subordinates) are expected to accomplish the work and give feedback, and the audience is the group that benefits from the goal attainment. In the case of health care, the audience is the patient. Unless you consider all three elements, your leadership will be ineffectual.

LEADERSHIP PRINCIPLES

1. Know your profession and be able to teach it.
2. Know yourself and seek self-improvement.
3. Know your staff and look out for their welfare.
4. Keep your staff informed.
5. Set the example.
6. Insure that the task is understood, organized, supervised, and accomplished.
7. Train your staff as a team.
8. Make sound and timely decisions.
9. Seek responsibility and develop a sense of responsibility among subordinates.

55

10. Employ your command in accordance with its capabilities.

11. Take responsibility for your actions.

These principles of leadership are merely rules or guides used by leaders to influence their own actions and the actions of their subordinates. Adopt those rules, and you are well on your way to successful leadership—but do not become a slave to them. Remember, flexibility is a primary trait necessary for leadership. The leader who is able to function within the broad guidelines of these leadership principles—but still maintain creativity and originality—is the best kind of leader.

THE NATURE OF LEADERSHIP

There are two common theories concerning leadership: (1) the trait theory and (2) the situational theory.

The Trait Theory

Until the middle of the 1940s, the study of leadership centered around the traits possessed by successful leaders. Leaders were carefully studied, and the traits that each possessed in common were considered necessary "equipment" for the good leader. Traits such as honesty, drive, objectivity, judgment, initiative, and the like were thought to be absolutely necessary to the leader. People who did not have some of these attributes felt that they could never be effective leaders.

The fault of this theory lies in the assumption that the process of leadership is a "thing" that you either have or do not have. The theory implies that, if you are born with these traits, you will be a leader; if not, you are destined to be a follower for all of your professional life.

Simply relying on leadership traits, however, and assuming that others will follow your guidelines are dangerous mistakes. You must know your group, know your organization, and be willing to adapt your techniques to each situation presented. Even trait theorists who studied leaders noticed that not all good leaders possessed the same traits. In some situations, leaders who did not follow the traditional guidelines of the trait theory were very successful, because the best leaders are able to use these traits as an action orientation. They are able to judge each situation individually and to practice leadership as a *process* of guiding and directing.

The Situational Theory

The situational theory emphasizes the existence of leadership roles and skills that are evoked by situations or contexts. This entirely action-oriented theory assumes that, given the proper training in problem solving and leadership principles, anyone can be a leader.

The fault in this theory is that it fails to consider the fact that leadership is a complex process in which the traits of the leader *do* play a part. Adapting to each and every situation is important, but the really successful leader must also develop the traits of a leader: honesty, drive, objectivity, judgment, initiative, and so on.

You must learn to consider both theories as necessary to leadership. A good blend of the two is the key to successful leadership. Nurse/leaders are not blind followers of particular leadership styles. They are able to choose the method that they consider most appropriate for a given instance and, using the traits of a good leader, lead others to the accomplishment of goals.

GRADATION OF LEADERSHIP BEHAVIOR

There are several types, or levels, of leadership. Each has its own merits, and each can be an effective tool in directing others toward goal attainment.

Leader Makes a Decision and Announces It

In this most autocratic type of leadership behavior, the leader gives no opportunity for the group to express its opinions or thoughts. This brand of leadership is usually reserved for an emergency situation or in a teaching situation.

Leader "Sells" a Decision

The leader recognizes the feelings of subordinates, accepts some feedback, but basically is still in control of the situation. The leader attempts to persuade the group to accept his or her plan of action. This approach is usually employed when leaders feel that they are more aware of the overall plan and have the knowledge and experience necessary to make the best decision. It can be a very effective way of teaching others the proper method of solving problems. The wise leader is able to use a rational plan for problem solving and can teach the group to use the same system. Once the group is proficient in the methods of problem solving, they can be more independent. The steps in problem solving are:

1. State the situation and determine objectives.
2. Assemble all pertinent facts.
3. Analyze the problem in light of the facts determined.
4. Set up a tentative conclusion.
5. Check your conclusion by asking yourself, "Will this decision satisfy the first three steps?"
6. Put your plan into action and check the results.

Once your staff has learned to apply these steps, you have to rely on "selling" your decision less and less. As your group becomes more independent and participative, they become more committed to the goals of the organization.

The Leader Presents Ideas and Invites Questions

This sort of leadership incorporates a degree of participation. As the leader, you may still have an idea in mind, but you may be open to modification of your original plan. Depending on the level of control you have in your group, this can be an effective way to practice problem-solving techniques. If, as the leader, you have great control over the group, this method does not give the results that you desire. The group invariably chooses not to question your decision, because of fear, and resentfully goes along with your plan of action. If you are using this method, you must make it clear to the group that you are indeed willing to change if the situation warrants. Without this assurance, the group will not feel committed to the project.

The Leader Presents a Tentative Decision

This is the midpoint in the development of true participatory problem solving. The leader still defines the problem and works out the initial solution, but the group is well aware of the fact that this is only a possible solution. The leader makes it clear that he or she is very flexible and open to feedback.

The Leader Uses Suggestions to Make a Decision

In this method, the leader presents the problem, gets suggestions from the group, and then makes a decision based on these suggestions. You approach the group without first making a decision. This method invites the input from the group and allows them to solve problems and find facts. This is not total participatory leadership, however, because you, as the leader, are still defining the problem and making the final decision. This method is usually employed when the leader knows the problem, understands the organizational limitations, and seeks possible alternative action from the group. It is very effective when you do not really know how to reach the goal you must reach. Often, the actions decided on by a group as possible alternatives are not workable because of time or money limitations. The leader can inform the group of these limitations while still allowing their participation.

The Group Makes Decision
Within Set Limits

In this type of problem solving, the leader defines the limits and asks the group to make a decision. The leader takes less of an active part than in any other approach. Not only is the group allowed the freedom to define the problem, they are allowed to make the decision based on the limits set by the organization or by the leader. This method is usually applied to the health care setting. It is not often that a decision can be made without limits. There are always organizational considerations and limitations. The function of the leader is to express these limitations without crushing the creativity of the group.

The Group Functions
Within Broad Limitations

The leader permits the subordinates to function within the broadest limitations, thus allowing the maximum degree of subordinate participation. The subordinates are allowed to function as far as the limits of your authority as the leader. You allow your group to function as you, yourself, are able. No person who functions within the framework of an organization is able to perform totally indepedently, but you allow the group to function with as much independence and authority as the organization permits.

YOUR PERSONAL STYLE
OF LEADERSHIP

The best nurse/leaders are able to understand each of these gradations, and they are able to use the most participative method possible under a given set of circumstances. The method of choosing your own personal leadership style depends on three elements:

59

1. the organizational environment,
2. the personalities of the organization's members, and
3. the similarity of the group's and the organization's objectives.

The Organizational Environment

As an organization becomes more complex, the leadership usually becomes more authoritarian. In health care agencies, many departments and units must work together for the common good of the client, an effect that involves much interaction on all levels. This degree of communication can be accomplished only if all members of the group feel personally committed to the common goals. The task of the nurse/leader is to achieve the goals of the complex organization through participative leadership rather than authoritarian leadership. While this is a much more time-consuming and difficult process, the results of staff commitment and dedication are worth the effort.

The Personalities of the Organization's Members

Nurse/leaders must know their groups and their group members' personalities before selecting a style of leadership. Your personal style is affected by the personalities and expectations of your subordinates. Nurses and trained health care workers are characteristically motivated from within. They receive a great deal of personal satisfaction from the achievement of the goals of good patient care. As a result, they expect participation in problem solving, and they are motivated by this type of leadership. Trained nurses respond to the recognition of their knowledge and skills and are more effective, efficient, and satisfied if this is allowed to occur.

The Congruence of Objectives

When the goals and objectives of the organization are very similar to the goals and objectives of the group, a less formal structure is permissible. If the group feels that they are a team, working for common goals, they can be allowed much freedom in participating in decisions that affect their work situation. If the group does not feel that their goals are the same as the organization's, problems occur, and a more formal or authoritarian method of leadership must be employed.

THE PERFECT(?) SUPERVISOR

Some observers argue that leaders are born, not made—that various successful leaders use quite different methods. Their wide difference in styles, however, does not prove that they are "born leaders." Rather, it proves only that, since their personalities are different, they have adopted methods that suit their personalities and the personalities of their group.

Some leaders succeed in spite of obvious faults because they are outstanding in other aspects. For example, one supervisor is impatient and extremely critical, but she gets good results because she is decisive, because she gives orders and answers promptly, and because she freely and openly admits mistakes. She appears to be disliked but respected. Her staff tolerates her shortcomings because they have confidence in her. How much better it would be to use that self-confidence to develop the same feeling in her staff.

Yet any leader can do a better job by eliminating faults. For example, another supervisor may be openly contemptuous of mistakes, but so brilliant and hardworking that his staff respects him. By eliminating his faults, this leader could be more effective. Instead of establishing respect by productivity, he could gain even more respect by teaching his staff to be as proficient as he is. This change does not reduce his leadership effectiveness, but enhances it.

No one is, or can be, a perfect supervisor. Supervisors sometimes fail to observe all the rules of good leadership, because no one can always remember all of them and because no one has enough self-control to avoid occasional mistakes. All supervisors, however, can become better by following a program of improvement, which consists of:

1. becoming conscious of as many shortcomings as possible and trying honestly to correct each of them;
2. taking full advantage of every opportunity to use good leadership tactics; and
3. developing a reputation for possessing one or more leadership characteristics to an outstanding degree by practicing them constantly.

Practicing good leadership helps counteract the mistakes. Time and effort are required, but good practices are easy to follow. The results are better performance from subordinates and greater job satisfaction for both supervisor and subordinates.

HOW LEADERSHIP IS ESTABLISHED

Leadership is established by winning the respect, the confidence, and the loyalty of subordinates. In a sense, leaders must "sell" themselves to their staffs.

How to Win Respect

You must have the respect of your subordinates, for people do not give loyalty to, nor do they have confidence in, a person they cannot respect. Lack of respect for a supervisor may mean lack of respect for his or her instructions.

ENCOURAGE FREE SPEECH   No one consciously wants subordinates to be robots. Yet, by their attitudes toward objection and criticism, too many supervisors encourage or require their subordinates to obey them without feedback. This attitude causes you to lose:

1. the benefit of independent ideas;
2. information on operations or areas that require attention, correction, or improvement; and
3. the respect of your subordinates.

As the supervisor, you should welcome suggestions and criticisms, consider them fully, and, if necessary, take action. If suggestions or criticisms are not offered, you should seek them.

FINISH WHAT IS STARTED   Inaugurating a new plan or campaign involves doing three things:

1. adding to the work of subordinates;
2. attempting to improve efficiency; and
3. putting a plan and instructions to a test.

Failing to follow up a program has two ill effects: For one, it wastes the time, effort, and energy spent developing it, and second, it permits subordinates to disregard instructions. It may also encourage them to disregard other current orders and condition them to pay decreasing attention to future orders. Therefore, follow-up is necessary to win and hold respect. Keep track of what is started, and keep it going as long as a reason exists. If a better system is developed or if the need for the activity ceases, cancel the activity or project. The steps necessary to cancel a project are:

1. announce or publish the fact;
2. make it clear it was stopped because it was ordered stopped by a higher authority; and
3. give the reason for stopping.

KNOW WHAT IS HAPPENING   For proper management, you must know:

1. what kind of job is being done;
2. what kind of job the various individuals supervised are doing;

3. what job conditions are like;
4. what forthcoming changes may affect the unit;
5. irregular or improper habits or practices that may be developing among personnel; and
6. changes in operating procedures of related agencies that may affect the unit.

Statements, actions, or decisions that show you lack knowledge in an area are damaging to your subordinates' respect for you—particularly when the information is common knowledge, when "everyone knows but you." A lack of knowledge on your part makes it possible for subordinates to fool you. They may try to falsify charts, time cards, work short hours, take excessive time on breaks or on personal business, or misuse the organization's supplies or equipment.

To know what is going on, you must remain active and alert. Keep up-to-date on bulletins, orders, statistical analyses. Spend time with subordinates. Observe, ask questions, engage in casual conversation. Be alert for leads that require follow-up. Never violate the confidence of a person who gives you that information you should have. If a person is embarrassed, harassed, or criticized because you identified him or her, the source of future information is gone. You must be alert for information or leads in contacts with the public, business people, officials of related agencies, and others. Never seek to "save face" by pretending knowledge of affairs or brushing off further discussion of matters pertaining to the organization.

This sort of activity is merely another part of a supervisor's duties. Accept the fact that gathering information or intelligence about the organization is not "tale-bearing," "squealing," or "snitching." It is essential to good supervision. Both employees and the organization benefit from a system that brings difficulties to your attention. This is particularly true when conflict is found and corrected before dissatisfaction festers and spreads, or before misconduct damages the good name of the agency.

ASK ONLY NECESSARY QUESTIONS Request only work or activity that is really necessary and worth the time, effort, and expense it involves. Few things are as demoralizing as having to do work that is obviously of little value. Also, avoid unnecessary instructions. Where the desired action is clear, excessively detailed instructions arouse resentment and humiliation, by implying a lack of confidence.

EXPECT GOOD WORK AND CONDUCT Let your subordinates know that you have confidence in them and that you expect they will do their best. Don't accept work that is of poor quality. By accepting such a job, you are, in fact, approving it, and correction becomes that much more difficult. Tact and patience may be required to show the staff how the job should be done, but improvement comes no other way.

63

Set work standards as high as possible, and work toward them. Watch for the little errors, the small omissions, the insignificant oversights. Together, these add up to a poor job. People tend to perform according to what is expected of them. If standards are high and any substandard work returned for correction, the quality of work stays high—but keep a proper sense of proportion.

Be sure you supervise adequately. Don't permit errors to grow. Clear up questions and misunderstandings at once. An uncorrected error, repeated, becomes the fault of the supervisor.

Standards of conduct, as well as of quality, must be high. By your attitude and conduct, you—the supervisor—set the style for your staff. A supervisor whose habits are irregular, who is late for appointments, who is careless about facts, or who gets bored—this sort of supervisor imparts a similar attitude to the staff, and thus the staff reflect the same behavior.

You must have the initiative to investigate unsatisfactory work and conditions, along with the courage to take corrective action. Some of the most important facts of leadership are often overlooked or not understood. These facts are that:

1. people want to do good work;
2. morale is never a problem in an alert, progressive, efficient unit;
3. high morale is never found in a slipshod, substandard, easy-going unit;
4. high standards alone do not produce high morale, but high morale is impossible without them; and
5. "Our chief want in life is somebody who will make us do what we can [Emerson]."

ACKNOWLEDGE GOOD WORK   Praise stimulates good work. It is a far better stimulant than criticism, because building up a person's self-respect is preferable to tearing it down. Also, praise offsets necessary criticism, by appealing to the basic human desire to feel important.

Too little praise is a greater danger than too much. On the other hand, too much praise, or praise given uncritically, loses its value. Exercise care and good judgment. People properly crave the assurance and confidence that come from knowing that they stand well as members of the group to which they belong.

Yet it is the rare supervisor who goes to excess in telling the staff how well they are doing. Most supervisors, in fact, are too stingy with praise. They forget that it is part of their job. They fail to realize how important it is and how much it can accomplish. They fear it will make the staff self-satisfied, that they will relax their efforts. Some situations require criticism and correction, lest further harm be done, but the need for praise is seldom so obvious.

Praise publicly. Praise that others can hear has extra weight; it raises morale, standing, and self-confidence. People being praised have additional assurance that the praise is genuine—they have witnesses. Other staff members are put on notice that good work is observed, provided the praise given was earned, and that other deserving people are not overlooked.

Public praise may be either verbal or written. If it is a written commendation, it should be posted on a bulletin board or distributed. Use news media when appropriate. See that the facts are available for a good story, and let the person's name be used.

Praising need not be complex or difficult. In normal day-to-day activities, watch for opportunities to convey casual, verbal praise. Few supervisors realize how much people welcome a few honest words of admiration for their efforts. For example:

> That was a really good job of planning you did on the patient care.
>
> Your unit always looks terrific. How do you do it?
>
> That report was outstanding. After I read it I couldn't find a single point you overlooked.
>
> That patient was a hot-head, but what a good job you did of handling him.
>
> I've heard nothing but praise for that class you gave for in-service.

Praise is very important to morale, by improving self-confidence and giving people a deserved feeling of importance. It is evidence that a person's efforts are noted and appreciated. People just can't keep chips on their shoulders if you let them take a bow.

BE BUSINESS-LIKE IN ALL YOUR DEALINGS   Conducting yourself with dignity conveys assurance that your responsibilities are not taken lightly, but it does not necessarily mean being solemn. You can be cheerful, pleasant, and friendly, and still be business-like. On the other hand, levity or horseplay, particularly at inappropriate times, only causes loss of respect. Profanity, coarseness, and rudeness in speech are certainly not dignified and are inconsistent with leadership. People may be amused by clowns, but they do not respect them and do not accept their leadership.

BE CONSISTENT   Consistency is necessary to maintain the momentum of the organization. Most units operate after a fashion for a long time on sheer momentum. Policies, practices, assignments, and duties are known. Yet conflicting orders, abrupt changes, or obvious inconsistencies—with the supervisor's authority behind them—create confusion. The agency's effectiveness deteriorates much more quickly than without any supervision at all. Don't change orders without due thought, and then change them only when necessary. Don't overrule or modify instructions of subordinate supervisors unless absolutely necessary, and then do so only after adequate explanation. Don't change policies or practices without deep thought and good reason.

A supervisor who displays moodiness, or who is alternately optimistic and pessimistic, is not a leader. A supervisor who is affable and easygoing one day, but sullen and dour the next, is not a leader. Subordinates become cautious, not knowing which attitude to expect. They lose confidence in you and become bewildered.

BE PATIENT, CALM, AND SELF-CONTROLLED   The successful management of people requires learning and self-control. People do not always understand orders the first time. They may ask questions whose answers appear obvious to you. To a busy supervisor, the time spent in clarifying instructions or in listening to poorly organized arguments may be irritating to the point of producing an outburst of anger. Yet you cannot afford to let your emotions dictate your conduct. Calmness and patience are essential to good leadership.

Intolerance and impatience, the opposite traits, are disorganizing because they encourage undue haste, which means waste and confusion. Avoid such haste. This caution does not mean going slowly; rather, it means avoiding going faster than subordinates can or will go. Be slow to criticize or blame. Analyze, suggest, help, assist. Do not expect too much too soon. Set reasonable goals to avoid disappointment that results when unreasonable goals are not met.

Calmness is contagious. Subordinates will copy your attitude and manner, particularly in emergencies when people watch the supervisor closely. If you are calm, they will be too.

To stay calm, you have to fight your instincts. The human body is geared to jungle warfare. It has wonderful mechanisms to put up a good fight. When anger is aroused, the body's response is immediate—it is prepared to fight, and the brain is *not* prepared to think. However, fighting is usually impractical, and civilization does not permit it. So individuals must either "keep the lid on" but seethe inside, or "blow their tops" and say and do things they would never do normally. These things may never be forgotten, and permanent harm may be done.

There is no evidence whatever that anyone is born with a quick temper. Just as the control of temper is learned, losing your temper is also a learned behavior. Some people are actually proud of having a quick temper. What they are really proud of is the learned ability to stop thinking with their brains and to start thinking with their glands. The latter sort of thinking is, of course, *not* thinking at all; it is reacting. *There is no such thing as a good supervisor with a quick temper.*

Learn to control your temper. The first step is to *force* yourself to control it. Since control is learned, each success makes control easier the next time. The goal is never to lose your temper, no matter what the provocation. If circumstances make a loss of temper seem likely, politely but firmly refuse to continue the matter at hand, if it possible to do so. When dealing with an employee, this is a must. Defer the matter, even if for only a short time, until you gain control. A curious fact is that some supervisors know about this good tactic but refuse to use it for fear of tacitly admitting a lack of self-control. Yet how much more prestige is lost in the ensuing flare-up than would have been lost by postponing the discussion?

GIVE CREDIT FOR IDEAS   Many supervisors fail to give proper credit. Because they add to or improve upon an idea before passing it on, they believe they have the right to take full credit. This assumption is really wrong. When reward results, as from a merit award system, it is also legally wrong. Further, any respect gained from superiors by taking credit is far outweighed by the loss of respect from subordinates. Unselfishness in this respect stimulates trust and loyalty. Your staff becomes convinced that you are fair, square, honest, and appreciative.

TAKE PERSONAL RESPONSIBILITY FOR ERRORS   The responsibility of leadership, frequently a heavy burden, is always a dangerous burden for the person who is not prepared to assume it. Leadership calls for sacrifice, for prudence, for placing duty above personal gain and frequently above personal satisfaction. One of the basic principles of organization requires that supervisors must be given enough authority to perform the jobs for which they are responsible. This principle works both ways: Supervisors, since they are responsible for getting the job done, must be responsible for the use of their authority. They are responsible for any errors that may result from their instructions or for any other errors that the subordinate may make.

Some supervisors have an excessive fear of being wrong. They seem to believe that being wrong suggests they are not qualified to be supervisors. They seem to fear the loss of respect of both subordinates and superiors. To avoid the liability, they seek to blame anyone but themselves.

> I *told* him not to do that.
> I didn't know that could happen.
> I can't understand why she would order a thing like that.
> I didn't tell him to go that far.

Taking blame for errors or wrong decisions is essential to winning respect. No one expects supervisors to be perfect. You do not "lose face," as long as you are not wrong too often. Even if the mistake is only partly your fault, you should take all the blame rather than passing

67

it to a subordinate. Oddly enough, this measure increases the respect of your subordinates, and their awareness of the error is far overshadowed by their admiration for your courage and honesty.

In addition, you must be able to show by your voice and manner, as well as words, that you really do accept responsibility. A leader must have the ability to maintain poise under stress, even under actual criticism.

MAKE PROMPT DECISIONS   Supervisors who defer decisions are not leaders. They leave subordinates confused, not knowing what to do. Delay is frequently disadvantageous to the matter at hand, but the lasting effect of procrastination and indecision on subordinates is even worse. The clear inference from delay is that the supervisor lacks ability, knowledge, or courage.

Making decisions promptly does not mean making them hastily. Some delay may be necessary to get the facts. Sometimes you may not know the answer. Yet if you take action immediately to get the facts or to get the answer you need, subordinates will respect you.

Leaders may not let a faulty procedure or operation go on and on because they "don't have time" to work out something better. If you can't do it, you should assign someone else to do it. Ignoring a problem—hoping that it will go away—is not leadership.

BE COMPETENT PROFESSIONALLY   To lead, you must know the answers. You cannot bluff your way through all the time. You cannot hope that competent subordinates will carry you indefinitely. There is no substitute for exact knowledge. The supervisor must also give prompt, as well as correct, answers to job questions from subordinates. You cannot delay. You must know or find out promptly. Such questions concerning how to do various jobs or the correct procedures of the department must be promptly and correctly answered. To do so, you must have a good working knowledge of all subordinates' jobs, follow changes in policy, and generally keep up-to-date. You cannot supervise adequately unless you know the basics of the job supervised.

EXHIBIT HIGH PERSONAL INTEGRITY   Integrity is the observance of principles of conduct that are never subordinated to expediency. Leaders must be technically proficient in both their specialty and in leadership techniques, but technical proficiency alone is not enough. Before leading others, a person must learn self-control. Leaders must be mature persons with moral principles, standards to live by, and an aim and purpose in life. Leaders must do as they expect others to do, including areas such as:

1. obvious wrongs, such as misuse of department supplies or equipment;

2. work habits, such as promptness, dependability, courtesy, and industry; and
3. personal habits, such as neatness of dress and appearance, off-duty conduct.

People do not respect supervisors whose conduct and actions are not admirable, or those who attempt to enforce different standards for subordinates from those they adopt for themselves.

MAINTAIN GOOD PERSONAL APPEARANCE AND PHYSICAL CONDITION Appearance, manner, habits, speech, and social status do not make a leader, but noticeable weaknesses in any of these traits detract markedly. The importance of proper dress is very often overlooked. A nurse should be neat, clean, and well-dressed for all business or social occasions. For instance, a halter top and shorts—the "bare" look—are not acceptable dress for a social visit to the health care agency. The fact that most duty time is spent in uniform does not mean that a proper wardrobe of off-duty clothes is unnecessary.

Expecting proper dress is not unreasonable. Governmental employees, particularly those working in offices, are almost always well dressed. In fact, the average office employee spends more for clothes suitable for work than nursing personnel do for uniforms.

Keeping yourself in good physical condition is important for three reasons:

1. *Reaction of subordinates:* It is difficult for people to follow a supervisor who does not keep in good physical condition. The staff knows that their jobs require good health, and most nurses are in reasonably good shape. They resent a supervisor who is not in good physical condition.
2. *Reaction of the public:* The public has a rather glamorous opinion of nurses. They believe that nurses are gentle, but capable of heavy work if necessary. The public looks with disfavor on any member of the organization who is obviously not in good physical condition. This reaction is particularly true of supervisory personnel who, as leaders, should set the example. Furthermore, subordinates are embarrassed and resentful if supervisors do not look the part they play.
3. *Requiring staff to be healthy:* A supervisor who is not in good condition cannot expect subordinates to maintain themselves in good condition. This expectation poses an impossible dilemma: As a supervisor, you must require your staff to be healthy, yet, as an individual, you are not setting an example.

Supervisors who expect to be leaders should even exert the self-discipline necessary to control their weight. Excessive weight comes from just one thing: overeating.

All fat comes from food. There has never been a fat individual in the history of the world who could not lose if he followed a weight-reduction diet. Almost never are any of the glands of internal secretion associated with obesity. The only glands which seem to be involved are the salivary glands.[1]

How to Win Confidence

You must have the confidence of your subordinates. People do not give loyalty to a person in whom they lack confidence. You, as the leader, must take advantage of all opportunities to build confidence and guard against actions that destroy confidence.

INSIST ON HONEST, HONORABLE, AND PROPER METHODS AND PRACTICES   Reports on patient care must be honest. Admitting an error is far better than falsifying a report or giving false information. Comply with the intent of orders and policies. Do not attempt to circumvent them, and do not look for loopholes. Submit truthful reports even if they are unfavorable. Be truthful and factual in press releases, speeches, and statements. Shady or questionable practices or not-quite-true statements only destroy the confidence which you must have. Also, even tacitly permitting subordinates to do these things weakens your position as the leader.

FACE THE FACTS   A leader who faces facts gains the confidence of the staff. Subordinates know what the leader wants, they know where they stand, and they have no fear of bringing up problems or difficulties for advice or assistance. Frankness saves time. Do not beat around the bush, and encourage subordinates to be frank. Never be angered by a fact. Admit errors frankly and openly. Meet important issues squarely, and make a decision. Do not gloss over difficult assignments. Openly discuss the difficulties and how to overcome them.

KEEP SUBORDINATES INFORMED   Let the staff know what is going on. It is essential that staff be told as far as possible in advance of any changes that affect them. A proper presentation prevents the unrest that accompanies rumors, makes the staff feel they are part of the team, reduces the number of objections, and improves the likelihood of acceptance.

News of changes or proposed plans should be given to supervisors first. This procedure enables them to explain things intelligently to their staff and to the public. It prevents humiliation, moral demotion, or loss of respect, all of which occur when subordinates know more about operations than their supervisors.

[1] Edward H. Rynearson, M.D., "Obesity (The Overweight Problem)," *Police*, Vol. 1, No. 1 (September–October, 1956), pp. 56–57.

If supervisors cannot answer a question from a subordinate, they should not send the person to a higher supervisor to find out. The supervisor should go alone or with the nurse to find out.

Staff members must know more about operations of their agency than the general public. They will be asked questions regarding newspaper articles, radio and TV programs, announcements, and the like. If they are not familiar with the subject of the question, they may become embarrassed and resentful. They may feel they are not considered important by the agency, that they are not a part of the agency, or that their efforts are not appreciated.

When people are informed, efficiency is increased, in several ways:

1. they will think about problems and possibly have good ideas that can be used, and
2. they will avoid activities, statements, or operations that might conflict with the program.

AVOID CRITICIZING SUPERIORS Whether apparently justified or not, such criticism destroys the subordinates' confidence in the entire organizational structure—including confidence in the supervisor who is doing the criticizing.

Seek a constructive explanation for what might appear to be mistakes, oversights, delays, and the like. Do not say, "I tried to get this for you, but I couldn't get it through." This sort of statement is as good as admitting that your opinion carries little weight with your supervisors.

KEEP PROMISES The best way to avoid breaking promises is to avoid making them. New supervisors in particular are prone to make rash, impulsive promises that cannot be kept. Even some older supervisors never seem to learn the harm that can be done by making promises that are not kept.

The emphasis on keeping promises seems like much ado about a small matter. Yet some authorities in the personnel field believe that broken promises destroy morale more quickly than any other factor. Everyone has had experiences where promises were not kept. The memory and bitterness usually last for years. Confidence in the person who broke the promise is usually badly damaged or lost.

There is danger in people misinterpreting a statement so as to believe that a promise has been made. "I'll see what I can do" becomes "I'll do it for you if I possibly can" or "I'll do it." This misunderstanding can be avoided by clearly defining what you mean and what you will attempt to do. Disappointing the nurse immediately is better than compounding the disappointment later. In addition, besides disappointment, a lack of confidence in the supervisor results.

71

If you make a promise in good faith, you must keep it if humanly possible. If keeping it creates more work and difficulty for you than anticipated, that is the price that must be paid for making it.

If it is impossible to keep a promise, explain why at the earliest opportunity, in detail, to the nurse who was promised. If the promise was made in the presence of other staff members, see that they also know why the promise was not kept.

SUPPORT THE VALID INTERESTS OF SUBORDINATES   You must show that you have their interests at heart. If convinced of the justice of the situation, you should seek an equitable solution. You must demonstrate that you aggressively support the staff when they are right, that you support them when they *meant* to be right, but that do *not* support them in derelictions of duty, in deliberate violation of regulations, or in willful misconduct.

GET THINGS DONE FOR SUBORDINATES ON TIME   To win confidence, you must do your job both properly and promptly. If an undesirable situation develops and is discovered, correct it right away. If changes or improvements are promised, keep at it until the promise is fulfilled. Thoroughly accustom subordinates to the fact that your word is good. Promptness and decisiveness of action increase both respect and confidence.

HELP SUBORDINATES TO DO THEIR JOBS NOW AND THEN   Helping should be done not as a routine thing, but on occasions when the job is difficult and the person is obviously having trouble. It should be done with tact, never derision. If appropriate, let the person know the job is unusually difficult. You should show that you know the subordinate is capable of doing the job, but that this is nonroutine and may require two heads instead of one. You may let the person know that he or she cannot be expected to know how to do it without proper instruction. You should *help* the person, not do it all yourself. The self-confidence of the person is bolstered, and his or her confidence in your job knowledge is enhanced, provided a competent job of coaching is done. The tact used, along with the time devoted to helping, shows persons that you consider them important. This reaction invariably produces added confidence in the leader.

In addition to other advantages, helping out produces a greater acceptance of future orders and instructions, providing you actually did a good job of assistance and showed detailed job knowledge plus good judgment.

LISTEN TO YOUR SUBORDINATES' COMPLAINTS   The supervisor who readily receives complaints shows a real interest in the staff. If complaints and grievances are received reluctantly or deprecated, you show that you are not really interested in your staff or that you are trying to avoid hearing the trouble, fearing you may have to back up actions and policies or correct a difficult situation.

Welcoming discussion of complaints and grievances helps the supervisor keep in touch with what subordinates are doing and thinking. Discussion also helps supervisors detect dissension before it becomes serious.

APPEAR CONFIDENT   An attitude of success and assurance is contagious. It inspires self-confidence in the staff members, and it inspires the confidence of the staff in you. An attitude of worry, apprehension, and indecisiveness is also contagious. People lose their own self-assurance, lose confidence in the supervisor, and lose confidence in the department. They tend to view orders, ideas, and policies with doubt and suspicion.

Therefore, you must be something of an actor. Everyone has periods of depression when you are tired, worried, discouraged. You must learn to conceal your feelings and show a confident and assured face. You must have a strong belief in your own competence, as well as the ability to display self-confidence in a natural and acceptable manner.

RESPECT THE CONFIDENCE OF SUBORDINATES   Subordinates look to you for direction of their activities, for the authority to act, for approval or disapproval of their work. They expect to be told what their jobs are, what is expected, how well they are performing. This important subordinate–superior relationship often produces considerable anxiety to subordinates. Subordinates keep a good deal of their attention on "the boss," alert to anticipate your wishes, to avoid your censure, to gain your praise. They are often very sensitive to your moods; they analyze and seek hidden meanings in your casual gestures. If you casually question an action, does it mean you disapprove?

This sensitivity occasionally produces the problem of over-reaction to commands and the misinterpretation of requests—from what the supervisor ordered to what they *thought* you wanted. What you say has a special impact on your subordinates. An unintended inflection of the voice, a careless choice of words, and the bypassing of a subject a subordinate has brought up can all breed misunderstanding and insecurity that interfere with efficient work. Thoughtless remarks, forgotten in a flash by those who make them, cause multitudes of restless nights and frustrating days for those who hear them.

Unfortunately, most people are more concerned with what their own supervisors think about them than how they are regarded by their subordinates. They are reluctant to pass on unpleasnat news, glossing over or favorably slanting bad news. Many subordinates watch for favorable times and moods to present a request or to pass on necessary

73

information. When they do so, they create a channel of communication that works only by fits and starts. This channel modifies and distorts what passes through, and, unless circumstances are deemed just right, it may effect a complete stoppage. The result is that you are insulated— you have only a partial and highly interpreted picture of what is actually going on. On successively higher levels of command, this sort of insulation becomes more and more effective, since the higher commanders must rely on reports for most of their information.

Respecting the confidence of subordinates helps to solve this problem. Welcome any information or problem they may bring. If the matter is confidential and if revealing the source would be embarrassing, protect the individual.

Avoid moodiness, as well as fluctuations in attitudes and in receptiveness. Insist that all pertinent information be given promptly, and let the staff know their confidence is respected and appreciated.

How to Win Loyalty

Respect and confidence alone are not enough. People do not respond well to leaders who are cold and unfriendly. A friendly feeling toward the leader is usually essential to building personal loyalty. In emergencies, when fast and blind acceptance of instructions is required, loyalty is indispensable. This acceptance is particularly necessary when circumstances require subordinates to do what they think the leader would *want* done, where immediate supervision is absent and communications impaired. Many supervisors, on the other hand, refuse to develop friendly relations, fearing that subordinates will take advantage on the principle of "familiarity breeds contempt."

Loyalty is a feeling or attitude, more emotional than intellectual. It is induced in the subordinate by the same feeling in the supervisor. In other words, loyalty begets loyalty, and the supervisor wins loyalty in proportion to the loyalty that he or she gives. Loyalty is related to friendship; thus some form of a personal relationship is necessary. Being friendly does not mean being weak. It is possible to be both firm and pleasant, and the proper mixture of firmness and pleasantness must be adjusted to suit the temperaments of individual subordinates.

BE PLEASANT   Cheerfulness is friendliness. Cheerfulness implies and conveys a liking for others, whereas grouchiness implies and conveys dislike. Cheerfulness is stimulating, because it implies faith in self, in the department, in the job. It produces a pleasant environment where more work can, and will be, done. It helps overcome obstacles, produces more cooperation, smooths relations. Cheerfulness and friendliness can be developed consciously, but, like everything else worthwhile, they require some effort and self-discipline. Being pleasant is more difficult for some than for others, who have developed it as part of their personalities through the years.

Developing cheerfulness starts with a very simple muscular operation, a smile. A smile requires some acting if you are not really feeling cheerful, but it more than pays off in smooth relations. Cheerfulness and friendliness are not undignified. Some supervisors fear that they will detract from their prestige, yet most of the really important people in the world are cheerful and pleasant. Only the uncertain, apprehensive, and insecure supervisor is afraid to be cheerful and pleasant.

BE AVAILABLE   Be at hand, be ready to be of service, be approachable. A supervisor who is distant in manner and difficult to talk with does not encourage a friendly relationship. Furthermore, you must show that you welcome consultation on any problem or concern. You must have an easy conversational relationship with the staff, which is important so that:

1. a new idea may be offered casually, even if the person is not sure of its value and even if all the details are not worked out;
2. the channels of information so necessary to a supervisor will stay open; and
3. most important, the subordinate–supervisor relationship becomes easy, informal, and workable.

Several techniques and practices help the supervisor to seem available:

1. Have a cheerful greeting, a few easy words to show you are available, in both body and spirit.
2. Have the maximum possible personal contacts. Be present at shift changes and at other times, and try to have a few words with the staff, whether meeting them in the office or on the road.
3. When nurses want to talk over a problem at the office, consider not talking across a desk. A desk is a symbol of authority and may create a barrier to free discussions. Sitting on the "wrong" side of a desk creates a restraining atmosphere of homage.

BE SYMPATHETIC   Modern personnel administration regards empathy as absolutely indispensable to a leader. You must be sympathetic with the staff in their troubles. When having personal or business difficulty, everyone craves sympathy. By simple transference, they come to like those who sincerely sympathize with them. Conversely, when people feel they deserve sympathy, they resent those who fail to sympathize. Supervisors must therefore never become so preoccupied with duty that they fail to respond to troubles of subordinates. *Any trouble that is important to a subordinate must be important to the supervisor.*

RECOGNIZE THE STAFF AS INDIVIDUALS　Employees are people. The department hires the whole person—complete with hopes, plans, financial worries, domestic problems, personal history, training and experience, likes and dislikes, special abilities and deficiencies. You can direct the activities of nurses while knowing little about them, but doing so is *not* leadership. Developing cooperation and job enthusiasm in nurses requires appealing to their beliefs and interests, and these can be learned only by having a real interest in them, drawing them out tactfully.

　　To produce loyalty, there must be liking. To produce liking, there must be interest. To produce interest, there must first be interest in the person on the part of the supervisor. Leaders who are really interested in the staff always find that the nurses are interested in them. Ambitious people have always made it a point to take interest in and be informed about the things that their superiors were interested in. The obvious purpose, of course, is to produce liking and possible favorable consideration for advancement. The same thing works in reverse. Subordinates develop a liking and work better for a leader who is interested in them as individuals in the same things they are.

　　Show a real interest in the ideas and suggestions of the staff. The reasons should be obvious: The thoughts may be of value; the interest you show stimulates future thinking by the staff; and it is an easy way to further friendly relations.

　　Interest and friendliness must be sincere. Insincerity is detected and produces dislike. You must not only feel real interest, but show it. Some techniques are: using first names, knowing and asking about families, holding short and informal "bull sessions" at intervals, and having lunch together on occasions.

WATCH HEALTH AND SAFETY　Concern for health and safety, a supervisor's duty, prevents economic loss to the organization through lost time, through the training of new employees, and through destroyed or damaged supplies and equipment. It also gives supervisors a splendid opportunity for developing loyalty, if they are positive but tactful in their methods and if they show that they are genuinely concerned with the well-being of their personnel.

　　You should protect your employees' health. Do not let them work when they are ill. Doing so is not good for the individual, and it is not good for others working with them or for their patients. For example, the "heroic" employee who comes to work with a bad cold is prolonging the illness, increasing its severity, and infecting co-workers and patients. Encourage and assist employees to get adequate medical care.

Also take necessary action to insure healthy working conditions in your department, such as fresh air, controlling draft, proper temperature, cleanliness (including wash rooms), proper sanitary supplies (soap, towels, and the like), good lighting, freedom from unnecessary noise. Anything that affects the employee's efficiency during working hours is the supervisor's business, particularly in the case of nursing personnel, where dulled reflexes or vision on duty can cause disaster. Watch for excessive drinking, insufficient sleep, excessive fatigue from outside employment, and drug abuse.

Consider health factors in making work assignments. Try to distribute the workload as evenly as possible, and schedule work to avoid "rush jobs." When tension is added to a heavy workload, fatigue is greater. Where possible, assign people to work they like to do. They will not get nearly so tired.

Insist employees relax when possible. Check to see that they take their lunch hours and coffee breaks. Long study has proven the value of rest periods in maintaining health and improving efficiency. Give vacations at the best possible times for employees, considering the needs of the organization.

Watch your personal attitude. A cheerful and encouraging supervisor has the same kind of people. A job well done and appreciated by the supervisor is the best health tonic an employee can have.

Protect employees from accidents by regular inspections and proper maintenance of the facilities and equipment, and watch for unnecessarily unsafe practices, correcting them immediately. Promote safety by using prepared posters, through discussions at meetings and conferences, and by observing and counseling individuals.

BE COURTEOUS, TACTFUL, AND CONSIDERATE   Courtesy, tact, and consideration are essential in winning friendship, without which loyalty is impossible.

Courtesy consists of polite behavior and thoughtfulness for others. It is a great defensive tool, because it begets courtesy, increases self-control, and produces respect. Courtesy is not deference; people in the highest positions are courteous to subordinates. Always be as courteous to subordinates as to superiors; always be as courteous to subordinates as to strangers. Subordinates should not be interrupted when talking any more than strangers should. The same expressions of courtesy used with strangers should be used with subordinates: "please . . . thank you . . . may I—. . . could you," and so on.

Make it a point to speak pleasantly and courteously to subordinates and their families whenever appropriate. Remember names. Although remembering names becomes increasingly difficult as you attain higher rank, because you have more subordinates, it also becomes increasingly important. One whose name is remembered feels important; one whose name is forgotten feels unimportant, discouraged, sometimes resentful. Failure to remember a name is a discourtesy.

Tact is regard for another's personality. Tact is selecting approaches, words, and phrases that appeal to positive moods and feelings (loyalty, duty, justice, fairness, courtesy, liking). Tact is avoiding approaches, words, and phrases that provoke negative moods (hatred, suspicion, fear, resentment, anger). Tact is not the avoidance of unpleasant subjects. It is not side-stepping disagreeable, distasteful, or disappointing subjects.

Considerate leaders put themselves into their subordinates' places before making decisions affecting them. They recognize the problems of their subordinates, both official and personal, and they know that their staff members have pride and self-respect, characteristics that are assets unless trampled upon.

BE IMPARTIAL   Try to avoid prejudices. Prejudice is arriving at conclusions or opinions on insufficient evidence or allowing preconceived ideas to color your attitude. Do not form an adverse opinion of a subordinate without good and complete cause. Do not let a single action of a subordinate create a prejudice. If you have to make a decision affecting an individual subordinate and if you have any reason to believe yourself prejudiced, you should discuss the problem with an impartial individual whose judgment you respect.

Avoid favoritism. Favoritism is giving an individual a greater number of privileges than his or her performance or position warrants. Supervisors are much more frequently accused of favoritism than they deserve. The reason is that they fail to justify their choice for desirable assignments when such assignments are first made. Supervisors may certainly have the authority to make a choice without explanation, but they may damage morale if they use that authority arbitrarily.

The solution is to discuss your reasons for selection at the appropriate time, such as at meetings or conferences. You may also post or distribute your reasons in the written order for assignment. Or you may discuss the reasons with key subordinates whose opinions carry weight with the staff, the "natural" leaders.

Be open-minded. In disciplinary situations be willing to see both sides. Get all the facts, seek the cause. Be willing to look for faulty instructions, poorly conceived procedures, inadequate supervision. Consider the long-range welfare of the individuals concerned, as well as the immediate good of the organization.

HANDLE SOCIAL FRIENDSHIPS WITH SUBORDINATES CAREFULLY   Many supervisors are wary of social contacts with subordinates. In general, they are right. You should be able to develop the right sort of friendliness during business hours, while maintaining the necessary barrier. Supervisors who are too familiar with subordinates have thrown away a very valuable supervisory advantage. It is difficult to snap back to a business relationship after a period when all the barriers are down. The supervisor must guard against the appearance of favoritism. Considerable social mixing with one or two out of a group is resented by others. *A rule: Be one with, but not one of, the staff.*

Certain exceptions must be recognized and require special care. Whenever the entire group gathers socially you should attend. You may leave early or when good judgment indicates. You must maintain reasonable decorum, but a failure to appear hurts you. The usual reaction of subordinates to the nonappearance of the supervisor is that you are not friendly and do not care for them, and that feeling is reciprocated.

Relationships with subordinates at a level close to yours require the recognition that there is no clear-cut middle ground to the problem of social friendships. The best policy is to go as far as seems safe, stopping short of the point where subordinates threaten to presume on the relationship. Supervisors who are close to, or very friendly with, a subordinate several levels below must confine their relations entirely to off-duty times. Otherwise they are placing their intermediate supervisors in an awkward position.

The most effective practical technique for maintaining the necessary barrier is to insist on being addressed by title in any official relationship, when either is on duty or when you are discussing business. Always being addressed by title has the psychological effect of subtly reminding both parties of their relationship.

DISCUSSION QUESTIONS

1. How is leadership established?
2. Why is it vital to have the respect of your subordinates?
3. Why is it a sound practice to give praise publicly?
4. In what ways is consistency important in supervision? Why?
5. How do supervisors go about retaining control of their tempers? What is wrong with "blowing off a little steam" now and then?
6. Who should be held responsible for errors? Why? Can you "pass the buck" for mistakes?
7. What are the qualities of a good supervisor? Why is each important?
8. How should supervisors go about winning the confidence of their staffs? Why is confidence important?
9. Why is it important to keep subordinates informed? What happens when a supervisor fails to keep the staff informed?
10. Under what, if any, circumstances should a supervisor support the staff? Should the supervisor support management against

the staff, right or wrong? If not, what should he or she do about a conflict?

11. What is so important about an attitude of confidence?

12. How should the nurse/supervisor handle social relationships on the job?

APPLICATION: LEADERSHIP CHECKLIST

This checklist is for use by all supervisors. Next to each question, place a check in the appropriate column. If you feel you are doing quite well in the areas indicated by the following questions, place a check under HIGH. If you consider your performance average or generally adequate, check under MIDDLE. If you find that you are doing little or if you are not satisfied with your performance, check under LOW. If you have had no occasion to perform in an area, try to estimate how you would act if the occasion arose.

Responsibility for Staff and Results

Do you:	LOW	MIDDLE	HIGH
• accept responsibility for the performance of your staff?	___	___	___
• know the duties and responsibilities of your immediate superior and try to anticipate events?	___	___	___
• perform all tasks to the best of your ability?	___	___	___
• give a day's work for a day's pay, while insisting on the same from your staff?	___	___	___
• maintain your physical fitness, mental alertness, and correct uniform? (Are you ready for each day's job? Is your efficiency unimpaired by a lack of sleep? Are you careful about your health? Are your clothes clean? And so on.)	___	___	___
• maintain an optimistic attitude?	___	___	___
• avoid bursts of rage?	___	___	___
• avoid vulgar language?	___	___	___
• avoid talk that "glamourizes" or appears to condone immoral or improper conduct or actions?	___	___	___
• cooperate with your superiors in spirit as well as in action? Are you loyal to the administration as well as to the staff?	___	___	___
• avoid loose criticism and careless grumbling? And do you take positive steps to prevent derogatory remarks of seniors by juniors?	___	___	___
• share the dirty work as well as the pleasant assignments?	___	___	___
• keep your superior informed of personnel problems as well as of material problems?	___	___	___

	LOW	MIDDLE	HIGH
• habitually follow the chain of command and require others to do the same?	———	———	———
• insist on loyalty downward as well as loyalty upward?	———	———	———

Knowing Your Staff

If you can answer all the following from memory, check HIGH. If you are not sure or if you are in error about several, check MIDDLE. If you draw a blank or almost a blank, check LOW.

Do you know:	LOW	MIDDLE	HIGH
• how many people there are in the department?	———	———	———
• their last names?	———	———	———
• their first names?	———	———	———
• their approximate ages?	———	———	———
• their level of education?	———	———	———
• marital status?	———	———	———
• number of children?	———	———	———
• ambitions and hobbies?	———	———	———
• how many of your people are taking college training or correspondence courses?	———	———	———
• the educational background of your staff?	———	———	———

Knowing Your Job

Lasting respect and confidence in leaders are based on their level of technical competence as well as on their honesty, fairness, and integrity. Check HIGH, MIDDLE, or LOW, according to your estimate of your success in the following areas.

Do you:	LOW	MIDDLE	HIGH
• make sure the staff gets the right answers from you? Or do you have to refer them to another person?	———	———	———
• regularly carry a notebook and use it to help keep a record of your staff, their assignments, jobs to be done, and so forth?	———	———	———
• read and interpret the instructions and manuals, and figure out how the equipment works or what the procedures are?	———	———	———
• study new operating manuals or procedures, and then explain their import to the staff?	———	———	———
• know the work and equipment in your charge as well as, or better than, any person under you?	———	———	———

81

	LOW	MIDDLE	HIGH
• keep up with new developments so that new equipment or procedures are no surprise to you?	_____	_____	_____
• assign people according to their ability?	_____	_____	_____
• delegate authority where possible and proper?	_____	_____	_____
• rotate assignments of disagreeable and of agreeable tasks among your group?	_____	_____	_____
• make sure a relief is trained and prepared for every job?	_____	_____	_____
• know what college courses are being offered and encourage your staff to attend?	_____	_____	_____

Training and Informing Your Staff

If you are doing well in the following areas, check HIGH; if just mediocre, check MIDDLE; if poorly, check LOW.

Do you:	LOW	MIDDLE	HIGH
• regularly review nursing publications and note information of interest to pass on to your staff?	_____	_____	_____
• have a regular "pass-the-word" session with your staff, in which they can ask questions about matters that concern them?	_____	_____	_____
• regularly (at least monthly) review progress in college or correspondence training courses?	_____	_____	_____
• keep an up-to-date bulletin board?	_____	_____	_____
• watch for people eligible for advancement and encourage them to prepare themselves for such programs?	_____	_____	_____
• always arrive on time for a report?	_____	_____	_____
• help people of low education improve themselves?	_____	_____	_____
• help people of ability get ahead faster?	_____	_____	_____

Thinking About Your Evaluation

Add up your check marks in the three columns. The number of LOW and MIDDLE check marks are guides to areas in which you need improvement. Why not write down your score of check marks and the date, and then, in three to six months, see what progress you can record?

DATE	NUMBER OF CHECK MARKS		
Now: _____	_____	_____	_____
Three months later: _____	_____	_____	_____
Six months later: _____	_____	_____	_____

APPLICATION: LEADERSHIP/FOLLOWERSHIP

1. Think of a person in your group whom you would, under most circumstances, feel most comfortable following. Describe that person in whatever terms are relevant to you.

2. Think of someone you would feel least comfortable following. Describe.

3. Assuming you are the leader, think of a person in your organization whom, under most circumstances, you would most like to have as one of your followers. Describe that person in whatever terms are relevant for you.

4. Think of someone you would least like to have as a follower. Describe.

5. Where do you think your leadership style fits between these types?

1	2	3	4	5	6	7

Leader I do not   Leader I like
like to follow   to follow

6. List some people you would be most likely to choose as a leader in the following situations:
  a. In a military battle? Why?
  b. Host at a party with people you have not met before? Why?
  c. Starting a new business? Why?
  d. Running an existing business? Why?

7. In which of the preceding four situations do you think you would make the best leader? Why?

REFERENCES

LATEINER, ALFRED, *Modern Techniques of Supervision.* New York: Lateiner Publishing Company, 1965.

LEAVITT, THEODORE, "The Managerial Merry-Go-Round," *Harvard Business Review* (July–August 1974).

MASSIE, JOSEPH L. AND JOHN DOUGLAS, *Managing: A Contemporary Introduction.* Englewood Cliffs, N.J.: Prentice-Hall, Inc., 1973.

PAYNE, BRUCE, *Long-Range Planning.* New York: McGraw-Hill Book Company, 1963.

RENSIS, LIKERT, "Motivation: The Core of Management," in *Human Elements of Administration,* Harry R. Knudson, Jr. New York: Holt, Rinehart & Winston, Inc., 1963.

SPRIEGEL, WILLIAM R., EDWARD SCHULZ, AND WILLIAM B. SPRIEGEL, *Elements of Supervision.* New York: John Wiley & Sons, Inc., 1967.

5

Communication

THE IMPORTANCE
OF COMMUNICATING

Many studies have been done on what the active supervisor does during the work day. Unfailingly, most of these studies show that the average supervisor spends more than 50 percent of his or her time in one function, communication. As you move up the so-called "managerial hierarchy," this percentage tends to increase. Many top executives in health care spend 90 percent or more of their time communicating. At first glance, these percentages are awesome. However, when you stop to analyze exactly what you do, they are not so surprising. Most of the responsibilities of supervisors, after all, consist partially or totally of communication: assigning, evaluating performance, counseling, and training. In fact, communication is the supervisor's most important function—the one that overrides all the rest. Imagine what would happen to all your other functions—planning, organizing, delegating, controlling, and the like—if you were not able to understand others and make yourself understood. It's easy to see that a communication problem affects supervisory effectiveness far more seriously than any other problem.

The question is, how can you, as a supervisor, improve your ability to communicate? You have to understand the processes involved—understand what's happening and change your ways, if necessary. Communication processes all start with our bodies. Our eyes, ears, nose, and nerves convey messages from the world outside us. In a vast complex of bones, tissues, nerves, organs, muscles, glands, cartilage, and chemicals, various centers of thought act and react constantly. The problem is trying to communicate under these conditions of multiple stimuli. Specifically:

1. What can you do to communicate your needs to others in the organization?
2. How can you help others communicate their needs to you?

T–A–G OBJECTIVES

To get down to the basics, try looking at communication as a fast game of verbal "tag," in which the rules are important. At the start of the game, every communicator (the source) thinks he or she has ideas that are going to reach the intended receivers (readers, listeners, viewers). Whether or not these ideas can be "T" (translated into a persuasive message) is one question. Whether the message "A" (attracts the attention of receivers) is another question, and whether the communicator "G" (gets a reaction) is an important third question.

"T"—Translating Ideas

The first stage of the three-stage communications model takes place within the source or communicator, before a word is spoken or written. The source's primary objective is to translate ideas into a message. The primary problem of idea translation is the selection of accurate, meaningful, and persuasive words to represent the ideas. Some specific psychological variables come into play to block or affect the translation of an idea. These are:

1. education,
2. experience,
3. motivation,
4. prejudice, and
5. fear.

EDUCATION   The educational levels of both the communicator and the receiver are important because of the strong influence they have on word choice and word understanding. A well-educated person tends to use and comprehend more complex and sophisticated words than someone with little formal education. You must always consider the educational level of the person to whom you are communicating.

One of the biggest problems in communication, especially written communication, arises when you try to dazzle people with your intelligence. You should communicate to express, not impress. The purpose of communication is to convey your meaning, not to show your cleverness. Simple words, when they are adequate to express a thought, are best. Your communication should send a message. Keep all communication simple, to-the-point, and useful.

EXPERIENCE   Experience, like education, may vary widely between the source and the receiver. The communicator must establish a common ground of experience with intended receivers and speak in terms they understand. Use a different approach to a student nurse than to an experienced staff nurse. Never assume that your listener understands, and make sure that there is a real understanding.

MOTIVATION   When you use any form of communication, you have a reason for the communication. The people for whom the message is intended also have a reason for listening to your message. They may be listening just to please you, they may be seeking the answer to a question, or they may be trying to learn a new procedure. To communicate effectively, you must know why you are sending the message, and you must have a general idea of why the group is receiving the communication.

PREJUDICE   When people speak, we hear not what is said, but what we want to hear. Everything we receive is tempered by our own ideas and feelings. We assume that the words we use mean the same to the hearer as they do to us, but in reality this assumption is false. The same word may have an entirely different meaning to the communicator than it does to the hearer. The supervisor must communicate, not to be understood, but so as not to be *mis*understood.

Sometimes perfectly innocent words or phrases can be misinterpreted by the listener. For example, a man on a bus is greeted by a familiar looking woman, but he cannot place where he met her. She greets him very loudly with, "Aren't you the father of one of my children?" After many strange looks from bystanders and a few minutes of total embarrassment, he suddenly realizes that she is his son's teacher. We all say things without thinking how they sound to others. The problem is not with the hearer; it is with the communicator. Try to think how your audience will interpret your words or phrases. If necessary, say the words out loud to yourself to hear how they sound.

Other words are theoretically neutral, but in fact they have meanings that are colored by our own prejudices. Black, white, liberal, red, free, and female are words that can trigger feelings that have no relation to the idea being expressed. Prejudice is an admittedly difficult problem, so it is important for you as a supervisor to anticipate and avoid the words that can create problems.

FEAR   Many times listeners are not able to receive our messages because they are frightened. Your position of supervisor may trigger a fear response in subordinates, and they are rendered unable to understand what you are saying. Relieving the tension as much as possible in dealings with staff members reduces the fear and opens the door for better communication.

"A"—Attracting Attention

The second stage of communication involves the message. The purpose of the message is to attract attention. If it fails to do so, then the communication fails. In this phrase of the transmission, there are frequent breakdowns, which are usually caused by carelessness in the speech or writing habits of the communicator.

Using speech shortcuts frequently causes receivers to miss the message; their attention is not attracted. Using sloppy speech habits—such as saying, "shoppin" for "shopping" or "huh?" for "what?"—can cause problems. Most people get lazy in their speech habits because it is easier to use these shortcuts. Spend a day or so intently listening to your speech pattern. See how many shortcuts you use, and try to eliminate these sloppy speech habits. Another way to improve your speech habits is to tape record your conversations for a few days. Listen to the tape, and you will be surprised at how careless you can be if you do not make an effort to avoid shortcuts.

Say what you mean when you speak, and when you write. Even an error in punctuation can cause you to lose the attention of the receiver. The classic sentence to illustrate this is:

Woman without her man is nothing.

Try to punctuate this sentence to give two completely different meanings to the idea.

Woman, without her, man is nothing.

Woman without her man, is nothing.

Other problems in the "attention attraction phase" occur because of idiosyncrasies in our language. Why do we say "big bottleneck" when we know that bottlenecks are small? Why do we say "blow out the candle," when it is the flame that is blown out? To a foreigner, "entering speed zone" means that you are entering an area where you are expected to "speed." A hot water heater really heats cold water, doesn't it? Do we take a bus home, or does it take us? No wonder we have difficulty in transmitting our messages.

Remember, when you are trying to convey a message, your hearer must *hear* you, and your reader must be able to read what you write. Speak loudly enough to be heard and enunciate your words. Write legibly and in a vocabulary that is easily understood. The *Reader's Digest* would have you believe that a more extensive vocabulary makes a more effective person. Actually, the reverse is true; people are frightened by an overly extensive vocabulary. Some interesting statistics concerning our standard vocabularies are:

- we recognize 70,000 words, but use only 15,000;
- about 2,000 words are used in daily conversation;
- only 44 words comprise half of our conversation; and
- only 10 words are present in one-quarter of everything that is written: the, of, and, to, a, in, that, it, is, and I.

The environment must also be considered when sending a message. Is the room noisy? Is there much distraction? Circumstances such as these tend to cause a breakdown in the message transmission. Make sure that you are attracting the attention of your listener.

"G"—Getting a Reaction

The final stage of the transmission involves the receiver. The end to a successful communication process is when a receiver gets precisely the same meaning out of words that the communicator put into them. Select ideas appropriate to your purpose. Outline or structure these ideas into a meaningful message. Write words that best convey the ideas you want. Edit what you write to streamline your message and to assure proper impact. Finally, rewrite your message to incorporate your changes. If your message fails, go back to the three Rs: (1) rework it, (2) revise it, and (3) resubmit it. If you cannot rework it, throw it away and make a fresh start.

Make sure that your message is getting across. Watch out not only for verbal clues that your communication has been received, but also for nonverbal signals that the message was either received or lost. A wandering gaze or picking lint off a sleeve may indicate a lack of interest or the covering up of anxious feelings about your transmission. Be aware of the power of silence. In parliamentary procedure, the lack of a second is a powerful message—the significance of saying nothing.

Other danger signals may block understanding, such as "selling" an idea rather than "telling" it. Also avoid the use of the word "don't," a negative word that brings unpleasant associations. Try to tell persons what they can do, not what they cannot. For example, say, "If you move that piece of equipment, people will not stumble"—rather than, "You can't leave that cart there, people will fall on their face."

The success of communication is not in its form, but in its warmth; not in words, but in meaning; not in techniques, but in mutual understanding. When you are sending a message, use common sense. The family pet, the dog, is a perfect example of using communication to its best effect. Dogs can say nothing, but, no matter what emotion they want to express, they can do so with simple, easily understood communication.

LISTENING

One of the most important elements of communication for the supervisor is the art of listening. We tend to get so caught up in the transmission of messages and in the need to have these messages understood, that we forget we must receive messages also. Our staff is interested in conveying information to us, and the way in which we receive this information tells the staff much about how we feel about them.

Communication means exchanging. We should read as much as we write, listen as much as we talk. We, as human beings, spend more time listening than anything else, but it is the least taught skill. We spend much time hearing, but little time really listening. If listening is something that we do so much, why is it so hard to do?

Hearing and listening—in other words, *really understanding*—take concentration. While the average speech rate is 125 words per minute, the average person can listen to 250 words per minute. These statistics mean that we can listen to twice as much as what we hear; our minds are capable of that much. Since people do not talk faster to accommodate us, we tend to use that excess energy for other things. We let our minds wander, we doodle, we knit or sew, or we plan for what we are going to say when it is our turn to talk. All these activities interfere with our genuine listening and can cause problems in communication. When we are not giving our full attention to speakers, we mistake what they say, or we give our own interpretation to the words. Some examples of phrases that need complete attention and interpretation to be fully understood are: Is 32° freezing or beginning to thaw? Is a gray day "partly cloudy" or "partly sunny"? Is a glass half empty or half full of water? Unless we give our full attention to the communicator, we may mistake the meaning of the message.

While most people agree that communication is a "two-way" process, most of us practice it as a "one-way street." We concentrate on the meaning of the information sent rather than on a two-way exchange of ideas. We communicate within the framework of our own understanding. In a discussion, we tend to make ourselves the authority. We don't ask questions, we give answers. Generally, when someone agrees with us we respect them; if they disagree, we are critical. *Our* convictions are logical; *others'* are prejudices. These are just a few of the quirks of human nature that cause problems in communication.

When someone is speaking, listeners are constantly responding in some way. They may be using nonverbal communication, but they are responding. The goal of meaningful communication is to make sure that all communication is directed toward the desired outcome. Communication and listening do not come naturally; they are skills that need to be practiced and used to develop. The test of real communication is not in the telling, but in the understanding.

Dr. Abraham Kaplan of the University of Michigan has written a paper on the art of *not* listening. He cites as an example of people's poor listening habits the fact that when we are listening to a joke, we are rehearsing the joke we are going to tell next. Some people give obvious clues that they are not listening. For example, some people finish every sentence for you. Although they appear to be hanging on your every word, listening so intently that they know what you are going to say, in reality they are trying to hurry you up so that they can have the floor. Dr. Kaplan calls this lack of listening "duologues" rather than "dialogues." His example of a duologue is a situation where everyone talks, but no one listens. A cocktail party is a perfect example. For his "duologues," he lists specific rules:

1. You must give each person a turn.
2. You must give signals that indicate you are listening such as, "um, hum, yeah, etc.".
3. You must refrain from saying anything that matters to you as a human being.

If you do all these things, you are participating in a duologue. A nearly perfect example of a "duologue" is a person watching TV. The perfect example of a "duologue" is two TV sets facing each other.

PRINCIPLES FOR EFFECTIVE COMMUNICATION

1. *Clarity:* The quest for clarity is really an attempt at better manipulation and comprehension of language. Try to use simple sentences; avoid the use of jargon or slang terms.

2. *Consistency:* Messages must be consistent with one another.

3. *Adequacy:* The goal in communication is to insure the flow of the optimum amount of information—neither too much nor too little.

3. *Timing:* The same message is received or responded to differently by different groups at the same time. Know the psychological importance of good timing.

4. *Timeliness:* Out-of-date information is as bad, or worse, than none at all. The responsibility of supervisors does not end with issuing the memorandum; they must review and revise instructions to eliminate obsolescence.

5. *Distribution:* One of the most frequent causes of breakdown is the failure of information to reach the right audience. Make sure that your communication arrives at its destination.

6. *Adaptability and uniformity:* Try to achieve a happy balance between these two elements. For example, the use of standard forms for some types of communication may have a tendency to limit the initiative. Know when to use a standard form and when to be flexible.

7. *Interest and acceptance:* The purpose of any communication is to secure a positive response. If your message is not interesting, you will not influence your audience.

HOW TO COMMUNICATE TO SUBORDINATES

Success in communication depends on gaining acceptance of what is said. Therefore, you must carefully plan not only what to tell, but how to tell it. One of the best ways to gain acceptance is to give reasons that bear meaning to those being informed.

Where persuasion is needed, the oral word can be more effective than the printed word. A face-to-face discussion gives an opportunity to observe reactions and to adapt the presentation to gain the required end. If the details are complex or if the employees do not want to believe the facts, you will undoubtedly have to follow up with a review and a retelling.

Keep the channels open both ways by inviting response from subordinates. Communications flow down more easily if a few observations and opinions flowing up are welcomed—even unpleasant ones. If planning to communicate, always seek more than one method. A written general order supplemented by a staff meeting to discuss it is much more effective than the order by itself.

What to Communicate to Subordinates

Informing subordinates properly removes the wonderment, anxiety, and aimless questions that make for confusion and indifference at work. Give them facts that make them feel as though they belong and as though they are informed and inseparable parts of their unit and their organization. Tell them the plans and decisions that give them a feeling of both opportunity and security. Select information that they

91

will take pride in knowing and that will satisfy their needs for attention, status, and the feeling of importance. Also tell subordinates all that they might eventually learn for themselves anyway. In this way the facts can be given truthfully and constructively, and thus you prevent distortion through a lack of information.

Information for exchange generally falls into three categories:

1. facts that should be told immediately,
2. those that should be told as soon as possible, and
3. those which *may* or may not be told.

INFORMATION TO BE TOLD IMMEDIATELY   These facts are things that directly affect nurses or their jobs: work assignments, methods of operation, rules and regulations, duties and responsibilities, quality of performance, and the like.

FACTS TO BE TOLD AS SOON AS POSSIBLE   These facts are a little less directly or a little less immediately connected with the physical operation and conduct of the agency. These facts affect the knowledge and attitudes necessary to coordinate each nurse's work with that of other people or units. They deal a little more with the future and with situations a little more distant from the job: policy matters, departmental organization, pay and fringe benefits, the place of the individual job in the overall scheme of organizational planning, expected standards of personal conduct, work expected, or anticipated changes in operational procedures, systems, or personnel that may influence the nurse, the job, or the unit.

FACTS FOR CERTAIN EMPLOYEES ONLY   Information that people at one level must know may become less essential for people at another level: Such information may deal broadly with the organization, future plans for growth and changes in organization, broad departmental policy, and other large-scale matters. No hard and fast rules dictate what to tell or whom to tell. Only good judgment and knowledge of what people want to know may serve as guides. For example, everyone who is directly affected by information should be kept well-informed on those matters. Telling someone who does not need the information is better than overlooking someone who does. People who are forgotten become resentful. In fact, employees have a broad and almost unlimited desire for information. Results of management surveys indicate that few employees think that they receive too much information.

In choosing who should communicate information, pick a person who is highly acceptable personally and has a record for communicating clearly and in an interesting manner.

THE IMPORTANCE
OF GOOD LEADERSHIP

Good leadership simplifies the task of giving orders or communicating, because no one can rely on the subordinates' high morale and good attitudes alone. Supervisors who have the respect, confidence, and loyalty of their staffs find that they have little difficulty in getting instruction and policies carried out. Staff members fail to carry out orders properly for three basic reasons:

1. They don't know what to do.
2. They don't know how to do it.
3. They don't want to do it.

It is your job to see that:

1. The staff know what to do.
2. They know how to do it.
3. They want to do it.
4. A check is made to see that it was done properly.

ISSUING DIRECTIVES OR ORDERS

TEST THE ORDER'S DESIRABILITY Before ordering a plan into action, no matter how minor, ask yourself:

1. Is it important, worth doing, necessary?
2. Is it practical? Will it work? Will it take more time than it is worth?
3. Can it be carried out? Is it both possible and reasonable?
4. Is there any conflict with other orders, policies, or practices—written or unwritten?
5. Will it require excessive instruction or training time?
6. Will it require excessive follow-up to insure compliance?

If you expect difficulty and if the plan is not really important, do not enact the plan.

USE COURTESY IN WORDING ORDERS Whether written or verbal, the phrasing of an order has a good deal of influence on its reception. Poor wording can arouse resentment and anger, even though the order is proper and legitimate. Use terms that are easily accepted, such as: "Would you . . .", "Please . . .", "I will appreciate . . . ." Avoid peremptory phrases that build barriers, such as: "Go and . . .", "I want you to . . .", "Get out to . . . ."

STATE INSTRUCTIONS CAREFULLY   Persons cannot do the job properly unless they receive clear, adequate instructions and understand the instructions. The greatest single reason for failure to carry out orders properly is a lack of understanding. Explain at the beginning what you want. Make your instructions clear, using simple, easily understood language and correct grammar. Be precise. State exactly what you want done, and break complex orders down into simple steps.

MAKE INSTRUCTIONS BRIEF   If you use more words than are necessary, you increase the possibility of misunderstanding. Say only what is necessary. Too much detail encourages scanning or skipping in written orders. Too much detail in verbal orders is boring, and you lose attention. Your listeners may also conclude that none of the order is worthwhile. If detail is necessary, use a brief preface to summarize it.

MAKE INSTRUCTIONS COMPLETE   Brevity is desirable, but not at the cost of being incomplete. The order should be clear on what is to be done, who is to do it, where it is to be done, when, how, and why.

BE SURE ORDERS ARE UNDERSTOOD   Orders are often misunderstood because the supervisor assumes that subordinates already know a great deal about the assignment, when in fact they may know absolutely nothing about it. Try to anticipate questions that might arise, and answer them in advance. Verify understanding. Discuss the task with the subordinate to make sure, and ask key questions for verification.

BE AWARE OF THE INDIVIDUAL'S PSYCHOLOGY   People react differently to words, phrases, and tasks. Some people catch on quickly, others slowly. Some anticipate, thinking they understand before they really do—and don't pay attention to details. Individual instructions must be tailor-made to fit the individual.

WRITTEN OR VERBAL ORDERS

Use verbal orders when:

1. the job is not complex, and confusion or misunderstanding is not probable;
2. the job has been done before and has become standardized;
3. handling emergencies; and
4. time is an important element.

Use written orders when:

1. orders are standing;

2. they are nonroutine;
3. they are complex enough that misunderstanding is reasonably possible;
4. several persons are involved, when all must have the same understanding, and when coordination is necessary; and
5. control and follow-up will be necessary.

Written orders force the supervisor to organize instructions systematically. They involve less possibility of overlooking an important item. When using written orders, all persons receive the same instructions and are more likely to have the same understanding. Written orders permit recipients to refresh their memories as to details, and they serve as a reminder if the activity is not to be done immediately. Follow-up is facilitated through the use of file copies, and, in the event of noncompliance, the copies also serve as evidence of the precise instructions given.

Whenever a person performs a job improperly due to failure to understand, the time required to clear up the misunderstanding is usually far greater than the time required to make the instructions clear in the first place. Using written orders prevents lost time and effort.

FOLLOW-UP ON ORDERS

Follow-up is an essential part of supervisory control, and the individual who gives an order must see to it that it has been properly executed. The consequences of failure to follow up are:

1. supervisory time and effort are wasted;
2. the subordinates' time spent in receiving and considering the order is wasted;
3. subordinates are confused and uncertain during the time the order is in effect but not being followed;
4. the supervisor loses prestige because of the failure of the instructions and his or her failure to secure compliance; and
5. it becomes more difficult for you to gain compliance with future orders.

Without a follow-up, you never know whether instructions have really been "sold" to subordinates. Subordinates may agree that the instructions are proper and desirable because they have found that you make it uncomfortable for them if they disagree. This acceptance, however, does not necessarily mean that they will comply. Their compliance may be dilatory, or they may put up passive resistance. Also, subordinates may agree with the instructions at first but object later when they have had a chance to think about them. They may comply at first but slack off later, particularly when they see no follow-up by you.

Follow-up demonstrates your interest in the matter. It serves to re-emphasize your belief that the orders are sound and important, and it provides the subordinate with a reasonable opportunity for compliance.

HOW TO FOLLOW UP Follow-up by inspections and reports may be accomplished in several ways. One way is to check standard reports and records that contain the desired information. If really needed, set up or require special reports; but remember that this adds not only to the workload of the staff but also to that of the supervisor in the preparation and reviewing of the special report. Be sure to discontinue special reports as soon as they have fulfilled their purpose. Make inspections at the level of immediate supervision, and take every opportunity to observe the operation and examine the work being done for compliance with orders.

The desirable frequency of follow-up inspections or reports varies. Some follow-up checks accomplish little because the intervals between them are too long. Checks should begin after instructions are given, as soon as at least partial compliance is possible, and they should be repeated at sufficiently close intervals to keep orders fresh in the minds of the personnel affected.

COMMUNICATION AND SUPERVISION

Supervision involves the transmission and reception of an idea from one person to another. Never-ending communication is inevitable for management and supervision, and it is an essential tool of management. Because social communication is concerned with the interactions of people, as individuals and in groups, the subject is interwoven with semantics, sociology, psychology, anthropology, education, and administration. The efficiency and morale of all of the personnel in an agency, from top management to the lowest levels, depend on the effectiveness of communication within the organization.

Administrators draw on all the available communication resources in their day-to-day work, with their organizations serving as a communication proving ground. That employees understand their job duties and how they are to be accomplished is of primary importance. Furthermore, employees must understand why they are doing something and how well they are doing it. Otherwise, their motivation may decline, with the result that grievances, accidents, waste, and other problems are quite likely to arise. The successful operation of any health agency is dependent not only on the effectiveness of its individual members, but also on the cooperation and teamwork that exists among them. For this reason, the role of communication in the development and functioning of the group structure deserves careful attention from supervisors.

DISCUSSION QUESTIONS

1. What is the importance of communication to management?
2. What are the essential elements of an act of communication? What is the significance of each?
3. What are the different types of communication? What is the significance of each?
4. What is the meaning and importance of positional communication?
5. What are some of the methods of communication besides verbal and written?
6. In which directions do communications flow within the organization? What sorts of items flow in each of the channels?
7. What are the basic principles of effective communication? How is each of them important in supervision?
8. What are some of the problems of communication in management? How are they overcome?
9. What are the essentials in giving orders? Why are these important?
10. How should the supervisor follow up on orders?

REFERENCES

DIEKELMANN, NANCY L. AND MARTIN M. BROADWELL, *The New Hospital Supervisor.* (Reading, Mass: Addison-Wesley Publishing Company, 1977).

DOUGLASS, LAURA MAE AND EM OLIVIA BEVIS, *Nursing Leadership in Action.* (St. Louis: The C.V. Mosby Company, 1974).

MAHLER, WALTER R., *Diagnostic Studies.* (Reading, Mass.: Addision-Wesley Publishing Company, 1974).

RUBIN, IRWIN M., RONALD E. FRY, AND MARK S. PLOVNICK, *Managing Resources in Health Care Organizations.* (Reston, Va.: Reston Publishing Co., 1978).

6
Decision making

Decision making is the core of supervision. All other parts of the administrative process are auxiliary to the making of decisions. James L. McCamy defines decision making as the complex of human associations, events, and words leading to, and including, any conclusion for a program of policy or operations. It is a process of people acting upon each other toward a conclusion.[1]

The study of decision making has changed substantially over the past few decades. In the past, most analyses of organizations have emphasised *horizontal specialization*. The earlier investigators considered the division of work to be the basic characteristic of organized activity. Luther Gulick, for example, in his "Notes on the Theory of Organization," says, "Work division is the foundation of organization: indeed, the reason for organization."[2] Current thinking in this field is primarily concerned with *vertical specialization*: that is, the division of decision-making duties between staff and supervisory personnel. This arrangement makes for a more integrated process.[3]

---

[1] James L. McCamy, "Analysis of the Process of Decision-Making," *Public Administration Review* (Winter 1947), p. 41.

[2] Luther Gulick and L. Orwick, *Papers on the Science of Administration* (New York: The Macmillan Co., 1947), p. 3.

[3] James N. Rosenau, "The Premises and Promises of Decision Making Analysis," *Contemporary Political Analysis* (New York: The Free Press, 1967), p. 195.

REASONS FOR VERTICAL SPECIALIZATION

There are three reasons for vertical specialization or decentralized decision making. First, since there is much horizontal specialization in health care, vertical specialization is essential to achieve coordination of personnel and operations. Secondly, just as horizontal specialization permits greater skills to be developed by the working group in the performance of their tasks, so vertical specialization permits greater skills in the making of decisions. Third, vertical specialization permits the operative personnel to be held accountable for their decisions.[4]

Good organizational behavior requires not only that correct decisions be made and adopted, but also that all members of the organization accept those decisions. By the proper exercising of influence, decision making can be decentralized so that, while a general plan governs all members of the organization, each person has the freedom to function and participate at his or her own level.

Subdividing the work of an organization is necessary so that all processes requiring particular skills are performed by persons possessing those skills. The responsibility for decision making must also be so assigned to insure that all decisions requiring a particular skill are made by persons possessing that skill. Subdividing decisions, however, is more complicated than subdividing performance, but it is essential to good organization.

The authority for decision making exercised by subordinate personnel is limited by policies determined by the administrative hierarchy. Within his or her assigned sphere, however, each administrator, supervisor, and staff member is constantly involved in the process of decision making.

FACTORS AFFECTING DECISIONS

Many factors affect decisions. The so-called "acts of God" and other nonhuman events certainly affect decisions. Floods, fires, and famines may cause public officials to take appropriate actions that affect health care. Political activity or world situations, such as the influence of an impending economic crisis or war, may also force decisions. These circumstances, although unusual, must be considered as factors in decision making.

No person ever makes a decision in administration alone. Since interpersonal relations are inevitable, persons always influence each other. Supervisors are therefore always influenced by other persons,

[4] Herbert A. Simon, "Decision-Making and Administrative Organization," *Administrative Behavior* (New York: The Macmillan Co., 1947).

whether present or not. Their decisions are the result of advice, affection, fear, hostility, envy, admiration, contempt, or condescension. All these factors are involved in the complex human relationships that permeate administration and affect decisions.

In some cases, the person who is actually responsible for a decision is not the decision maker. Instead the responsible party may be at any level in the organization, perhaps considerably lower in the hierarchy than the one officially responsible for the decision. Some people can bring about decisions by persuading those with authority to decide on their proposals. Some supervisors rely exclusively on those subordinates' proposals that they deem acceptable. Others favor proposals from their subordinates in order to evade the responsibility of deciding on their own. Competent supervisors do not evade this responsibility. They accept the influences brought to bear on them by others and consider new influences from their own level. They then make the decision based on these factors, together with whatever personal factors they are in a position to contribute to the decision process.[5]

To understand the process of decision making in an organization, you must go beyond the immediate orders given by supervisors to subordinates. You must understand how subordinates are influenced by such things as standing orders, by training, and by the review of their actions. Also, you must study the channels of communication to determine what information reaches them and how this information may be relevant to their decisions. As you broaden the operational discretion left to subordinates in decision making, you render their contributions all the more important.

Factors affecting decisions may be divided in several ways, but probably one of the best is into (1) personal factors and (2) organizational factors.

Personal Factors

Persons in every walk of life are continuously engaged in interpersonal relations. Competent supervisors constantly manage these interpersonal relations in a conscious process. They should be more conscious than the average person of what individuals want, and they should have the sense and courage to manipulate human conditions to achieve the organization's objectives. They should constantly analyze what motivates a person and attempt to modify that desire to suit themselves or their organizations. Good supervisors realize that staff members are people who have desires and feelings, and who are vitally involved in the current administrative problem or situation.

[5] McCamy, p. 43.

Organizational Factors

In addition to obtaining information about the persons involved in a decision-making process, the administrator must gather organizational factors as a background for the decision. James L. McCamy suggests that the following factors be considered:

1. events in the field of the agency's work;
2. knowledge from research and analysis;
3. the expectations of individuals or groups to whom the decision makers are responsible;
4. the reputation of the agency;
5. the security of the agency;
6. the resources available; and
7. the legal conditions that affect the decision.[6]

METHODS OF INFLUENCING DECISION MAKERS

An organization's influence over its decision makers is exerted in many ways. A subordinate decision maker is influenced by:

1. command;
2. organizational loyalties;
3. by his or her efforts to achieve "efficient" courses of action;
4. by training;
5. by the information provided; and
6. by the advice that is transmitted through the organization's lines of communication, informal as well as formal.

Command or Authority

C. I. Barnard has stated that subordinates accept authority whenever they permit their behavior to be guided by a decision reached by another, without independently examining the merits of that decision. When exercising authority, the supervisor does not seek to convince the subordinates, only to obtain compliance.[7]

One important function of authority is to permit a decision to be made and carried out even when agreement cannot be reached. If, however, you attempt to carry authority beyond a certain point, disobedience follows. Barnard calls this the "zone of indifference,"[8] and

---

[6] McCamy, p. 46.

[7] Chester I. Barnard, *The Functions of the Executive* (Cambridge: Harvard University Press, 1940), p. 163.

[8] Barnard, p. 169.

Simon uses the term "zone of acceptance."[9] However it is worded, it means the same. Authority can only be exerted to the level of the staff's acceptance.

The "lines" of authority, as represented on an organizational chart, do have a special significance. They are commonly used to end debate when it proves difficult or impossible to reach a "meeting of the minds" on a particular decision. These formal lines of authority are usually reinforced by informal authority relations in the routine work of the organization.

Organization Loyalties

Members of an organization tend to identify themselves with that organization. In arriving at decisions, their loyalty to the organization and to its members leads them to evaluate alternative decisions in terms of their probable effects on the group as a whole. This approach has one important value: As a supervisor, you could not possibly evaluate your decisions in terms of the whole range of human values. By considering the decision only in the light of organizational aims, your task may fall more within the range of your abilities as a human being. This concentration on a limited range of organizational values also makes it possible to hold the supervisor responsible for these decisions.

Organizational loyalties, however, have certain disadvantages. The principal one is that they prevent the supervisor from making proper decisions in situations where organizational values must be weighed against personal or staff values.

Efficient Courses of Action

Supervisors are also influenced in their decisions by the "criterion of efficiency."[10] To be efficient means to take the shortest path and the cheapest means toward the attainment of the desired goal. The efficiency commandment is a major influence on the decisions of all supervisors.

Training

Training is an influence that prepares decision makers to reach proper decisions on their own, without the need for the constant exercise of authority or advice. Training, combined with experience, contributes most to decision making whenever the same elements are involved in a large number of decisions. Training also makes possible greater decentralization of the decision-making process by providing subordinates with the necessary competence to make decisions for themselves.

[9] Simon, p. 12.
[10] Simon, p. 14.

Information

The information provided to the decision makers greatly influences their choice of alternative actions. Whether correct or incorrect, any information obtained colors the thinking of the group and directs their thought processes. You must be sure that any information you receive or give is accurate and allows an open-minded approach to the decision process.

Advice and Communication

Many of the influences that the organization exercises over its members are of a more informal nature. Information and advice flow in all directions within an organization. The facts necessary for making a decision change rapidly and are obtainable only at the moment of decision. Sometimes these facts are known only by subordinate employees. The extent of the influence exerted by staff members depends on the desire of the decision maker for advice, the prestige of the subordinate, and the skill with which the advice is offered.

The group process of sharing communication and advice is always present. The supervisor should use these formal and informal communications to assess the group's position and to analyze how it affects the expected outcome of the decision-making process.

PROCESSES FOR INSURING CORRECT DECISIONS

Many processes can be used to insure correct decisions. They are:

1. planning,
2. review,
   a. diagnosis,
   b. influence,
   c. correction,
   d. enforcement, and
3. operations research.

Planning

Planning is the process in which a whole program is worked out in advance before any part of it is carried out. This process is extremely important because a great amount of detail can be included in the plan and because wide participation can be obtained in its preparation. Planning permits the participation of many experts without imposing any difficulties by the lines of authority.

Review

Review enables supervisors to know exactly what their subordinates are doing. It may be directed toward the results of the subordinates' actions, toward the tangible product of their activities, or toward the method of their performance.

Review may perform four different functions:

1. diagnosis of the quality of the decision;
2. influence on subsequent decisions;
3. correction of incorrect decisions; and
4. the enforcement of controls so that subordinates will accept organizational authority in making their decision.[11]

Operations Research

Operations research is essentially a process of learning by trial and error.[12] A health care agency or organization consists of a group of related activities which, when put together, produce predictable patterns of operations. These operations are generally repetitive enough to make it possible to create models of systematic behavior. These models are sets of patterns and situations showing relationships and how they change under varying circumstances.

To discover what the patterns are, how they work, or what they should be, a researcher might adopt different approaches: observation, theory, experimentation, and, finally, testing in actual situations. All testing does not have to occur in your own agency. Much can be learned by the study of other agencies' responses to the same problem.

THE SUPERVISOR
AS A DECISION MAKER

The decision-making role of a supervisor is essential to smooth operations in an organization. The basic characteristics of successful decision makers are:

1. They don't shrink from deciding, even though it means taking a chance.
2. They strike a practical balance between the need to sift the facts and the limitations imposed by time.
3. When they adopt another's suggestion, they put their full authority behind its execution.
4. They rely on a combination of reason and instinct.

[11] Simon, p. 28.

[12] "Making Decisions by Math," *Business Week* (November 13, 1954), p. 104.

5. In affairs outside their own specialized knowledge and experience, they consider the counsel of others, while accepting full responsibility for the decision.
6. Out of several conflicting considerations, they pick the one that is vital.
7. They accommodate their decisions to fact and circumstance.
8. They don't let stubborn pride keep them from reversing bad decisions when they are shown to be bad.[13]
9. They find the right answer to the right problem.
10. They make the decision at the appropriate time. Postponing a decision may in fact result in action, hence a decision has been made. Making a decision too soon may be as much of an error as making a decision too late.
11. They make decisions that result in action.
12. They look at decision making as an opportunity, not a problem.

STEP-BY-STEP PROCESS OF DECISION MAKING

The basic plan in any decision making is to move from situation to solution in a logical design or pattern. Using the steps of decision making enables you to look logically at each step and to take the appropriate action. Not all decisions can be made using these lengthy steps, but, if they are used frequently enough, they become almost automatic. The goal is to know the pattern so well that you can use it easily, even when the decision is made quickly. The steps are:

1. defining the problem,
2. finding the critical factor,
3. defining expectations,
4. gathering facts,
5. developing alternative solutions,
6. choosing an alternative,
7. using the decision, and
8. evaluation.

Defining the Problem

The first step is to understand the problem exactly. At the start of any decision-making experience, you usually see only the symptoms, not the problem. If you relieve the symptoms, you gain temporary relief, but, in the long term, the problem still exists. For example, a surgical

---

[13] Fred DeArmond, *Executive Thinking and Action* (Chicago: Lloyd R. Wolfe Company, 1952), pp. 110–124.

ward in a hospital was having trouble with its laboratory work. Whenever the staff looked for a laboratory report, they found that the work had not been done. When they called and questioned the laboratory, the lab staff told them that the work had not been done because there was not enough time or staff to do the work. After considerable thought and problem solving, the hospital administration decided that either the laboratory had to be enlarged or the staff increased. Both answers involved a considerable expense to the hospital. Due to the cost factor, the hospital administration decided to review their findings and look for an alternative solution.

In the review of the situation, the administration found that their error had been made not in the solution, but in the decision-making process itself. The administration had found the right solution, but the wrong problem. They were working with symptoms rather than with the actual problem. After gathering more data, the administration found that the problem was not in the laboratory staff at all. The staff was adequate, and the lab was large enough to service the hospital. The real problem was that the staff physicians were anxious to have their laboratory work done and on the charts in time for their visits. For this reason, they were ordering all work done STAT. Naturally, the laboratory could not finish the routine work, because their work was constantly being interrupted by these so-called STAT orders. When the problem was viewed in this way, the solution was easily seen. The doctors were instructed on the approved criteria for STAT work. Without the pressure of the immediate work, the laboratory had sufficient time to finish the routine work, and all the tests were done. This was a simple, inexpensive solution to what seemed to be a major problem.

Finding the Critical Factor

The critical factor is the one thing that must be changed, removed, or moved before anything else can be done. There is not always a critical factor, but, if there is one, it must be identified and handled. Too often, the decision-making process ignores this step, and the decision cannot result in action.

As an example, a hospital was having trouble with staffing a department. The position they were trying to fill was that of head nurse. The turnover rate in the position was high. Every time the personnel director hired a nurse for this position, she would work for several months and then leave. These were skilled, experienced head nurses, and there was no evident reason for them to leave. In this case, the problem was identified correctly as "filling the position of head nurse." The temptation was to continue the search for qualified applicants and hiring yet another head nurse, in the hope of finding one who would stay. Since this alternative had been tried three times with no success, the administration felt that they may have overlooked some possibility.

The decision-making group looked back over their thought process and found that they had neglected to take into consideration the possibility of the existence of a critical factor. To find the critical factor in this case, they interviewed the former head nurses in the department.

In doing so, they found that the nurses all had one problem in common, the reason that caused them to resign. They all cited the same situation, one that they were reluctant to discuss at their exit interview: That is, the supervisor directly responsible for them was unwilling to give up any of her control of the department. The head nurses had the responsibility, but no commensurate authority. The head nurses, feeling trapped, figured their only solution was to leave. The hospital had now found the critical factor—the supervisor. Now the solution was to deal with this employee, not to hire new nurses.

Defining Expectations

Although the next step in a decision-making process is usually to gather the facts, we will insert one more step. If you gather all the facts necessary to make a decision, with no idea of your expectations for the final solution, the job would be overwhelming. Defining expectations *before* gathering facts simplifies and speeds the process.

Defining expectations simply means that you decide at the beginning of the decision-making process what you want to have happen at the end. You set your goals, expectations, and objectives so that you can have a clear idea of the paths you should take. Only by making a decision based on future outcome are you able to review the results and see if you have reached a successful conclusion. Once you have thought through what you expect to have happen, you can see which facts you need to support the decision.

Gathering Facts

Now is the time to gather all the facts needed to support your expectations. If you need to buy a piece of equipment for the department, for example, and one of your expectations is that the instrument costs less than $500, gather information only on equipment costing less than $500. This expectation makes the task considerably easier.

Developing Alternative Solutions

The important part of this step is the letter "s" in "solutions." At this stage of the operation you need to allow for creativity and free thought, which are stifled if you spend your time looking for the "one right solution." The best way to handle this stage is to allow the group to "brainstorm" or use the "creative fifth dimension." As a leader, you accept any and all suggestions from the group, writing them down on a blackboard, flip chart, or a piece of paper. You must, as the leader, insist that the group offer no support or criticism of each statement or solution. Simply write the solutions down with no comment.

The reason for not allowing any comment is to maintain the free atmosphere of the meeting. A person who feels that his or her solution will be criticized is hesitant to offer it. But, if there is the assurance that no comments will be allowed, the group feels less inhibited, and their creativity emerges. Many times the very strange, seemingly impossible idea is the one that is the final choice. These unusual ideas are never expressed if you neglect this stage of the decision-making process by allowing comments or criticisms of the possible alternatives.

A case that points up the value of this approach quite well is a hospital that was having trouble staffing the eleven-to-seven shift. A group was appointed to look into the situation and come up with recommendations to relieve the severe shortage of staff. As the group worked through the process, they found the problem to be, indeed, staffing the eleven-to-seven shift. They found no critical factor, in that no one thing had to be changed before anything else could be done. Their expectation was to have the night shift adequately covered.

As the group reached the alternative solutions stage, the leader was very forceful and made sure that everyone knew that this was to be a brainstorming session—no comment or criticism would be allowed. Because of this supportive, free atmosphere, one of the nurses came up with what seemed to be a very strange idea. She suggested that the night shift differential be taken away and that the night nurses work four nights per week and be paid for five nights. Now this idea seemed unworkable, and the temptation was to speak up and say something about the possible problems in implementing this idea. The leader followed the process to the letter, though, and no comments were made.

At the end of the decision-making process, it was found that this was, indeed, the best possible solution. The staff had less sick time because of the extra sleep day. More people were willing to work the shift because of the benefits. No more staff had to work overtime, and no registry help was called in. All in all, this strange solution was the cheapest and most efficient—and the one implemented. This hospital has used the plan for several years now, and the administrators are still quite satisfied with the results. None of these benefits would have happened if the leader had not allowed free, creative thought.

Choosing an Alternative

With all the possible alternatives listed, the next step is to choose which alternative is best for your situation. At this stage, criticism and comment are not only encouraged, they are necessary. All the pros and cons of each solution should be explored. Do not ask the members of the group to choose which of the alternatives they feel is best. Ask for discussion on each alternative.

Above all, do not stop the process here and ask everyone to go back to their duties, think about the alternatives, and choose one. If you do so, all members of the group will think over their own solutions, perhaps even discussing them with their staffs. Each group then makes up his or her own mind and becomes emotionally committed to one solution. As the leader, you would then have two tasks: first, to talk them out of their decision and, second, to make the final decision. In such cases, even the staff may be disappointed, too, because *their* solution was not chosen.

During the discussion of alternatives, try to avoid the use of the word, "obviously." Any statement that starts out with this word should be questioned. If the subject is so "obvious" then why are you discussing it in the first place? Usually speakers are not talking from facts, but from their own prejudice. They feel that it is "obvious" to them, but it is not obvious to the rest of the group.

As a group, you must remember that you will never find the "perfect" solution. No solution can be perfect because decision making is always based on future events. Even if a decision is made and everything is worked out perfectly, who is to say that you failed to think of an even better solution? The goal of this stage is to find the best possible solution under the circumstances.

The way to arrive at the choice of alternatives from the list of possibilities is up to you as the leader. Perhaps just discussing the factors about each alternative will point up some new thinking, and the group will arrive at consensus through this discussion. The group members may talk each other into a possible choice of action, or you, the leader, may steer the group into the course you feel would be best.

One method of making the final decision could be to vote on the listed alternatives. In the case of voting, you must find out how committed each group is to its own ideas. If the group votes, and the side that loses does not go along with the plan, then the voting process is pointless. If the issue is very sensitive or important, one in which 100-percent participation is necessary, then, before any vote is taken, you must poll the group to see if they will follow the dictates of the group. If you are voting on switching to a ten-hour workday, for instance, and those opposed to it refuse to work the new hours, then you must find an alternative solution. There is no point in voting on an issue that will never be put into action.

The method of choosing the final decision is up to the leader. You know your group, and you are the one sensitive to their feelings. Try to use a method that puts as little pressure as possible on the group. The goal is to have the group reach consensus with little or no conflict.

Using the Decision

After the decision has been made, the next step is to use the decision, to implement it. This stage is ignored too many times. If, for some reason, you are unable to convert the decision into action, you must tell the group why. If you simply let the matter drop with no explanation to the group, they lose their faith and trust in you. The next time you ask this group to work together to make a decision, they will refuse. Nothing is more frustrating than to work very hard on a problem, make a recommendation, and then be ignored.

Evaluation

The last step in the decision-making process is evaluation. In our process we have a "built-in" measurement of its effectiveness. Evaluation simply consists of looking back at the expectation stage. Does the decision meet our expectations? If so, the decision is a good one. Notice that you do not say that the decision is perfect, or even the best. You merely evaluate whether the decision meets the expectations. If the problem is relieved and the expectations met, that is all you are looking for. Second guessing any course of action only leads to frustration, anger, or confusion.

The Reason for a Rational Plan

These steps may seem laborious, but they are well worth the time and effort. In some cases, they may even be time-savers. Trying to repair the damage that a poor decision may have caused usually takes more time than using a rational, well-thought-out decision-making process. Making a decision is never without risk, but using this process greatly reduces your risk of failure.

Decision making is a vital part of your job as a supervisor, and, for this reason, it demands much study and thought. If you can improve the quality of your decision making, you improve the quality of your supervision. Using a rational plan for decision making results in:

1. better decisions,
2. clearer decisions,
3. easier decisions,
4. faster decisions, and,
5. decisions that result in action.

THREE APPROACHES TO DECISION MAKING

Three basic approaches to decision making are commonly used in the health care setting. You should be familiar with the advantages and disadvantages of each. They are, as defined by Herbert A. Simon:

1. the rationalistic approach,
2. the incrementalistic approach, and
3. the mixed scanning approach.

The Rationalistic Approach

According to this method of decision making, the leader is in total control. The leader feels that he or she knows the problem, can establish a goal, and choose an alternative. This type of problem solving is very unrealistic, because it requires much greater resources and knowledge than the average supervisor possesses. Usually, it fails because the group has not set or agreed upon the objectives or values. Avoid using this method because it presumes that your group blindly follows the dictates of you or your health care agency. Because no group is that obedient, this method is unrealistic and unworkable. Ironically, this system is used the most.

The Incrementalistic Approach

This approach takes into consideration the limitations of the group and of the leader. The leader proposes a few, limited alternatives to a situation, and then allows the group to choose from these alternatives. Again, this system is not the best, because the leader is presupposing the fact that the goals of the group are the goals of the organization. Usually, this assumption results in a decision that is remedial, much like putting a band-aid on the problem. The symptoms may be relieved, but the problem remains. Although this method is the method of choice in some situations, it cannot deal with complicated or abstract problems. If there are severe limitations on the range of alternative action, the leader may be forced to choose this approach, but it should never be used exclusively.

Mixed Scanning

Actually a combination of the first two approaches is the method of choice in most situations, and it is the method used in our step-by-step plan for decision making. This approach provides information and allows the group to set their own goals and objectives. Because the group reaches a decision on the basis of a mutual thought process, it is more committed to the implementation of the decision.

As the supervisor, you must choose the alternative that best meets the needs of the particular situation. Knowing the possible choices gives you more flexibility in planning your decision-making activities.

111

DISCUSSION QUESTIONS

1. What is the role of the supervisor in the decision-making process?

2. What effect does vertical and horizontal specialization have on decision making?

3. How is decision making related to public relations?

4. Which factors influence the group's decision? Which factors influence the supervisor's decision?

5. How can you, as a supervisor, be assured of making the best possible decision?

6. What are some of the problems or pitfalls in the decision-making process? How can they be corrected?

7. What are the advantages and disadvantages to each of the three decision-making approaches? Give an example for the use of each approach.

APPLICATION: CASE STUDY OF ADMINISTRATIVE DECISION-MAKING EXERCISE

Objectives

- To define the problem.
- To find the critical factor, if any—the one thing that must be changed before anything else can be done.
- To define expectations and to find relevant facts.
- To develop alternative solutions.
- To make a decision.
- To implement the decision.

Directions

Read the case studies and then make an appropriate decision for each one. Be prepared to discuss the decision, and to defend the reasons behind your decision.

Statement of Problem No. 1

The supervisor of a two-operating-room surgical unit is expected to provide operating rooms and adequate staffing for fifty staff surgeons. Several of the physicians have complained that they can never get on the schedule when they want to.

Relevant Facts Concerning the Situation

The surgical unit is in a small one-hundred-bed community hospital in a prosperous, primarily residential city. The hospital is fairly new, having been functioning about five years. At the present time a city-wide fund-raising drive is on to raise money for the institution. All staff members are being asked to participate through gifts and increased bed tax.

Numerous physicians have complained that whenever they schedule a patient, they have to wait an unreasonable length of time, or they are bumped at the last minute.

The supervisor has always tried to accommodate everyone and, using a triage system, to make provision for emergencies. She does notice that most space is taken by the same ten surgeons, but they do the bulk of the surgeries.

More and more, the OR staff is noticing cases added as emergencies that are really elective. Some doctors are waiting a month to book an elective, while the ten most prominent doctors are booking daily.

If one of the main surgeons is told there is a delay, he complains to the administrator. As past records are reviewed, it seems as though, many times, the doctors threatened to send cases to other hospitals, although none was actually ever sent.

Statement of Problem No. 2

The planning commission of a city council has been given a federal grant of $30 million to improve medical facilities in the city. The only guidelines are that the project chosen must benefit most of the people in the community. The city council, citizens groups, senior citizens council, college district, and state agencies are at odds to decide which facilities to build.

Relevant Facts

The background of the city is as follows: The city is newly incorporated with a population of 25,000. The city is primarily residential, with some businesses located on two main through streets. The population for the most part is employed in the industry of surrounding adjacent cities.

There is no hospital in the city. The nearest hospital is a county facility located approximately thirty miles from the city. The hospital is a major unit with teaching facilities and a thousand beds. The communities have grown rapidly around the hospital, and it is severely overcrowded.

Five years ago, a multi-million dollar senior citizen's retirement community was built on the outskirts of the unincorporated area. This has now been incorporated into the city: Indecision, California.

Recently, there has been an increase in multi-dwelling apartment units to provide housing for the nearby university.

Expecting a population increase of 35,000 within the next decade, builders have been developing moderately priced tract homes catering to the young families with income ranges from $14,000 to $17,000 per year. These homes are 20 percent occupied.

Three elementary schools, one junior high, and one high school serve the area. One part of town is occupied primarily by very low-income migrant workers who work the local farms. These families are predominately Spanish speaking, and many are eligible for welfare benefits.

Indecision is a beach-side community with a large state beach and many recreational areas. The five surrounding communities are of the same size, and they use the recreational and shopping facilities of Indecision and would be using the medical facilities also.

Possible Decisions

1. The very powerful senior citizen's council would like a major medical center, providing medical and surgical facilities with the emphasis on gerontology research, home health care, and ambulatory care facilities.

2. The PTA is asking for a small community hospital to provide for the medical needs of the community. They feel that the building of a major facility would strain the resources of the city and increase its educational needs. They feel that Indecision should use the money to build a unit to meet the city's needs, and let the other communities do their own building.

3. The Homeowner's Association is asking for small satellite hospitals, one in each community to meet a specific medical need— one for geriatrics, one for pediatrics, one for obstetrics, one for research, and so on.

4. The university would like another major teaching facility to meet the clinical needs of its students.

5. The civic organizations such as Boys Club, Scouts, and YMCA feel there is a need for a large hospital with adjacent meeting rooms and a large pediatric center for the use of the children.

6. A corporation has approached the council with a plan to provide $400 million to help offset the cost of a large health care center. This center would be a private facility, serving the clients of its prepaid medical care plan.

7. The state agencies are pushing for a facility that would take care of the needs of the indigent patients and provide health care for those unable to pay for it.

The Decision

Assume that you are the city planning council. Devise a plan for using this money in the most appropriate manner, taking into consideration all the interests of the various groups. Make a very clear presentation of the building plans for the city. Try to frame out the plan in a logical sequence of building, year by year, over a ten-year time frame.

REFERENCES

BRISTOW, ALLEN P. AND E. C. GABARD, *Decision-Making in Police Administration.* Springfield, Ill.: Charles C. Thomas, 1961.

DRUCKER, PETER F., *The Practice of Management.* New York: Harper & Row, Publishers, Inc., 1954.

————, "The Effective Decision," *Public Administration News Management Forum,* Vol. XVII, No. 2 (May 1967).

EBERT, R. AND T. MITCHELL, *Organizational Decision Processes: Concepts and Analysis.* New York: Crusk, Russad, 1975.

GLUECK, W., "Decision Making: Organization Choice," *Personnel Psychology,* 27 (1974).

HARRISON, E., *The Managerial Decision-Making Process.* Boston: Houghton Mifflin, 1975.

KASSOUF, S., *Normative Decision-Making.* Englewood Cliffs, N.J.: Prentice-Hall, Inc., 1970.

MACCRIMMAN, K. AND R. TAYLOR, "Decision Making and Problem Solving," in *Handbook of Industrial and Organizational Psychology,* ed. M. Dunnette. Chicago: Rand McNally & Company, 1976.

ROSENAU, JAMES N., "The Premises and Promises of Decision-Making Analysis," *Contemporary Political Analysis.* New York: The Free Press, 1967.

SIMON, HERBERT A., *Administrative Behavior: A Study of Decision-Making Processes in Administrative Organization,* 3rd ed. New York: The Free Press, 1976.

7

Motivation

No one really motivates another. Supervisors do not "motivate" others; they merely set the climate so that workers in the organization can be motivated. As the supervisor, you do not make anyone do anything that he or she does not want to do. The notion of actually "motivating" others only gives supervisors the additional role of being "cheerleaders."

This assertion may be only a question of semantics, but it is also a way of easing the burden of supervision. Most supervisors cite motivation as one of their major problems, and too many supervisors are willing to take the entire blame for the lack of it: "I can't get my staff motivated," is a frequent lament. Granted, the most difficult tasks of the nursing supervisor are understanding the motivations of workers and channeling those motivations into the goals and objectives of the organization. Yet the best way to deal with these tasks is to understand immediately that *you* cannot motivate. Get rid of that defeating attitude, and use your energy to find out *what does motivate* your staff. Then set a climate that encourages them to feel satisfied while achieving the goals of the organization. Every person works for a multitude of reasons, and each and every person presents a different set of motivational problems. Trying to deal with each of these situations calls for an astute understanding of human nature and the background of behavior. Knowing your employees and meeting their needs within the context of the organization sets the climate for the employee to be motivated.

PRINCIPLES OF MOTIVATION

Industry and the social sciences have provided us with set patterns and plans—guidelines, if you will—for motivation. These are standard methods for dealing with staff members, and they must be considered only as a rough guide for the general handling of motivational problems. The "rules-and-regulations" approach does not work in dealing with human beings. The best supervisor is able to interpret these basic principles in terms of individual cases and work with the person as a unique entity. Although these guidelines have proven successful in business and industry and although they can be applied to health care, they are not guaranteed to work in all cases. Yet they are a good starting point for understanding motivation. If you, as a supervisor, practice these principles, your staff will be motivated toward the same goals to which you and the organization are directed. The guidelines are:

1. encourage self-involvement,
2. give freedom but keep control,
3. help subordinates identify with you and with others,
4. give credit,
5. show confidence,
6. assign blame, and
7. instill fear.

Encourage Self-Involvement

Allowing as much freedom of choice as possible encourages motivation. As a supervisor, you encourage self-motivation by allowing workers to choose their methods of operation for any given task. Persons work more effectively—and more efficiently—and get more satisfaction from doing a job that they themselves want to do than from one that they are told to do. Basically, staff members give more of themselves and try harder at the jobs that they enjoy doing. Individuals who feel competent at a particular duty try harder and accomplish more.

People are not robots. They enjoy the challenge of establishing their own experience and knowledge, and a good supervisor draws on that experience, allowing workers to enhance the organizational goals with their unique approach. Staff members who are expected to carry out duties in a prescribed and routine way eventually withdraw their commitment to the goals of the health care agency. In effect, they will carry out tasks with little or no personal involvement. This is the lack of motivation that most supervisors complain about.

Training is an important part of encouraging self-involvement. If staff are properly trained in their duties, they can be allowed the freedom to use their own creative talents. Doing a job that they have planned and coordinated is much more satisfying than simply carrying out someone else's orders.

Should you take this approach, your duty as a supervisor is to set the standards for acceptable behavior and make sure that all subordinates understand these standards. By your example and by the rules and regulations of the health care agency, you simply show the staff what the organization expects of them. If they understand why certain policies are enforced, they are more willing to accept the bureaucratic limitations. Once the staff understand the basic parameters of the work situation, you can encourage them to be creative and innovative in their methods. You should see yourself as the person who plants the seeds in the minds of staff members. You can give suggestions and recommendations, but you should avoid giving orders or instructions that are too specific. Very few individuals can be enthusiastic about doing a job that is assigned if they have no understanding of why it is being done.

If at all possible, assign staff members to work situations in which they are proficient and feel capable. This arrangement benefits the employee, the patient, and the organization. Try to find out what each individual staff member likes to do and does well, and then tailor assignments to include as much of that work as possible. In allowing workers to have this degree of control over their work situations, you are setting the climate for efficiency and involvement. This accommodation does not mean that workers should do only what they feel comfortable doing. The efficient supervisor plans for a specific program of developing new skills in staff members and strengthening weak areas. Employees must learn to have a tolerance for tasks they dislike. This attitude can be established by assuring them that the bulk of their work will be in areas of their own personal interest.

Allow staff members to voice their complaints and criticisms of work that they feel is too routine or that does not meet their needs. Perhaps some change in the overall plan can be initiated. The feedback from your staff may help you to see the overall perspective of the faults in the organizational system, and some changes can be made. If no change is possible, the staff at least feel that they had the chance to express their opinion and that their suggestions were taken seriously. Tell staff members why the change is not possible, and allow them to express their feelings, either positive or negative. This permissiveness opens the door to free communication, and it prevents resentment and anger.

A few practical ways that a supervisor can encourage self-involvement in subordinates are as follows:

1. Allow staff members to participate in planning.
2. Rotate assignments that are disagreeable or routine.

3. Assign staff members to their own area of specialized interest or training, such as obstetrics, ICU, CCU, emergency room, and the like.

4. Have a good general plan for in-service education so that each person can be trained to do all the tasks necessary to meet the organizational goals. A competent worker is a more satisfied worker.

5. Encourage the staff to seek outside educational programs to broaden their scope of expertise.

6. Give adequate time for sharing feedback and for listening to the ideas and opinions of subordinates.

7. Take action on some of the specific areas of improvement or change suggested by staff members.

Another way to encourage self-involvement is to make sure that all employees know the total outcome of their work assignments. Many times persons perform only a small function in an overall plan. If they do not understand the final outcome, they see themselves as insignificant and unimportant. Make sure that all workers understand how important their own personal function is to the final outcome.

In situations where there is no time to allow feedback or the reporting of the overall objective, such as in emergency situations, the staff responds quickly to your directions if they understand that this is the exception rather than the rule and that you use this technique only when the situation warrants it. A staff who is constantly "ordered" to perform in set methods does not respond as efficiently in an emergency situation. Trust your staff members, and they will trust you. When the emergency situation is over, tell the staff members the results of their actions, and praise them for their activities during the situation. Knowing the final result encourages staff members to follow your directions in the future and helps them to understand the need for total compliance in these types of situations.

Give Freedom but Keep Control

As the leader in a health care setting, you are in control of the situation. Yet you can maintain control and still allow the individual worker to have some freedom. When you delegate a responsibility to subordinates, you are showing faith in them to do the best job possible. They feel confident and give you their best effort. Always give employees a chance to grow by delegating responsibility, by teaching, by allowing initiative and creativity, and by demonstrating your faith.

Many new supervisors are in the habit of carrying out certain tasks themselves. Although they are really tempted to do so in the interest of time or efficiency, rather than delegating, they are defeating their own purpose by doing everything themselves. The staff never learn to do the work expected of them, and their own supervisory tasks suffer. Remember, you must accomplish work through others; do not do the work yourself.

Another mistake is to assume that you should demonstrate your nursing proficiency to your staff by doing the work yourself. They admire your expertise for a short time, but later they learn that they do not have to do anything because you do it all for them. They resent your interference and accomplish less than they did before. If you, as the supervisor, are going to do the work yourself, why is a staff necessary? You must take the necessary time to teach staff members to do their jobs. If every person holds up his or her own part in the organization, the health care agency will be efficient, and staff members will be motivated.

Allowing staff members to make their own mistakes is difficult. Supervisors are sometimes too quick to jump in and prevent an error. The best supervisors know when to give advice to prevent a major error, but they are also willing to accept minor problems as learning situations. If you take over and prevent the staff from trying to think for themselves, they never learn or grow. It is hard to watch things go wrong when you are trying to be an effective supervisor, but it is sometimes necessary to prevent further problems. If an error occurs, talk to the staff and make sure that they understand why the error occurred and how to prevent it in the future. You must allow this freedom so that your staff develop the necessary self-confidence. A supervisor who is able to give this "freedom to fail" in situations that do not jeopardize the safety or care of patients is rewarded by a more effective and independent staff.

Too many supervisors feel needed only when their staffs are totally dependent on them. They meet all the needs of the staff and make all decisions for them. Then they wonder why they are so busy that they cannot accomplish all the necessary supervisory tasks. Staff that have become dependent on their supervisor cease thinking. They automatically turn off their brains and wait for you to come and bail them out of a situation. If you are not immediately available to solve the problem, the staff do nothing or make a decision that is not based on experience or good judgment. When a staff member approaches you with a problem, the best first response would be, "What do you think should be done?" In this way the staff member is allowed to try out new approaches or plans without the threat of an error. You have a perfect opportunity for giving advice without the impression of dictating to the staff. Teach your staff to think of possible alternatives and to weigh the merits of each one. Help the person choose the best alternative, and encourage the independent thought process.

Delegation of authority should never be viewed as a threat to your position. Sure of yourself and your abilities, you must not feel threatened by the opinions or actions of subordinates. Your staff's independence does not make the job of leadership unnecessary. Good supervisors delegate responsibility only after setting up controls that enable them to take corrective action if things go wrong.

In order to delegate effectively, the supervisor must be sure that several conditions are met:

1. The staff must be properly trained for the responsibility and understand fully what is expected.
2. Subordinates must be given the responsibility in the proper dose. Do not give responsibility in a step-by-step kindergarten approach. On the other hand, do not simply give broad generalizations that leave the staff member feeling threatened or confused. Know how much responsibility to give in each stage, and maintain that proportion.
3. Give staff members progress reports. Tell them of successes and also of areas of concern as the project is underway.
4. Stay on top of the situation to prevent serious or irreversible errors and to prevent them before they occur.

Help Subordinates Identify with You and with Others

Staff members work harder and more effectively when they like the supervisor and feel that he or she likes them. They are more productive in a work situation that allows them to make friendships and good working relationships with other members of the staff. Encourage this social exchange by being interested in your staff members and in their outside activities. Allow time for the staff members to make social friendships, and be aware of the best combinations of staff members. Whenever possible, allow people who are compatible to work on projects as a team.

Acknowledge the individuality of your staff, and make an effort to know each person as a human being. Spend time discussing their family, friends, and other interests. Show your staff that you care about them as persons and that you are interested in what makes them happy. Make sure that no one is lost in the crowd, and show a sincere interest in the people who make up the organization. Do not become overly involved in the lives of staff members, but know what is going on in their minds. Be friendly and warm, but do not allow your social relationships to cloud your professional judgment.

Give Credit

When a responsibility is delegated, the task is to be now accomplished by another person. If the job is well done, the person who did

121

it deserves the credit. Make sure that all praise and recognition go to the staff members.

Human beings have a great need to be recognized. Recognition may take the form of praise, reward, promotion, or the satisfaction of a job well done. Staff members who are recognized for their contributions to the goal attainment of the organization are motivated employees. Be free with sincere praise. The few minutes spent praising a person reap many rewards for you and the health care agency. Persons who feel good about themselves accomplish more, and they are more comfortable in the work situation.

Praise does not cause staff members to relax their efforts and bask in your approval. Actually, the opposite is true. The more praise that individuals receive, the more effort they expend to receive more of this positive reinforcement. Praise freely and publicly. If an employee has done a good job and deserves credit, make an appropriate comment in the presence of others. Nothing feels better than to be told of a job well done in the presence of peers. Do not be so effusive as to embarrass people, but show by your actions that you are pleased and want the other members of the work group to share in this pleasure. This reaction motivates others to try harder to receive the same type of recognition. Everyone likes to be told when he or she is succeeding, even if the individual already knows. The praise makes the feeling of pleasure even greater.

Show Confidence

Confidence breeds confidence. A real leader may often give subordinates courage that they otherwise would not have. If you indicate by your words and actions that you trust your staff, they rise up to the challenge.

The staff need to have security in their leadership. So you must make sure that you are confident of yourself and of your actions so that the staff trust you. They need to know that you are there to help and guide them and that your decisions will be correct. Give your staff this security by being open to them and by displaying enough self-confidence to overcome their doubts and fears. You are their leader, and they want to know that you will come through for them when they need you. Independence is good, but you must also show that you can provide for their needs when the situation calls for strong leadership.

Assign Blame

Just as positive feedback, in the form of praise or reward, is a useful motivational tool, so is negative feedback or blame. Praise shows the employee what is going right; blame or discipline shows the staff member how to correct a situation or what is going wrong. Both types of feedback are essential. Subordinates need to know that they will be informed about errors or about areas of concern, and that you are available to assist them in correcting these problem areas. If you delegate a responsibility, staff members must feel that you also expect positive results from their actions. If persons know that they will receive constructive criticism from a supervisor, they will trust you and give increased effort. If a job "belongs" to a person—bad or good—that worker is personally involved and does his or her best to see that the project succeeds. The staff need to know where they stand with you. They need to know that they will be praised for a job well done, but that they will also be corrected for an error made.

People know when they are not doing the best they can and they actually expect a reprimand. If you do not comment and try to solve the problem yourself, they feel that you do not care, and they do not correct their own behavior. Also, if you are very free with your praise, but never criticize staff members, they may not feel that your praise is genuine.

Instill Fear

Although a strange leadership concept, the ability to instill fear is a useful motivational tool. Fear is not caused by the threat of physical or verbal abuse. Rather, it is evoked by the knowledge that when you, the supervisor, become aware of certain actions of your staff, you are willing and able to take the necessary steps to ensure compliance with organizational objectives. A certain look, a scowl, silence—these are all ways of showing displeasure with the activities of subordinates. If your staff know that you will carry out necessary disciplinary actions, they will respect you and work more effectively. You show by your actions that you mean what you say.

Trying to have everyone like you is an impossible goal for a leader. Avoiding unpleasant situations is natural, but leaders must be brave enough to use the authority that the organization gives them. The staff may be unhappy when you reprimand them, but they feel secure in the knowledge that you do not tolerate any infractions on their part. This assumption assures a smooth working group and gives the staff the security of your control.

WHAT IS MOTIVATION?

In a simple definition, motivation is "encouraging subordinates to perform organizational objectives because they want to perform." It means appealing to their needs and matching these needs with the duties and responsibilities of the organization. If staff members perform a task because it fulfills a personal need, they are more willing to do the task. They are motivated.

Motivation is not something that you do to people; it is something that they do themselves. Putting pressure on staff members, or "cheerleading," does not increase motivation. Actually, as you put more pressure on staff members to produce, their motivation is lowered. Studies have shown that most individuals function at only 10 percent of their potential. The other 90 percent represents the untapped resources that a good supervisor can use simply by setting the climate for motivated employees.

CONCEPTS OF MOTIVATION

Of the many concepts of motivation, each delves into an aspect of the psychological makeup of the human personality. Each concept has merit, and the best supervisor is able to understand and apply each of them to individual workers.

Reward and Punishment

This concept is based on the supposition that a supervisor can increase the motivation of employees by balancing rewards and punishments. In other words, if people do a good job, they are rewarded; if they fail, they are punished. This very simplistic explanation of motivation assumes that people do a good job to gain approval or reward and to avoid punishment. The idea is to balance the positive with the negative. For example:

Positives	Negatives
A job	Termination
Advancement	No promotion
Salary increase	No raises
Prestige	Nonrecognition
Security	Insecurity

The assumption is that all individuals seek the positive recognition and are thus motivated. Yet psychology has shown us that people receive as much, if not more, recognition for negative behavior as they do for positive behavior. If individuals cannot succeed and receive positive recognition, they engage in negative behavior, such as acting out, just to be noticed. Relying on people to invariably seek out positive behavior characteristics does not result in motivation. You must understand the needs of the individual and meet those needs.

Maslow's Theory of Motivation

In 1954 Dr. Abraham Maslow wrote a book called *Motivation and Personality,* which has had a profound influence on management thinking in the area of human relations. In this book, which is based on his extensive research developed through the study of people in their daily lives, he outlines his concept of man's needs. His study avoids persons getting psychiatric treatment and concentrates on the average or "normal" person pursuing daily work.

Maslow said, "Man is motivated to act by interrelated and interacting needs that are hierarchical in character reflecting a span that ranges from bodily needs to those of self-actualization." In other words, human needs, desires, urges, and drives can be classified or arranged in levels or steps. When certain basic "needs" are relatively satisfied, the "needs" on the next level begin to press for fulfillment. Dr. Maslow has divided man's drives or needs into five main levels. These five broad needs appear in man's life in the following sequence:

1. physical needs,
2. security and safety needs,
3. social needs,
4. ego needs, and
5. self-fulfillment needs.

The five basic needs are not separate and detached; they are all within us at the same time in a hierarchy of strength. In Figure 7–1, a triangle is used to represent the relative power of each level of needs. By their very nature, the lower needs on the scale are the stronger ones. The lower levels must be satisfied first before needs on the next level become important and press for satisfaction. Dr. Maslow says, "For the man who is extremely and dangerously hungry, no other interest exists but food." Only when one has satisfied his body needs, his security needs, and his social needs, will one need his "ego" uplifted. (See Table 7–1.)

TABLE 7–1
Examples of needs on Maslow's scale

LEVEL 1—PHYSIOLOGICAL NEEDS (Physical–Body)

Survival	Sleep/rest	Comfort	*Acquired Needs:*
Air	Sex	Freedom from	
Water	Clothing	pain	Cigarettes
Food	Shelter	Health	Liquor
Elimination	Warmth	Mobility	Drugs
		Weapons	

TABLE 7–1 (cont.)

LEVEL 2—SECURITY NEEDS (Safety–Protection)

You	Your Job	Money	Community
God—Faith	Your position	Insurance	Organized world
Mental attitude	Company	Savings	Economy of
Goals	stability	Home	country
Education	Company new	Investments	Politics
Experience	business	Fringe benefits	Armed Forces
Skills	Company	Part-time work	Laws
Talents	reputation	Spouse works	Courts
Social groups	Job performance	Credit rating	Police & fire
	Recognition	Budget	protection
	Leadership		Scientific
	Policies &		progress
	procedures		Medical progress
	Seniority &		Charities
	unions		
	Retirement		

LEVEL 3—SOCIAL NEEDS (Communication–Response)

Love	Belong to Groups	Recreation	At Work	Miscellaneous
Family	Clubs	Sports	Conversation	Contribute to
Friends	Civic	Parties	Work groups	society
Sweetheart	groups	Dancing	Coffee break	Help your fellow
Spouse	Business	Drinking	Telephone	man
Children	groups	Theater	Meetings	To be alone at
Pets	Church	Card	Lunch	times
	Political	playing		
	groups			
	Night			
	school			

LEVEL 4—SELF-ESTEEM NEEDS (Ego–Self-Confidence)

Self-Respect	Respect from Others		
Must "like"	Acceptance	Praise	Reputation
yourself	Appreciation	Prestige	Respect
Be expert in your	Attention	Promotion	Seek your
field	Courtesy	Raise in pay	advice
Have skills and	Fair dealing	Recognition	Status
talents			Understanding
Have "positive"			
qualities and			
characteristics			

LEVEL 5—SELF-ACTUALIZATION NEEDS (Fulfillment–Realization)

Fulfilling one's potential	Reaching towards one's potential
Using one's capabilities	Seeking new knowledge

TABLE 7–1 *(cont.)*

Positive Characteristics	Negative Traits
Loves the challenge	Different
Dedicated to work	Nonconformist
Loves to work	Reserved
Highly objective	Unfriendly
Has ability	Forgetful of minor details
Is creative	Detached from daily happenings
Has sense of humor	
Enthusiastic	
Flexible	

Figure 7–1. Maslow's theory of motivation and human needs.

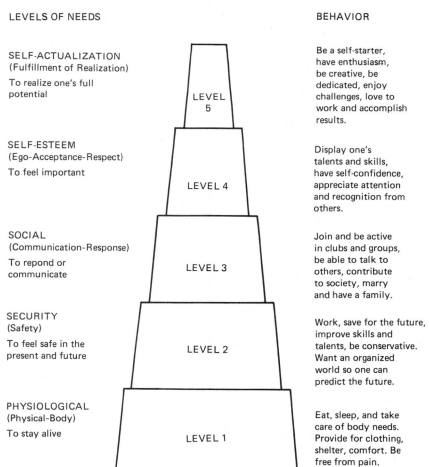

LEVELS OF NEEDS

BEHAVIOR

SELF-ACTUALIZATION
(Fulfillment of Realization)

To realize one's full
potential

LEVEL 5

Be a self-starter,
have enthusiasm,
be creative, be
dedicated, enjoy
challenges, love to
work and accomplish
results.

SELF-ESTEEM
(Ego-Acceptance-Respect)

To feel important

LEVEL 4

Display one's
talents and skills,
have self-confidence,
appreciate attention
and recognition from
others.

SOCIAL
(Communication-Response)

To repond or
communicate

LEVEL 3

Join and be active
in clubs and groups,
be able to talk to
others, contribute
to society, marry
and have a family.

SECURITY
(Safety)

To feel safe in the
present and future

LEVEL 2

Work, save for the future,
improve skills and
talents, be conservative.
Want an organized
world so one can
predict the future.

PHYSIOLOGICAL
(Physical-Body)

To stay alive

LEVEL 1

Eat, sleep, and take
care of body needs.
Provide for clothing,
shelter, comfort. Be
free from pain.

The following four points are extremely important in understanding human nature:

1. Man is dominated by unsatisfied needs.
2. Man is an ever-wanting person, never completely satisfied.
3. Satisfaction is always short-lived.
4. Needs change according to time and circumstances.

Maslow has made an important contribution to our understanding of people. His five-way classification of needs is somewhat artificial because in a real situation all needs interact within the whole person, but it does provide management with a convenient way of understanding which type of need is likely to dominate one's drives in a certain situation.

As a nursing supervisor, you must understand Maslow's hierarchy of needs in dealing with staff members. For example, a nurse who is trying to support her family alone and is constantly worried about how she is going to feed her children cannot be expected to seek higher education to better use her ability and thus fulfill her needs for self-gratification. When the staff are hungry or tired, they do not respond to an in-service program to increase their skills. The best supervisor is constantly aware of the needs of the group and seeks to meet the needs as they are presented.

Motivational and Maintenance Factors

A significant development in motivation was the distinction of motivational and maintenance factors in the job situation. The original research was based on interviews, conducted by Frederick Herzberg[1] and his associates, of two hundred engineers and accountants in the Pittsburgh area. Their approach was to ask each employee to think of a time when he felt especially good about his job and a time when he felt particularly bad about it, and then to describe the conditions that led to these feelings. They found that employees named different types of conditions for good and bad feelings. For example, if a feeling of achievement led to a good feeling, the lack of achievement was rarely given as a cause for bad feelings. Instead, some other factor such as company policy was given as a cause of bad feelings.

Herzberg concluded that the absence of some job conditions operates primarily to dissatisfy employees, while their presence does not motivate employees in a strong way. These potent dissatisfiers are called "maintenance factors" in the job, because they are necessary to maintain a reasonable level of satisfaction in employees. They are also

[1] W. J. Paul, Jr., K. B. Robertson, and F. Herzberg, "Job Enrichment Pays Off," *Harvard Business Review* (March–April 1969).

known as dissatisfiers or as "hygienic" factors because they support employee mental health. Although many such factors are traditionally perceived by management as motivators, they are really more potent as dissatisfiers. In this instance, the perceptions of management are just not the same as the perceptions of employees. As an example, for many years managers wondered why their fancy personnel policies and fringe benefits did not increase employee motivation on the job. The distinction of motivational and maintenance factors helped answer their question, because fringe benefits and personnel policies were shown to be primarily maintenance factors.

The orginal Herzberg study included ten maintenance factors:

1. status,
2. interpersonal relations with supervision,
3. interpersonal relations with peers,
4. interpersonal relations with subordinates,
5. technical supervision,
6. company policy and administration,
7. job security,
8. working conditions,
9. salary, and
10. personal life.

Another set of job conditions operates primarily to build strong motivation and high job satisfaction, but their absence rarely proves strongly dissatisfying. These conditions are known as "motivational factors," motivators, or satisfiers. The original Herzberg study included six motivational factors:

1. achievement,
2. growth potential,
3. responsibility,
4. work itself,
5. advancement, and
6. recognition.

The results of the study show that motivation is based on job content and what employees do. Employees are unhappy if they have significant dissatisfiers. Correcting such dissatisfiers does not make unhappy employees happy, but it helps to keep employees from being unhappy. As an analogy, a good clean working situation keeps people from being unhealthy, but it won't make them healthy. Another example is pay: If employees see pay as a maintenance factor (in other words, if the lack of pay makes them unhappy), then increasing their pay does not motivate them. Yet if they see pay as a form of recognition for good performance, they are motivated to perform more effectively. To increase motivation, increase the satisfiers or intrinsic factors, while decreasing the dissatisfiers or avoidance factors. (See Figure 7–2.)

A composite of the factors involved in causing job satisfaction and job dissatisfaction, drawn from samples of 1,685 employees, is shown in Figure 7–2. The results indicate that motivators were the primary cause of satisfaction, and that maintenance or hygiene factors were the primary cause of unhappiness on the job. The employees, studied in twelve different investigations, included lower-level supervisors, professional women, agricultural administrators, men about to retire from management positions, hospital maintenance personnel, manufacturing supervisors, nurses, food handlers, military officers, engineers, scientists, housekeepers, teachers, technicians, female assemblers, accountants, Finnish foremen, and Hungarian engineers. They were all asked which job events in their work had led to their extreme satisfaction or extreme dissatisfaction. Their responses are broken down in the chart into percentages of total "positive" job events and of total "negative" job events. (See Figure 7–2).

"Theory X" and "Theory Y"[2]

Management's attempts to harness human energy to organizational requirements may be regarded from essentially two viewpoints: "Theory X" reflects the authoritarian point of view, and "Theory Y" recognizes the interdependence of managers and employees. Other terms for these theories are "traditional management" versus "inspirational management." (See Table 7–2.)

There are three cornerstones of Theory X:

1. Most people just do not like to work.
2. Some kind of "club" has to be held over their heads to make sure that they do work.
3. Ordinary mortals would rather be told what to do than have to think for themselves.

The world, in other words, is supposed to be full of peons, and managing them is largely a matter of vigilance, catering to their security needs with various fringe benefits and keeping the implied threat of unemployment handy in case it is needed. McGregor stresses that this set of assumptions, obsolete as it is, continues to have a very broad influence in American industry. Much of the literature on principles of organization, with its emphasis on centralized authority and controls,

[2] Douglas McGregor, *The Human Side of Enterprise* (New York: McGraw-Hill Book Company, 1960).

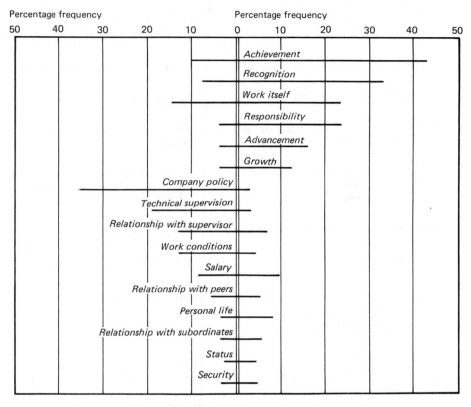

FACTORS OF JOB DISSATISFACTION   FACTORS OF JOB SATISFACTION

Figure 7–2. Herzberg's factors affecting job attitudes.

TABLE 7–2
Assumptions of X and Y theories compared

"THEORY X" (TRADITIONAL MANAGEMENT)	"THEORY Y" (INSPIRATIONAL MANAGEMENT)
1. People are lazy.	1. People are motivated by many factors.
2. People do not want to work.	2. People want and enjoy work.
3. People are prone to error. The organizational structure is designed to detect and correct these errors.	3. People try to do an excellent job with minimal errors.
4. People are somewhat dishonest and must be constantly watched.	4. People are fundamentally honest and can be trusted.

TABLE 7–2 (*cont.*)

"THEORY X" (TRADITIONAL MANAGEMENT)	"THEORY Y" (INSPIRATIONAL MANAGEMENT)
5. People need tight controls.	5. People work better with light controls.
6. People work mainly for money.	6. People work for many reasons.
7. People are not very bright and do not care to learn.	7. People are willing to learn, to develop, and to change.
8. People are concerned with their needs and not concerned with the company needs.	8. People see the attainment of their own needs linked with the goals of the company.
9. People are units of production.	9. People are human beings with many wants, needs, and desires that must be fulfilled.

seems to take these assumptions for granted. More importantly, so do many experienced managers.

Theory Y holds:

1. People do not like or dislike work inherently, but rather they develop an attitude toward it based on their experiences with it.
2. While authoritarian methods can get things done, they do not constitute the only method. There is nothing inevitable about them, and their undesirable side effects do not have to be tolerated.
3. People select goals for themselves if they see the possibility of some kind of reward, be it material or purely psychic. Once they have selected a goal, they pursue it at least as vigorously as they would if their superiors were trying to pressure them into doing the same thing.
4. Under the right circumstances, people do not shun responsibility but seek it.

At the conventional extreme, management can be "hard" or "strong." The methods for directing behavior involve coercion and threat (which is usually disguised), close supervision, and tight controls over behavior. At the other extreme, management can be "soft" or "weak." The methods for directing behavior involve being permissive, satisfying people's demands, achieving harmony; workers then become tractable and accept direction.

The conditions imposed by conventional organizational theory and by the approach of scientific management for the past half-century have tied people to limited jobs that do not utilize their capabilities. They have discouraged the acceptance of responsibility, encouraged passivity, and eliminated meaning from work. People's habits, attitudes, expectations, and their whole conception of membership in an industrial organization are conditioned by their experience under these circumstances. As a result, people today are accustomed to being directed, manipulated, controlled in industrial organizations and to finding satisfaction for their social, egotistic, and self-fulfillment needs away from the job. This attitude is true of management as well as of workers.

In other words, Theory X places exclusive reliance on the external control of human behavior, while Theory Y relies heavily on self-control and self-direction. This difference is the difference between treating people as children and treating them as mature adults. After generations of the former treatment, you cannot expect a shift to the latter overnight.

HOW TO MOTIVATE SUBORDINATES

1. *Help people achieve more.* Assist people who like to excel in quality and quantity. Generally, the key to higher achievement consists of improved methods rather than greater effort.

2. *Give your people personal recognition.* Routine pay increases are a small recognition. Pay based on specific performance can be a motivator. Use nonmonetary means of recognition such as compliments and awards. How often do you operate under the attitude, "If you are not doing a good job, I'll tell you so"?

3. *Help make work interesting.* Help people to identify with your goals and to see that your operation is worthwhile. People find work interesting when they are given responsibility for making their own decisions and for establishing methods to accomplish their goals.

4. *Give your people responsibility.* Assign tasks that have some importance and that require a certain level of knowledge. Delegate authority by providing job enrichment, not job enlargement. Try to eliminate highly repetitive tasks in areas such as reports and the like.

5. *Help people grow and advance.* Grow or go—become promotable or get out. Because subordinates need help in gaining new knowledge, supervisors must promote training activities and an annual program of individual growth.

6. *Try to eliminate dissatisfiers,* especially in such areas as pay or working conditions. Elimination of dissatisfiers in the job environment does not motivate your people, but their presence can prevent your

133

people from being motivated. Pay, working conditions, policies and procedures, and interpersonal relationships all play a part.

Practical Measures
That Motivate Employees

You can take many small steps every day on the job to enhance the environment for motivation:

1. Help each person achieve the highest job level he or she can as soon as possible.
2. Give careful attention to compensation plans, to be sure that they are up-to-date.
3. Help people build on formal education with the practical advice you can give them.
4. Invite and use their ideas whenever practical.
5. Encourage them to question you when they believe they have some good reason for doing so.
6. Let them know you expect only as much loyalty as you deserve.
7. Show them how they can get diversified experience and responsibility within your organization.
8. Make sure your people know what their fringe benefits are, but stress the job content and opportunity they have.
9. Help them balance the needs and opportunities of the agency against their family obligations and interests.
10. Counsel each of them about the results they are to achieve and qualifications they need if they are to be promoted.

The one best way to motivate people is to help them, one by one, define and attain what they want from their jobs. Annually, find out the responsibility they seek within the next one to five years, what they would like to learn, and how they think the content of their jobs can be improved. Help them individually to define and determine programs of personal growth, reading courses, planned experience, and their own objectives.

Your Personal Role

You must be an intelligent, successful, human relations expert. You have to understand why people act as they do, and you must expect certain kinds of behavior in different situations. Try to see problems from the employee's point of view. These talents enable you to set the climate for motivation and to make each person productive. Remember these suggestions:

1. Employees like competent and colorful leadership.
2. Supervisors must do things that are worthwhile.

3. Supervisors give employees an opportunity to tell what, how, and when to do their jobs.
4. When supervisors must correct an error, they do so in a way that helps employees keep their self-respect and sense of personal worth.
5. Supervisors must earn and keep the respect, confidence, and cooperation of their employees.
6. Supervisors help employees demonstrate their capabilities.
7. Supervisors boost their employees' morale.
8. A supervisor is given authority from above but must earn respect from below. Use your position for displaying your knowledge and abilities effectively.

DISCUSSION QUESTIONS

1. How do you get a person "involved" in performing a disagreeable job?
2. In what ways is recognition important to people under your supervision?
3. What forms might this recognition take in the health care field?
4. Why is self-confidence so important to the supervisor?
5. Why is fear a factor in motivation?

HOW DO YOU RATE?

1. How good is your motivational climate?
2. What is good about the motivational climate in your organization? How can you improve the situation?
3. What is bad about the motivational climate in your organization? How can you improve the situation?

APPLICATION: TEST FOR IMAGINATION

Objective

- To create ideas and situations from pictures seen briefly.

Procedure

1. Write out a brief story for each picture.
2. Make a continuous story; don't just answer the questions, which are only guides for thinking.
3. Spend only 5 minutes on each story.
4. Don't simply describe the picture—tell the story.

135

5. Look at the picture for 10 to 15 seconds, and write what first comes to mind.

6. Work rapidly. Do not spend over 5 minutes on each story.

7. When you have written your stories, read the introduction.

8. Using your score sheet, score your stories.

Questions

These questions apply to Figures 7-3 through 7-8. Answer the questions on a separate piece of paper.

1. What is happening? Who are the people?

2. What has led up to this situation? That is, what has happened in the past?

3. What is being thought? What is wanted? By whom?

4. What will happen? What will be done?

When you have finished your story or when your time is up, look at the next picture. If you have not finished, go on anyway. You may return at the end to complete your story.

Introduction

Job satisfaction among nurses is a major concern of nursing supervisors. However, identification of elements that affect job satisfaction in nursing is a difficult and complex task.

The purpose of this exercise is to explore the extent that a person's motivation relates to his or her level of job satisfaction. David McClelland of Harvard has used this imagination test as a way of identifying dominent themes of basic motivation. The stories are a tool to record thoughts and concepts. From these stories, you can see a dominant theme, which can be compared to your personal job satisfaction.

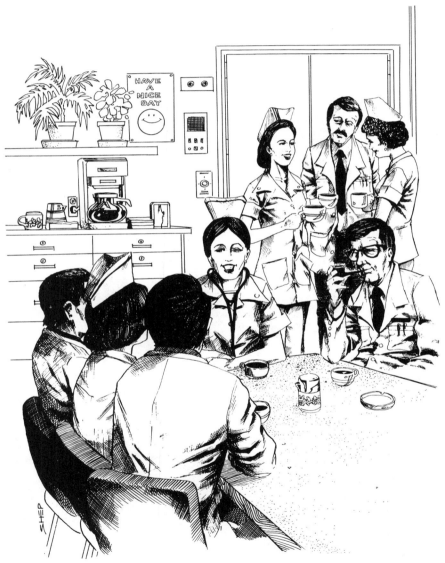

Figure 7–3.

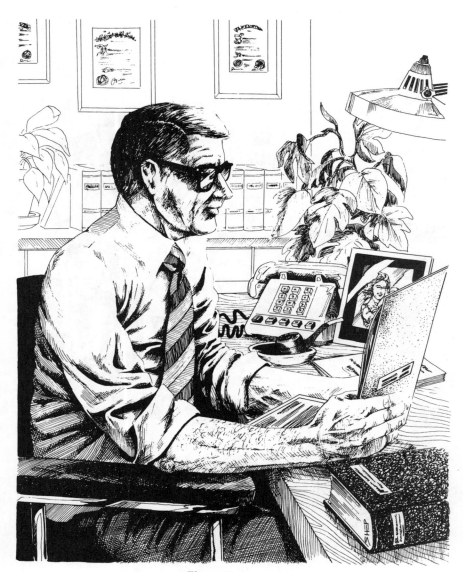

Figure 7–4.

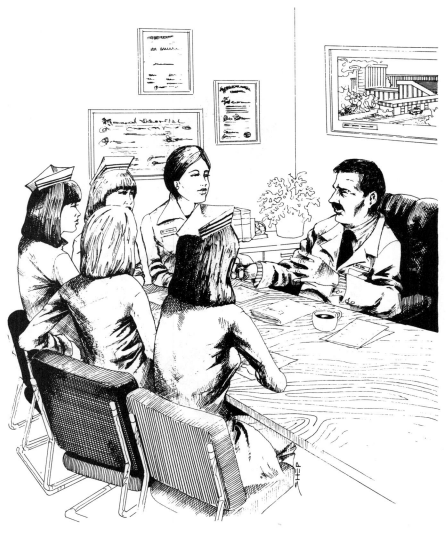

Figure 7–5.

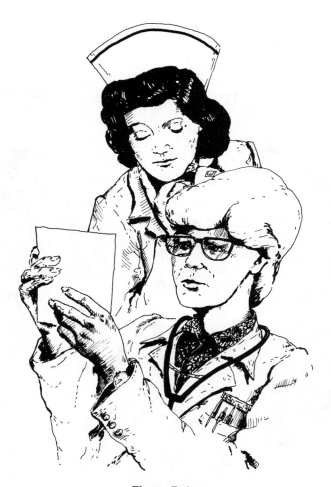

Figure 7–6.

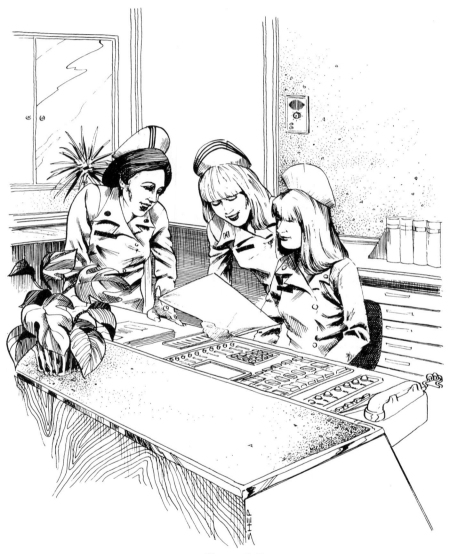

Figure 7–7.

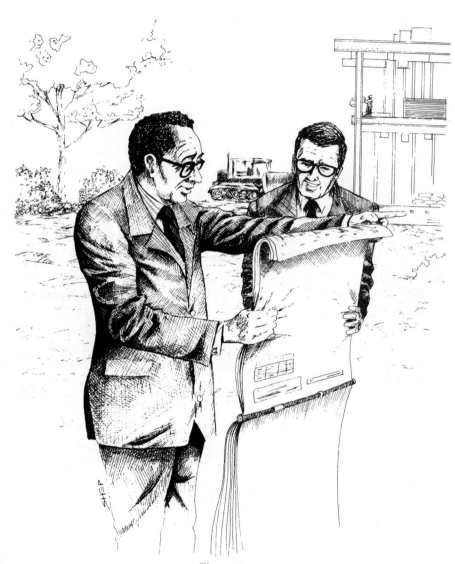

Figure 7–8.

Motivation is unique to an individual's personality. These personality differences account for much of the variation of individual behavior in organizations. These differences may be defined as needs: for achievement, for affiliation, and for power. Each person possesses these needs in different amounts and strengths.

We score the stories to find the need that emerges as most dominant. As you read your stories, look for subtle clues that indicate one of the needs. Every time you make a statement that indicates one of the needs, mark it on your score sheet (Table 7–3). After you have scored all your stories, add up the scores and find the motivation that is most dominant.

TABLE 7–3
Individual scoring form for test of imagination

Circle the motives present in each story, and indicate other motivational concerns in the space provided.

	PRIMARY SOCIAL MOTIVES	OTHER MOTIVES PRESENT
Story 1	Achievement Power Affiliation	
Story 2	Achievement Power Affiliation	
Story 3	Achievement Power Affiliation	
Story 4	Achievement Power Affiliation	
Story 5	Achievement Power Affiliation	
Story 6	Achievement Power Affiliation	
Summary	Total Number of:	
	Achievement Power	Affiliation

Scoring

Look for any dominant themes, such as:

1. aggression,
2. a need for security,
3. sex,
4. hunger,
5. happiness, or
6. fear.

Primary Social Motives

Achievement motivation is present if:

1. Someone in the story is concerned about *standard of excellence.* Look for someone who:
   a. wants to win,
   b. sets performance standards,
   c. is involved in goal setting, or
   d. uses words such as "good" or "better."
2. Someone is involved in *unique accomplishment.* Look for:
   a. invention,
   b. innovation, or
   c. artistic endeavor.
3. Someone is involved in *long-term goals.* Look for:
   a. specific career or
   b. being a success in life.

Power motivation is present if:

1. Someone is concerned with getting or controlling *influence* over a person. Look for someone who is:
   a. winning a point,
   b. dominating,
   c. convincing, or
   d. wanting to teach, inspire.
2. Someone is doing something to *control.* This person might be:
   a. arguing,
   b. forcing, or
   c. commanding.
3. Someone plays *culturally defined power role.* Look for a:
   a. boss–worker relationship, but

b. a parent–child relationship does not count.

Affiliation motivation is present if:

1. Someone is concerned with a *positive emotional relationship.*
   Watch for:
   a. friendship,
   b. a father–son relationship, or
   c. lovers.
2. Someone *likes or wants to like another person.*
3. Any affiliative activity, such as:
   a. parties,
   b. visits,
   c. reunions, or
   d. small talk.

Interpretation

Now that you have found your dominant motivation, see how it applies to the job that you now hold. Ideally, the position you hold meets your needs. If so, you are probably very satisfied. If not, you must analyze the job itself and try to tailor it to meet your needs. Personalities cannot be changed, but environments can.

As a supervisor, you can also try to analyze the dominant motivational needs of your subordinates, and change the climate to meet those needs. Persons who are satisfied in their jobs are more highly motivated.

ACHIEVEMENT MOTIVATION If your highest score is in achievement motivation, you are the type of person who assumes personal responsibility for finding solutions to problems, takes calculated risks, and seeks concrete feedback on how well you are doing. You set realistic but high goals for yourself. You would be best suited to work in research, in an in-service operation, as an independent nurse practitioner, in discharge planning, or in overall planning and coordinating functions. You are very comfortable in a high-level supervisory position and like to assume the responsibility for long-range planning.

AFFILIATION MOTIVATION If this is your high scoring area, you are the type of person who relates positively and affectionately to others, who is concerned about being liked, who helps others, and who pays attention to others' feelings. You are seen as a good leader, a "helper." Your staff likes you, respects you, and enjoys working for you. You may have a tendency to "buck for your staff," and you are never comfortable working in the highest levels of health care. You would be very unhappy working in a situation that was independent of contact with others.

POWER MOTIVATION   If this is your highest area, you are concerned about your influence over others. You like to win arguments, and you enjoy having authority and status. As a supervisor, you would like strengthened structure, order, status, a narrowed span of control, clearly defined position responsibilities, and conformity to standards. You may have some trouble dealing with people as individuals, but you accomplish a great deal of work. You are efficient, organized, and thorough—and you expect the same of others.

SUMMARY   Ideally, you show a combination of all of these motivations. If you do, you are probably a good nursing supervisor and very satisfied in your job. Basically, high-achievement and affiliation people are comfortable in high supervisory positions, whereas power motivation is best met in direct leadership roles with clear-cut role models.

The work situation creates a "climate," which helps to determine the kinds of worker motivations that are actually aroused—that satisfy workers' motivational needs for achievement, for affiliation, or for power. Ideally, then, employees would be matched with a work climate that is most suited to their motivational personalities, so that job satisfaction is enhanced. For example, if a worker's motivational need pattern is predominantly affiliation-directed, he or she would be most satisfied working in a job that allows warm, friendly relationships, socialization, and group effort. That is an "affiliation" climate.

REFERENCES

CLELLAND, DAVID I. AND WILLIAM R. KING, *Systems Analysis and Project Management*. New York: McGraw-Hill Book Co., 1968.

DORSEY, JOHN R., JR., "A Communication Model for Administration," *Administrative Science Quarterly*, 2:307–324 (December 1957).

FAYOL, HENRY, *General and Industrial Management*, trans. Constance Storrs. London: Sir Isaac Pitman and Sons, Ltd., 1949.

GROSS, BERTRAM M., *The Managing of Organizations*. New York: The Free Press of Glencoe, 1964.

KATZ, DANIEL AND ROBERT L. KAHN, *The Social Psychology of Organizations*. New York: John Wiley & Sons, Inc., 1966.

LIPPITT, R. AND R. K. WHITE, "An Experimental Study of Leadership and Group Life," in *Readings in Social Psychology*, ed. G. E. Swanson, T. M. Newcomb, and E. L. Hartley. New York: Holt, Rinehart & Winston, Inc., 1952.

LOCTHLISBERGER, F. J. AND W. J. DICKSON, *Management and the Worker*. Cambridge: Harvard University Press, 1939.

LONGEST, BEAUFORT, JR., *Management Practices for the Health Care Professional*. Reston, Va.: Reston Publishing Co., 1976.

MCCLELLAND, DAVID, *The Achieving Society*. Princeton, N.J.: D. Van Nostrand Company, 1961.

MARCH, JAMES G. AND HERBERT A. SIMON, *Organizations*. New York: John Wiley & Sons, Inc., 1958.

NEWHAUSER, DUNCAN, "The Hospital as a Matrix Organization," *Hospital Administration* (Fall 1972).

SCHEIN, EDGAR H., *Organizational Psychology*. Englewood Cliffs, N.J.: Prentice-Hall, Inc., 1963.

TAYLOR, FREDERICK W., *Shop Management*. New York: Harper & Row, Publishers, Inc., 1911.

URWICK, L., *Elements of Administration*. New York: Harper & Row, Publishers, Inc., 1943.

WEBER, MAX, *The Theory of Social and Economic Organization*, ed. Talcott Parson, trans. A. M. Henderson and Talcott Parsons. New York: Oxford University Press, Inc., 1947.

YOUNG, STANLEY, *Management: A Systems Approach*. Glenview, Ill.: Scott, Foresman & Company, 1967.

8

Concepts of managerial duties and responsibilities

LIVING UP TO RESPONSIBILITIES

Supervisors direct and control the work of others. They therefore have a great deal of responsibility. Only through a constant study of your own supervisory responsibilities can you obtain the high quality of supervisory behavior that is essential in a modern health agency. To better understand the responsibilities of the supervisory job, you must learn some of the duties and responsibilities common to most supervisors. While nurse/supervisors must continue to improve their technical skills and knowledge of the nursing process, they must also learn the skills of the professional manager. The tasks of supervision are very complex, and you must have a strong educational foundation in the supervisory skills to function efficiently.

This chapter focuses on the *concepts* of managerial duties and responsibilities rather than on the specific task-behavior necessary in day-to-day functioning. Task-behavior, such as scheduling, budgeting, auditing, and setting policies, differs from one health agency to the next. These specific and relatively simple procedures can be learned through in-service education, once they are explained. The difficult part of the supervisory role is in the attitudes and activities necessary to become the leader of a staff. The problem is not how to do the tasks; it is how to work within the management framework.

Most of the questions asked about supervision deal with personnel relations, attitude adjustment, and areas of authority. Supervisors' specific areas of responsibility are therefore explored, as well as their related duties. No matter what level of supervision you achieve, the predominant responsibilities do not change, of which there are three main levels:

1. administration
2. supervision, and
3. training.[1]

ADMINISTRATION

This area of responsibility is concerned mainly with the preparation for accomplishing work and the maintenance of an organized environment. The specific areas within administration are:

a. planning,
b. organizing,
c. staffing,
d. directing, and
e. coordinating.

Planning

To accomplish work in an organized and rational manner takes much planning and forethought. Although most organizational planning takes place on the higher levels of administration, everyone in a supervisory role takes part in the planning stage in one way or another. The planning function is essential to start the flow of creative movement. Supervisors must plan the implementation of departmental policies and procedures. The staffing patterns and patient care ratio must be planned and implemented. Also included in the planning function are the in-service requirements and long-term goals and objectives. Even if a nurse's role is not one of direct leadership, the planning stage is important. Arranging the workload for the day, planning the nursing care, and planning methods of organizing patient care all fall into this responsibility.

Organizing

Once the basic plan has been made, organization is necessary to put it into effect. Nursing is a process-oriented profession. Actions and activities are necessary to accomplish the tasks necessary to achieve the organizational goals, which all boil down to meeting the needs of

---

[1] Joseph L. Massie and John Douglas, *Managing: A Contemporary Introduction* (Englewood Cliffs, N.J.: Prentice-Hall, Inc., 1973).

the patient. The organizational function of supervision enables the staff to achieve these goals with the maximum ease and efficiency.

Staffing

Usually listed as one of the major problems in supervision, this area causes much concern. The careful planning of future staffing needs helps to eliminate some of the concern. In nursing, we find that the quick turnover in staff brings an almost constant problem of understaffing. To assist in the hiring of competent staff members and to make the staffing responsibility of supervision an easier one, try to anticipate the needs of the health care agency and analyze the training or educational needs of your staff.

Nurse recruitment has become a major specialty in health care. Many health care agencies are using a staffing coordinator who relieves the supervisor of this function. This position, which may be filled by a nursing or non-nursing staff person, is a valuable addition to the organization. No supervisor should spend the majority of duty time on the telephone arranging for staffing, as is so often done. This task is easily delegated to a specially trained person to free the supervisor for more important work.

Directing

Effectively using the authority of your position enables you to accomplish work through others rather than doing the work yourself. The best managers are able to delegate authority and responsibility to others so that their function becomes one of directing others to achieve organizational goals. As a supervisor, your goal should be to allow others the freedom to accomplish work in their own way, using their own creative thought and initiative, while still remaining within the limits of the organization. In the directing function, it is up to the supervisor to set these limits and see that they are enforced. As a movie director sets the tone and mood for a film, so too the supervisor sets the tone of the health care agency. Given the same script and the same actors, two directors achieve totally different results because of their personal styles. Neither may be better than the other. Each experience is unique, with its own merits. Likewise, two supervisors in health care may achieve different results through their personal styles, each using the same procedures and staff. Comparing one to the other is impossible. Each is effective and meets the needs of the organization.

Coordinating

A supervisor is responsible for many tasks and persons at the same time. The only way that the supervisor's staff can function efficiently is through careful coordination of activities. No two persons should be responsible for the same task, and no task can be ignored. Along with the coordination of activities goes the task of documenting this coordination. Clear, concise written reports are therefore an important part of the supervisor's duties and responsibilities. Many supervisors complain that they are drowning under a pile of paperwork, but, in reality, that paperwork is necessary to maintain the coordination of a health care agency. Without proper documentation, efficient operations cannot result.

SUPERVISION

In this area of responsibility, the supervisor is chiefly concerned with getting the job done, making sure that all the administrative functions are operational. Since plans and organization are effective only if they can be worked and implemented, the supervisor's task is to direct all this activity. If a process is not operational, the supervisor must find out the cause of the breakdown and remedy the situation. Discipline and the correction of errors insure that the plans of an organization are working on the operational level. First-line supervisors should be very sensitive to the suggestions of their staffs concerning the implementation of the administrative plans. Many times those closest to the operations are in the best position to assess and judge the merits of specific plans. Encouraging creativity and innovation makes supervision more effective.

TRAINING

This area of responsibility may be the most important of the three. Without proper training, staff members render your administrative and supervisory activities useless. Increasingly better training in a health care agency means an ever more efficient and effective staff. A health care agency is only as good as its employees: the better the staff, the better the care.

PRINCIPLES OF RESPONSIBILITY

The extremely important duties and responsibilities of a supervisor must be learned and practiced to be effective. Although every supervisor is different, bringing his or her own style to supervision, certain constant principles remain necessary tools for every leader.

There are eight principles of responsibility that the supervisor must know and practice.[2]

1. *Final responsibility cannot be divided.* At the end of the line, one person must take final responsibility for a task. If you are the supervisor, you must control and direct the work so that at the end of the task or process, your goals are met. There is no room for blaming others or for passing the responsibility. If the job was not done correctly, you should have seen the process going wrong and corrected it before completion of the task.

2. *Accept responsibility fully or not at all.* You cannot take responsibility for only part of a task or part of an operation, and not the entire operation. Too many times the excuse is, "Well, I wasn't in charge of that part." If you are going to accept the final responsibility, you should want to be responsible for all aspects of the job and how it is being done, so that you are assured of the quality of the work.

3. *Delegate responsibility, but do not relinquish it.* When you work through others, you delegate authority, but the final responsibility stays with you. Just because you have assigned the task to someone else does not relieve you of the responsibility.

4. *Responsibility should always be accompanied by commensurate authority.* Many supervisors complain that they "have the name but cannot play the game." To assign a task but to withhold the authority that goes with the task guarantees confusion, if not failure. For example, a head nurse might be given the responsibility for discipline on his or her ward, but none of the authority necessary to carry out the discipline: no authority to hire and fire, to give overtime, to grant days off without pay, to write reprimands, or to transfer employees. In essence, that supervisor has no "clout." The staff soon learns that no action is taken on discipline, and the supervisor loses respect.

5. *The responsible person should know what is expected and be accountable for the results.* A responsibility cannot be assigned in stages or parts. You must see the overall plan including the anticipated end result. When you know that you will be held accountable for your actions, you strive to achieve your maximum effort. If you know the expected outcome, you can concentrate your efforts toward achieving that goal.

6. *Delegate responsibility in terms of results expected.* Achieving a goal is impossible if you do not know the goal expected. The supervisor should make the objectives well-known, then give the freedom to reach those goals.

7. *Leave the method of reaching the goal to the individual.* It is a good procedure to delegate a responsibility in terms of the results ex-

[2] William B. Melnicoe and Jan C. Menning, *Elements of Police Supervision* (Encino, Cal.: Glenco Publishing Co., 1969), pp. 34–35.

pected and then allow individuals to reach the end product in their own way. Staff members are not robots, programmed to carry out the whims and desires of an omnipotent supervisor. They are thinking, feeling human beings with the intelligence to reach a goal using their own individual skills and talents in a creative way. Taking the creativity away from an individual takes away a great deal of the joy of the accomplishment as well.

8. *Assume no authority for work that is not part of your professional responsibility.* This seems to be easily understood: Don't do someone else's job. Often, however, it is abused. Watching over others and sticking our noses into affairs that are not our concern seem to be common human failings. Staying out of a situation for which we are not responsible is very difficult when we see an obvious problem. The only course of action in that type of situation is to speak tactfully to the persons directly in charge of the work, and try to help them solve the problem. Never try to correct things at the operational level. In other words, don't direct other supervisor's subordinates. This approach only leads to personnel problems and more errors.

DEFINING DUTIES
AND RESPONSIBILITIES

As a supervisor, how do you know when you are responsible for a goal, an operation, an area? How can you tell when you are not? How can you determine which of your subordinates is responsible for something well done or for an error? How would you know whether you are taking over someone else's job? How do you tell whether you should take action to correct something that is wrong?

All these and similar questions are answered if you have a written statement of your basic duties and responsibilities as a supervisor and if you have a similar statement for each position on your staff. With these statements, you know precisely what you are responsible for and what your staff may be held responsible for. With them, you can coordinate and plan more effectively, locate neglected duties, find overemphasized duties, evaluate the handling of your own job, gauge the efficiency of staff and equipment, and be aware of which jobs may be delegated and which may not. These statements are the basic tools of your supervisory assignment. As such, they are essential to the smooth operation of the health care agency and should be reviewed and updated at least once a year.

Written statements are composed of two documents: (1) the agency's organization chart and (2) job descriptions.

Organizational Charts

The first stage in making up a written statement of duties is the organizational chart of the health care agency. No matter how the agency is set up, there should be a chart showing the relationship of each employee to the others. All employees should know their superiors and subordinates. All should know to whom they report. The organizational chart also shows where each department fits into the overall plan of the agency. This chart eliminates confusion over responsibilities and gives the staff the security of knowing where they belong in the organization. Knowing your relationship to other staff members also avoids competition and complaints. If each level is written down on the general plan, no one can take responsibility for an area that is not in his or her authority. There is no excuse for pleading ignorance if everything is written down and understood at the beginning. Proper understanding of the organizational chart thus assures smooth communications in the hierarchy of authority.

Job Descriptions

The next step in the written statement is the job description. All employees in a health care agency should have job descriptions that define and explain in great detail *all* the duties and responsibilities expected of them. These job descriptions should include not just the task-behaviors expected of the classification, but the attitudes and psychological traits that are expected by the organization. Outlining the tasks for a nurse's aide, for instance, is not enough. You must also include the behaviors of team spirit, promptness, appearance, judgment, and so on. Ideally, the job description should be so complete that the employee knows that every expected task is included in it, and that anything not included on the job description is not part of his or her responsibility.

Most health care agencies have job descriptions as part of their policy and procedures manuals, and these should be routinely checked for accuracy. Job descriptions should be reviewed often with the employee to make sure that they are up-to-date and cover the jobs actually being done. If job descriptions need revision, employees should take part in the process of revision. Allowing employees to help write their own job descriptions makes them feel a part of the organizational structure and shows that the administration cares about their opinions. Participation in the writing of a job description also ensures that employees are fully aware of what is expected of them, and that the expected performance is physically possible.

Job Analysis

A job analysis is an even more complete job description. An analysis not only lists the tasks or duties performed and the required behaviors, but it also classifies them as to the type of responsibility. Examples of some of the items that might be found on a job analysis for a supervisor might be:

Type of Responsibility	*Duties Performed*
1. Administrative	1. Integration of functions
2. Supervisory	2. Control of staff
3. Instructional	3. Giving information
4. Personnel	4. Checking to assure that the work group fulfills the requirements of the organization
5. Research	5. New procedures, studying other agencies
6. Clerical	6. Charting audit, census
7. Custodial	7. Maintenance and purchase of equipment
8. Public relations	8. Dealing with the public and staff

DEFINING SUPERVISORS' AUTHORITY

One of the duties of the supervisor is to change existing behaviors of the staff—or to teach them new ones. A change in behavior is accomplished by the *influence* of the supervisor, which is a set of actions and behaviors initiated to bring about change. Any action that produces change or that effects a situation may constitute "influence."

A supervisor may have many reasons to influence behavior. One of the main reasons is to change or improve the behavior of others so that the supervisor's job is made easier. As the supervisor, you are responsible for all the actions of your staff, and your job is made easier if they are producing their maximum effort. The organizational goals are reached with maximum efficiency if you influence the staff to reach this goal in the best possible manner.

Supervisors may want to influence behavior for negative, personal reasons; one reason might be to widen their own power or prestige. Using influence simply to meet this end is an abuse of the authority of your position. You are not the "boss," you are the leader. There is a difference: A boss stands behind the horse and shoves; a leader holds the reins and guides the horse.

Change is basically uncomfortable for most people, even for those in the health care field. People resist change because it takes away the comfortable and familiar and substitutes the unfamiliar. As a supervisor, you may want to influence your staff to change for the better, but the final result is up to the employee. No amount of pressure influences an unwilling person. Successful supervisors know their staffs, and they do not demand too much of them. The staff should feel enough trust in their administration and in you, as their supervisor, that they do not feel threatened by change but are rather stimulated to develop their talents to the fullest with the guidance and support of the organization. Allowing staff members to participate in the planning for change eliminates some of the anxiety and resistance.

A supervisor influences the behavior or subordinates in many ways, all of which can be grouped into three categories of influence:

1. by authority,
2. by power, and
3. by motivation.

Influence by Authority

This sort of authority is defined as the *right* to command. In every organization, structure delineates the hierarchy of authority. This chain of command tells all employees where they fit on the organizational ladder. A person who is placed into a position of authority is given a job description defining his or her levels of authority. This written statement gives supervisors the *right* to command. If your name tag says "Head Nurse," you have the authority to direct and control the subordinates under your supervision.

Influence by Power

Power in this context is defined as the *capacity* or ability to command. Authority is the right to command; power is the capacity. Authority derives from the position, power from within the person. This sort of person controls every operation in the hospital, even though he or she may have no authority to do so. Power influence comes from knowledge, experience, or the ability to convince. No one can really say why a person has the power; it is just there, and everyone feels it. Hence you may have the authority to command, but lack the power to command.

People instinctively follow power whether they should or not. A study was done at a university in which students were asked to answer a mathematical problem. After each answered the problem correctly, he or she was subjected to a group of high-power people trying to change the student's mind. The power group insisted that the student's answer was wrong and should be changed. In 85 percent of the cases, the student changed his mind. The influence of power is also seen on juries, when eleven people collaborate, with great power, to change the mind of the one holdout.

The three types of power influence, as defined by Max Weber,[3] are:

a. traditional,
b. charismatic, and
c. rational–legal.

TRADITIONAL INFLUENCE   This brand of authority is founded on tradition or habit—for example, a monarchy or the parent–child relationship. A nonofficial traditional authority structure may be present in a hospital when one department "always" checks with another before taking action. There is no official need to ask permission of the department; there is no official authority. Yet traditionally this has been done, and so it continues.

CHARISMATIC INFLUENCE   This is present due to some emotional need or pressure, some hard-to-define emotional tie that causes behavior to change. A person who causes an emotional response, and thus influences behavior, is using charisma. Religion is an example of influencing by charismatic authority.

RATIONAL–LEGAL INFLUENCE   This authority is based on set rules and regulations. Supervisors are legally defined as being in an authority position, and, as such, they are able to influence behavior. In other words, a supervisor should be obeyed because legally and rationally it is the right thing to do.

Influence by Motivation

When a supervisor uses motivation to influence members of a group, they feel that they have changed on their own accord. In other words, the supervisor achieves *influence* by making the group want to change. If a supervisor can convince people that change will help them or their job, they will change themselves. People seek accomplishment, independence, and self-control, and they quite easily try to make their goals the same as the organization if it is to their benefit.

WHICH "STYLE" IS BEST FOR YOU?

Each of these methods of influencing has a place in supervision, and each one achieves a different type of behavior. Influence by au-

[3] William R. Spriegal, Edward Schulz, and William B. Spriegal, *Elements of Supervision* (N.Y.: John Wiley & Sons, Inc., 1967).

thority alone brings about minimally acceptable behavior. The group does only enough to follow the rules and regulations of the agency. There may even be hostility and competition. The high-pressure atmosphere of influence by power brings out a higher level of achievement, and it might even bring out a high level of creativity in the staff. Although the staff may be motivated by fear, they are constructuve. Influence by motivation brings out not only high quantity and quality, but spontaneous and innovative response. The group changes because they themselves want to do so. The anxiety level is very low.

The type of behavior you use to influence a group results in a predictable behavior response. As a wise supervisor, choose the response you want to achieve and then utilize the appropriate method of influence. For example, in an emergency situation, the supervisor would choose to influence by authority or power. This choice brings about the response of instant action; no questions asked—just the desired response. If you seek to stimulate creativity in your group, the appropriate method of influence is by motivation. Studying the methods of influence and the result of each gives you a variety of actions to choose from to get your desired response.

DISCUSSION QUESTIONS

1. Why is it so important that a health care agency have a written statement of duties?
2. Give an example of power without authority.
3. Of the three levels of responsibility, which is the most important? Why?
4. Using one of the methods of influence, how would you handle an over-aggressive person with good output, without diminishing his or her output?
5. How do you handle someone who possesses the power to influence your group, when you have the authority?

APPLICATION: JOB DESCRIPTIONS

Write a job description for an aide. (See examples in Tables 8–1 and 8–2 for some guidelines.) Include in your description:

1. the time and number of hours worked,
2. vacation, days off, and sick-leave,
3. the title of person to whom responsible,
4. the title of those for whom responsible, and
5. the duties for each shift.

TABLE 8–1
A team leader job description

JOB TITLE:	Team Leader
DIVISION:	Patient Care
DEPARTMENT:	Medical/Surgical Nursing
UNIT:	Medical/Surgical

JOB SUMMARY

Under general supervision of the Senior Team Leader, the Team Leader is responsible for providing nursing care to a specific group of patients on his or her tour of duty. Must be capable of planning work assignments for team members, in accord with patient needs. Must possess communication skills for effective relationships with patients, team members, supervisors, physicians, other personnel, and the public.

QUALIFICATIONS

EDUCATION:	Graduate of an approved school of nursing, registration in the state.
EXPERIENCE:	Six months as a team member preferred.
JOB KNOWLEDGE:	Must have up-to-date knowledge of nursing care and principles. Knows basic principles of supervision.

WORK PERFORMED

Receives and gives change-of-tour report. Visits and observes all patients assigned to team. Visits and observes all new patients within area of assignment. Makes rounds with the medical staff. Makes observations of signs and symptoms and reports to the physician. Assigns team members at the end of tour for the following day. Reviews assignments with team members at beginning of each tour. Conducts a daily team conference. Assist and supervises team members.

Gives direct care to patients. Evaluates patient's progress and assists in revising nursing care plans. Communicates with and prepares the patient and family for diagnostic procedures, treatments, or surgery. Encourages the patient in self-care. Utilizes community health and welfare resources. Assures that signals are answered promptly and that the patient's needs are met. Visits the patient at mealtime and confers with the dietician as indicated.

Sees that the proper nursing precautions are practiced, and is conscious of safety factors relating to patients and personnel. Assumes responsibility for the environment of patients. Knows fire plans. Knows hospital policies and procedures. Supervises care given by private duty nurses. Arranges for meal or break relief.

Participates in the orientation of new personnel. Participates in continuing-education programs. Assists the head nurse with personnel evaluations.

Assumes responsibility for the following records: nursing progress notes, medications, intake and output, verifying doctor's orders, diets, ordering drugs and narcotics, checking Kardex and keeping it up-to-date, preparation of patients for surgery and pre-op checklist, checking all requisitions for preparations for diagnostic work. Also takes responsibility for patient's condition, reports for the nursing team.

TABLE 8–1 (cont.)

JOB RELATIONSHIPS

SUPERVISED BY:	Head Nurse or Senior Team Leader.
WORKERS SUPERVISED:	Nursing team members, licensed practical nurses, nurses' aides as assigned.
PROMOTION FROM:	Nurse–Staff
PROMOTION TO:	Head Nurse

Table 8–2
Senior team leader job description

JOB TITLE:	Senior Team Leader or Head Nurse
DIVISION:	Patient care
DEPARTMENT:	Medical/Surgical Nursing
UNIT:	Medical/Surgical

JOB SUMMARY

Responsible for directly supervising nursing teams in providing care for patients on a single unit. This responsibility extends for one shift. Must plan and organize the activities of teams for patient care, and guide team leaders in developing patient care plans and conferences. Has responsibility for scheduling teams and delegating daily patient care assignments to the team leaders. Supervises, instructs, and counsels team leaders and team members. Uses initiative and independent judgment.

QUALIFICATIONS

EDUCATION:	Graduate of an approved school of nursing, registration.
EXPERIENCE:	At least one year as a Team Leader.
JOB KNOWLEDGE:	Has a thorough knowledge of principles and practices involved in nursing specialty. Knows how to organize and delegate nursing care and services, understands principles of supervision.

WORK PERFORMED

Visits and makes observations about all new patients. Assist Team Leaders in developing nursing care plans. Plans and conducts nursing team conferences. Evalutes nursing care plans. Counsels Team Leaders, team members, patients, and families. Visits all patients before discharge. Gives direct care to patients. Practices clinical skills. Assigns Team Leaders and members, assists Team Leaders in the assignment of members of patient care and services.

Makes nursing rounds. Makes rounds with doctors, and supervises carrying out the doctor's orders and plan of care. Supervises and evaluates the performance of Team Leaders and members. Assists in the orientation of new Team Members. Participates in planning and conducting programs of continuing education.

TABLE 8–2 (*cont.*)

Assists the Team Leader in evaluating environmental factors, including the supplies and equipment necessary for meeting the physical, spiritual, and emotional needs of patients and personnel. Knows hospital and division policies and procedures. Assists in interpreting hospital, medical, and nursing care to famiiles and visitors. Assists in interpreting the needs of nursing and coordinating activities with other divisions and departments.

JOB RELATIONSHIPS

SUPERVISED BY:	Supervisor
WORKERS SUPERVISED:	Team Leaders, LVNs, Nurses' aides, clerks.
PROMOTION FROM:	Team Leader.
PROMOTION TO:	Supervisor.

REFERENCES

BARRETT, RICHARD S., *Performance Rating*. Chicago: Science Research Associates, Inc., 1966.

INTERNATIONAL CITY MANAGERS' ASSOCIATION, *Municipal Personnel Administration*, 6th ed. Chicago: The International City Managers' Association, 1960.

KIRCHNER, W. E. and REISBERG, D. J., "Differences Between Better and Less Effective Supervisors in Appraisals of Subordinates," *Personnel Psychology*, 15 (Autumn 1962).

PFIFFNER, JOHN M., *Public Administration*. New York: The Ronald Press Company, 1946

YODER, DALE, *Personnel Principles and Policies: Modern Manpower Management*, 2nd ed. Englewood Cliffs, N.J.: Prentice-Hall, Inc. 1959.

9

Legal aspects of supervision

THE LEGAL BASIS

State law is responsible for establishing the titles of registered nurse, licensed vocational nurse, psychiatric technician, and nurse's aide. To understand the principles and practices that govern the activities of nursing personnel, nursing supervisors must first understand the legal basis for the profession. A *law* is a rule of human conduct established and enforced by a governmental agency. As far as nursing practice is concerned, four sources of law govern the actions of a nurse:

1. statutes,
2. regulations,
3. court decisions, and
4. Attorney General opinions.

Statutes

These laws are enacted by the state legislature or United States Congress to deal with issues and problems. Since 1974, the Business and Professions Codes and the Health and Safety Codes of many states have been amended to substantially change the definitions of registered nursing. Previous to these changes the statutes were so vague that there was little or no agreement on the scope of nursing practice.

Regulations

Once the state or federal legislature enacts statutes concerning a problem, they have the power to direct regulatory responsibility to a state-appointed agency, such as the Board of Registered Nursing. This agency then has the authority to adopt regulations that affect the activities and requirements of the particular profession it governs. This type of law, called *regulations*, is necessary to interpret statutes and to make them more workable for the particular profession. The state legislature has neither the time nor the manpower necessary to regulate every area of every profession. Neither does it have the ability to foresee problems of implementing statutes, the expertise to deal with every problem that may arise from the statute. Because of these problems, the regulatory agency is given the power to make all decisions concerning the profession, and to enact regulations to cover any problems that may develop.

For example, the state legislature enacts statutes establishing criteria for registered nursing. The legislature then names the State Board of Registered Nursing as the regulatory agency to set standards of training, requirements for licensing, relicensing, continuing education, and the scope of acceptable nursing practice. These regulations constitute a form of law and, as such, are as legally binding as a statute.

Each state's regulatory agency is responsible for setting these principles and practices, as well as for enforcing adherence to them. The regulations differ from state to state, and you, as a supervisor, should be thoroughly familiar with your state's principles and practices as defined by the State Board of Nursing.

Court Decisions

If a dispute arises over a problem, courts are often called upon to interpret statutes or regulations. The decision of the court is final, and it must be followed, because it is also a form of law.

Attorney General

If a member of a regulatory agency or of a public agency—or even a private citizen—has a question concerning a definition or clarification of legal statutes or regulations, this question may be directed to the Attorney General for an answer. The written decision of the Attorney General is treated exactly the same as statutes, regulations, and court decisions.

TYPES OF LAW

There are two basic types of law in the United States:

1. *Criminal law* deals with crime involving society. It prohibits any activity that is harmful to society. As an example, murder is harmful to society as a whole.
2. *Civil law* deals with individuals. It regulates behavior that is harmful to an individual. An example of a civil law is an action that harms one individual, but not society as a whole, such as an injury suffered in someone's backyard pool.

Nurses are concerned chiefly with criminal law, because performing functions that are not defined or authorized by their nursing licenses, or authorizing others to perform such functions, is a criminal offense.

THE LEGAL DEFINITION
OF THE PRACTICE OF NURSING

To understand the practice of nursing, you must first understand what is included in the practice of medicine, as defined by law. As a supervisor, you must study carefully the state's regulations concerning the legal definitions of the practice of nursing to avoid the possibility of criminal prosecution. Since each state has a different code, and since each code is worded slightly differently, it would be extremely helpful for you to send to your state capitol to obtain a copy of the Business and Professional Code to read the exact language. This document is public record and is available to anyone upon request. For the purposes of this text, we will briefly summarize the elements common to each state's regulations.

The Practice of Medicine

Basically, the Business and Professional Code states that a:

physician's and surgeon's certificate authorizes the holder to use drugs, or what are known as medical preparations, in or upon human beings and to sever or penetrate the tissues of human beings and to use any and all other methods in the treatment of diseases, injuries, deformities, or other physical or mental conditions. Any person who practices or attempts to practice, or who advertises, or holds himself out as practicing, any system or mode of treating the sick or afflicted in the state, or who diagnoses, treats, operates for, or prescribes for any ailment, blemish, deformity, disease, disfigurement, disorder, injury or other mental or physical condition of any person, without having at the time of so doing, a valid, unrevoked certificate as provided in the state's regulations, or without being authorized to perform such act by obtaining a certificate from some other provision of law is guilty of a misdemeanor.[1]

As you can see, this definition is very broad, and it sets no limitation to the practice of medicine by qualified physicians. The "practice of medicine" means that persons meeting the qualifications of their particular state are allowed to perform any function in any health care area. All other professionals in the health care setting must perform only those functions outlined in the regulations of their particular professional regulatory agency. In other words, only physicians have unlimited license in the health care area.

All health professionals, other than physicians, who perform an activity outside the guidelines of their professional regulatory agency, are guilty of practicing medicine without a license. This violation could subject the person to a fine and/or imprisonment, as well as discipline by the regulatory agency, which could include a revocation of license. It is therefore important to know the functions of medicine and of nursing so that you or your staff will not become guilty of the practice of medicine. If you are not perfectly clear on the definitions of the practices of medicine and nursing, it is easy to slip into the wrong area of practice and be guilty of a misdemeanor.

The Practice of Registered Nursing

The definitions of allowable activities are defined by the regulations enacted by the state's regulatory agency, the Board of Nursing. Most states have enacted legislation, such as Nursing Practice Acts, that regulate these activities. Some states have done little or nothing to change the existing laws, and some of the Nursing Practice Acts have not been changed for years. As a result, the laws are vague and do not accurately describe or define the activities in which nurses are actually involved. For example, in California a 1939 law had not been changed until 1974 when it was substantially altered. One important statement was added—the first *legal* recognition of the fact that the practice of medicine and the practice of nursing often overlap. Now some functions and procedures, formerly allowed to be performed only by physicians, can be performed legally by nurses under a physician's immediate di-

[1] Medical Practice Act (a summary) Business and Professions Code (New York, 1979).

rection and supervision. At one time, for example, breaking a patient's skin was considered to be the practice of medicine; hence it could not be considered a nursing function. This definition has been changed by the codes established by the regulatory agencies of registered nurses, and it has now been included in the scope of nursing responsibilities. As another example, before the change in New York's Nurse Practice Act, nurses' duties included the broad generalization, "nurses may do any procedure to assist in an emergency."[2] Another statement found in a state's Nurse Practice Act says, ". . . nurses may do any procedure ordered by a physician."[3] Such statements may seem clear at first, defining well the duties of a nurse as an assistant working under the guidance and direction of the physician. Yet they do not limit nursing in any way. Such vague statements are open to any type of interpretation, and they cause great problems in regulating the activities of nurses. They can be interpreted to mean anything from handing instruments to a physician to performing surgery. If you took a very liberal interpretation of these statements, you could interpret them to mean that the nurse could perform any diagnosis or treatment, including prescribing medication, if so directed by a physician.

Because of the unclear nature of these Nurse Practice Acts, the question remains, where does nursing end and medicine begin? Nurses have traditionally followed the guidelines of Florence Nightengale's Pledge, which states that you will not ". . . diagnose and treat." At the time of Florence Nightengale, physician's training was not as extensive as it is today. Far from it. Nurses were, in some cases, nearly as knowledgable as physicians, and the doctors felt threatened by this new group of health care professionals who knew almost as much about patient care as they did. To relieve this fear, Florence Nightingale assured the physicians that nurses were never going to usurp their power, that nurses were content to be assistants and would not seek more authority.

Today's nurse feels "boxed in" by this guideline. Not only the militant nurse seeks greater autonomy and clearer definitions of nursing scope; every nurse is concerned with the legal status of nursing. The increased level of training and the increased responsibility placed on nurses make it a concern of every nurse to understand clearly and completely the contributions they are allowed to make to the care and treatment of patients. Nursing has a great deal to offer to health care, much more than the function of assisting the physician.

As more and more health care agencies give increased responsibility to nurses, the problem seems to grow. With no clear-cut guidelines, nurses are limited only by their own knowledge and ability. For some nurses this freedom is exciting and challenging; others feel that

[2] *Medical Practice Act: Business and Professional Code* (State of New York, 1961).
[3] *Ibid.*

nurses are doing procedures that should remain medical practice and are thus becoming "pseudo-doctors." No matter how you feel, personally, about the problem, it must be faced, and the situation must be remedied as soon as possible.

State regulatory agencies are working on specific guidelines and on clear definitions of nursing practice, not only to protect nurses in their practice of nursing care, but also to allow registered nurses the freedom to use the extensive training they possess to broaden their scope of practice. Nurse Practice Acts are necessary to every practicing registered nurse. Regulations are the guidelines of our profession, and they must be as up-to-date and correct as possible. You should write to your state capitol for a copy of your particular Nurse Practice Act so that you are aware of the exact language of the definition of registered nursing in your state.

Amending Nurse Practice Acts

Let us examine an example of a current Nurse Practice Act, amended in 1974, that recognizes the increased value of registered nursing to the health care profession. Its statutes, as written by the Board of Registered Nursing, outline in great detail the scope of the activities and practice of nursing:

> Recognizing that nursing is a dynamic and continually changing field, the practice of which is continually evolving to include more sophisticated patient care activities, the legislature amends this Nurse Practice Act to provide clear legal authority for functions and procedures which have common acceptance and usage.
>
> The practice of nursing within the meaning of this statute means those functions involved in helping people cope with difficulties in daily living which are associated with their actual or potential health or illness problems, or the treatment thereof, which require a substantial amount of scientific knowledge or technical skill, and include all of the following:
>
> **1.** Direct and indirect patient care services that insure the safety, comfort, personal hygiene, and protection of patients, and the performance of disease prevention and restorative measures.
> **2.** Direct and indirect patient care services, including, but not limited to, the administration of medications and therapeutic agents necessary to implement a treatment, disease prevention, and rehabilitative regimen prescribed by a physician, dentist, or podiatrist.
> **3.** The performance, according to *standardized procedures*, of basic health care testing and prevention procedures, including, but not limited to, skin tests, immunization techniques, and the withdrawal of human blood from veins and arteries.
> **4.** Observation of signs and symptoms of illness, reactions to treatment, general behavior, or general physical condition. Determination of

167

whether such signs, symptoms, reactions, behavior, or general appearance exhibit abnormal characteristics; implementation, based on observed abnormalities, or appropriate reporting, referral, *standardized procedures*, or changes in treatment according to *standardized procedures*.

Standardized procedures are policies and protocols developed through collaboration among administrators and health professionals, including physicians and nurses, by an organized health care system. Such policies are subject to any guidelines set by the State Agency of Medical Quality Assurance and the State Board of Registered Nursing.[4]

To summarize the revised Nurse Practice Act, divide the definition of the practice of nursing into three parts:

1. why the Nurse Practice Act is being amended;
2. a definition of nursing practice, and
3. a definition of standardized procedures.

REASON FOR AMENDMENT   Every state's Nurse Practice Act should be amended to express the complexity of the nursing profession to give legal authority for tasks that are currently being performed by registered nurses, and to acknowledge the existence of the overlapping functions of medicine and nursing.

DEFINITION OF NURSING PRACTICE   This statement should include all procedures and functions that are to be legally included in the nursing function. The definition may include, but is not limited to:

1. an assessment of patient needs to form a nursing diagnosis,
2. developing a plan of action,
3. activating that plan of action by initiating those treatments necessary to carry out the plan, and
4. evaluation of the plan's effectiveness in meeting the patient's needs.

Included in this definition, there must be a statement concerning the responsibility of supervision. "Patient care services," as defined by law, include the supervision by registered nurses or licensed vocational nurses, licensed practical nurses, and unlicensed persons caring for patients. The supervisor is legally considered to be engaged in patient care services. Registered nurses can be disciplined for authorizing untrained persons, no matter what license they hold, to perform tasks that the supervising registered nurse knew or should have known they lacked the competency to safely perform.

[4] Nursing Practice Act (a summary), California Business and Professional Code, Sections 2700–2837 (1974).

DEFINITION OF STANDARDIZED PROCEDURES   When an organized health care system wants its registered nurses to perform functions and procedures considered to be the practice of *medicine,* the physicians and nurses within the system can collaborate to develop what are considered to be standardized procedures. Registered nurses following standardized procedures do *not* need a physician's order to perform these functions, nor does the physician have to be present for these procedures to be performed.

Some of the medical functions that can be done by nurses under the umbrella of standardized procedures may be: deciding whether a patient needs to have a skin test, be immunized or have blood drawn without the direction of a physician, electrocardiograms, glaucoma screening, pap smears, pelvic examinations, throat cultures, urinalysis, the formation of a screening procedure for patients to decide which patients should be seen by a physician, and the recognition of a need for, and initiation of emergency procedures.

The use of these standardized procedures means that a registered nurse using these standing orders or procedures can diagnose a patient's condition and render certain types of treatment without a physician's order or without the patient having to see a physician. The ramifications of implementing this regulation are farreaching. Nurses would be able to act in an emergency, diagnosing and treating patients without the fear of legal prosecution for practicing medicine without a license. Nurses would have the authority to treat patients needing cardiac care functions, including fibrillation, without waiting for a physician. Nurses could treat patients with common conditions such as pregnancy, arthritis, diabetes, and hypertension using standardized procedures. Added to the scope of nursing practice, under standardized procedures, would be suturing minor lacerations and inserting fetal monitoring devices.

In formulating standardized procedures, licensed health care facilities (which include acute care hospitals, acute psychiatric hospitals, skilled nursing homes, intermediate care facilities, and special hospitals) can follow any format they wish. The standardized procedures they institute are not subject to guidelines of the State's Board of Medical Quality Assurance or the Board of Registered Nursing. Any other type of organized health care system (such as clinics, home health agencies, physician's offices, and public or community health services) must meet the guidelines of the State Board of Quality Assurance and the Board of Registered Nursing. These guidelines are not difficult to meet, but they do put some limitations and controls on the health care agencies.

The supervisor should be aware of the difference between standardized procedures and nursing procedures. *Standardized procedures* are those procedures that normally fall under the heading of practicing medicine, and they can be performed only by nurses after the

169

formulation of a written standardized procedure. This statement is written through a joint effort between physicians and nurses. *Nursing procedures* are procedures that are commonly performed by nurses and always have been considered part of the practice of nursing. The procedures are written by a particular health care agency only to standardize the task, not to allow nurses to practice a procedure that overlaps medical practice. Nurses who perform standardized procedures are considered to be working more independently and are thus expected to perform to a higher degree of efficiency than nurses working under the direction of a doctor's orders.

The formulation of a Nursing Practice Act does not automatically allow nurses to perform increased or more difficult tasks. It merely defines the scope of nursing practice allowed by law. It legally covers nurses in the practice of their profession. Any individual health care agency can choose not to honor the Nurse Practice Act and take a more conservative stance as far as nursing is concerned. Just enacting the legislation does not give the nurse the right to do certain procedures; it is up to the individual employer to set the standards of practice for that institution.

Even with the changes in the Nurse Practice Acts in many states, there is no complete agreement as to what constitutes "nursing." An example is the nurse anesthetist. By law, a registered nurse may not administer a local, spinal, epidural, or regional anesthetic without the immediate supervision of a physician. There is no licensure act for nurse anesthetists. Individual licensed health care facilities have established standardized procedures to cover these nurses. The Organization of Nurse Anesthetists, however, is seeking to have anesthesia included in the scope and practice of nursing, enabling them to function in any health care setting without standardized procedures. "Nurse practitioners" constitute another example. As the law is now written, nurse practitioners have the same scope of practice, legally, as any other registered nurse. In essence, nurse practitioners are registered nurses using a title to perform standardized procedures. These and many other questions remain unanswered and must be evaluated and reviewed as to their individual merit. Each state must review its statutes concerning the practice of nursing and change the regulations as they see the need.

As you can see, a great deal of information is necessary to define the practice of nursing. Many factors must be considered, and the supervisor must be aware of this legal definition, as well as of the definitions of the practice of the allied health personnel.

As a supervisor, you must be aware of the qualifications of those persons engaged in the practice of nursing. Anyone who practices nursing, or anyone who authorizes a subordinate to practice nursing, without a valid license is guilty of a misdemeanor and may be punished by fine and/or imprisonment. Certain categories of persons are exempt from this law. In other words, they may practice nursing without a valid registered nurse's license. These individuals are physicians, friends or servants performing gratuitous or incidental nursing in the home, persons practicing nursing in a public disaster, psychiatric technicians (with nursing supervision), students of an accepted school of nursing, and nurses who practice in connection with a religion. The nursing these individuals perform is generally only physical care or ministerial service. They are not allowed to perform technical or skilled nursing tasks. A very important fact for the supervisor to remember is that practical nurses, unlicensed graduate nurses, nurse's aides, orderlies, and unlicensed persons attending patients may *not* perform services requiring special skill or knowledge *even though such services are requested by oral or written order of a physician*. Any person performing an act that constitutes the practice of professional nursing is guilty of a misdemeanor and subject to fine and/or imprisonment.

Prescribing Medication and Writing Prescriptions

A legal question that arises frequently in health care is the legality of prescribing and dispensing drugs by health professionals other than physicians. By law, no person other than a physician, dentist, podiatrist, or veterinarian can prescribe or write prescriptions. Registered nurses, even if they are working as nurse practitioners or physician's assistants, may *not* write a prescription.

Physician may, under legal authority, authorize any person to orally transmit their medication prescriptions. In other words, it is perfectly legal for the physician's receptionist to call an order in to the pharmacy or to the hospital staff. The pharmacy or the nursing staff may legally accept such an order and dispense or administer the medication. The doctor is accepting the responsibility for the transmission of the order. The doctor is allowing the employee to act in his or her behalf. In some health care agencies, a written policy prohibits the acceptance of medical orders transmitted by any person other than the doctor. This policy varies from agency to agency. The law clearly states that this nonmedical transmission is legal; whether or not the health care agency allows this practice is entirely up to them.

You should know the policy of your health care agency concerning the verbal transmission of medication orders. If your institution allows this practice, every person who accepts an order, either verbally or over the telephone, should carefully document the name of the person conveying the medication order. Nurses accepting orders who feel that there is some error in an order, either in the amount or type of medication, should refuse to administer the medication and ask to speak to the physician. In no circumstance is it acceptable to administer a medication that, in your estimation, could be harmful. If you do not question the order and injury results, you are liable.

In some health care agencies (for example, clinics, physician's offices, and out-patient health care services), nurses are called upon to dispense drugs to patients. A registered nurse may *not* dispense drugs upon a prescription from a physician, dentist, podiatrist, or veterinarian. To "dispense" means to furnish a drug to a patient by any means, sale or otherwise. The only exception to this rule is the procedure by which a nurse takes a small amount of medication from a hospital supply or pharmacy, for the express purpose of giving a specific patient a dose of the prescribed medication. This procedure is the administration, not the dispensing, of medication and is allowed by law. In selected cases, nurses may assist the physician in the dispensing of drugs under specific conditions. These conditions are:

1. A registered nurse, *under the supervision of a physician,* may reduce a bulk drug prescribed by a physician into a smaller container, label it, and dispense it to the patient if a *specialized procedure* has been written.
2. Any physician who engages in the practice of packaging and labeling drugs for patients' use at some time in the future, is practicing the "manufacture" of drugs. Anyone participating in the manufacture of drugs must follow the specific manufacturing techniques outlined by the Food and Drug Administration. Any registered nurse who assists in this process must meet the same stringent criteria.

In other words, in specific situations, with the direct supervision of the physician, the registered nurse is allowed by law to dispense drugs. It is a dangerous practice, though, and it should be avoided if at all possible. The best solution to this problem is never to engage in the practice of prescribing or dispensing medication.

Assisting Women in Childbirth

Basically, the assisting of women in childbirth is a medical procedure. Persons unlawfully assisting in the delivery process can be prosecuted by law. The two exceptions to this rule are: nurse midwives and physicians. A registered nurse who is not a trained midwife is *not* allowed to assist women in childbirth. Of course, the law recognizes that emergency childbirth is often attended only by registered nurses or even by lay persons. The law does not intend to stop this practice, and assistance in the emergency delivery of a child is entirely legal by any lay or professional person. The intent of the law is to prohibit the routine care and assistance of delivering women by persons other than physicians or trained nurse midwives.

GOOD SAMARITAN LAWS

Many states have enacted legislation to protect the nurse from civil liability in cases of emergency assistance at the scene of an accident or injury. This immunity does not apply if the emergency occurs at the nurse's place of employment or if the nurse is *grossly negligent*. Basically, the intent of the law is to encourage nurses and other citizens to come to the aid and assistance of their fellow human beings without the fear of civil liability. The law states that the registered nurse who stops at the scene of an accident or injury is only expected to act as the average lay person would act, not as the average *nurse* would act. The nurse acts as a private citizen and is expected only to offer care and aid that the average person could offer. The courts do not take into consideration the fact that the nurse, with additional training and expertise, *should* act in a different manner if an error occurs. The fact that a person is a nurse is not considered. In fact, the law does not even require that persons giving aid identify themselves as nurses. This statute is a great legal protection for nurses and encourages them to offer themselves to aid others.

Nurses can be held responsible for errors committed at the scene of an accident *only* if they are considered to be grossly negligent. "Gross negligence," as defined by law, is the exercise of *so little* care that one's actions could be interpreted to be almost careless or indifferent. The nurse who functions at a level below that of the average lay person can be called grossly negligent. For example, the average citizen knows that a person complaining of severe back injury should not be moved. A nurse who stops at the scene of an accident and moves a patient who insists that his back is broken can be judged grossly negligent. This action makes the nurse liable for civil litigation if the patient suffers further injury as the result.

This law is very important to the nurse, because it gives much needed protection as long as the nurse stays within the parameters of the law. First aid, of the type that would normally be given by the average citizen, is all that is covered by the Good Samaritan Act. Trying to perform skilled or technical tasks at the emergency scene may lead to error and thus to gross negligence.

You should know the law in your state, and understand to what extent the law covers your behavior. If you have a Good Samaritan Act in your state, and if you travel to another state, you may or may not be covered under your own state's act. The laws differ from state to state, and it is very important to never assume coverage.

Good Samaritan coverage is also applicable to firefighters, police officers, and mobile ambulance attendants, as long as their actions are not grossly negligent. The only person who may give aid, without the fear of being grossly negligent, is a lay person. Lay persons have Good Samaritan coverage, whether or not their actions constitute gross negligence.

Nurses are also immune from civil liability when:

1. they are giving emergency instructions to paramedics or to emergency personnel,
2. when a patient refuses their assistance, and
3. when they are a part of a legally constituted medical rescue team, such as a cardiac code team in a hospital or a mobile ambulance team.

REPORTING REQUIREMENTS OF NURSES

Under certain conditions, the nurse is required by law to report certain illnesses or conditions to the appropriate authorities. As a supervisor, you must be aware of your state's reporting requirements. Usually, the basic requirements are that registered nurses must report:

1. their current addresses to the Board of Registered Nursing,
2. any case of child abuse or suspected child abuse to the legal authority,
3. certain contagious diseases, such as venereal disease, to the Public Health Service, and
4. ophthalmia neonatorum to the Health Department.

Nurses failing to report diseases and/or conditions that are required by state law are subject to a misdemeanor conviction, punishable by fine.

THE LEGAL SCOPE OF PRACTICE FOR LVNs/LPNs

In your job as supervisor, you must also know the scope of practice for other health care providers. This scope also varies from state to state, but it is fairly consistent in some areas. Usually, an LVN or LPN is allowed to:

1. perform nursing functions that any LVN or LPN usually performs,

2. withdraw blood from a patient,
3. give some types of intravenous therapy, and,
4. immunizations, injections, and skin tests.

Performance of Nursing Functions

The routine nursing procedures that LVNs or LPNs may perform are those procedures and functions for which they have been trained in a State-accepted training program for licensed vocational nurses or licensed practical nurses. The training programs have different requirements in each state, but, whatever the requirements, LVNs or LPNs must meet these requirements and hold a valid license in order to perform simple nursing functions.

The licensing of LVNs and LPNs is done in one of two ways. An LVN may be a graduate of an approved school and take an examination following completion of his or her studies. Upon successful completion of the examination, the nurse is licensed to practice in that state. The second way to obtain licensure as an LVN or LPN is by waiver. In some states, a person who has consistently demonstrated expertise in the skills and knowledge of an LVN or LPN, and who has been performing these functions with a great deal of skill, can apply to the state licensing bureau for a license by waiver. If all the state-required conditions are met, the nurse is awarded a license by waiver.

Blood Withdrawal

Licensed vocational or practical nurses may, by law, withdraw blood from a patient under the following conditions:

1. if they have received special training in the procedure,
2. if they have demonstrated competence in the procedure, or
3. if they do the procedure following accepted standardized procedures.

Immunizations, Injections, and Skin Tests

The law authorizes licensed vocational nurses and licensed practical nurses to administer medication, including injectable medication, under the order and direction of a physician. The physician does not need to be physically present during the administration of this medication, but he or she needs only to have ordered the medication, immunization, or skin test.

THE FUNCTIONS OF NURSE'S AIDES OR ASSISTANTS

A nurse's aide may do many simple nursing procedures that an LVN or LPN is allowed to do. The state usually sets requirements of training for individuals functioning in a nurse's aide role. These requirements range from in-service education to a prescribed period of classroom instruction time with supervised patient care practice.

THE FUNCTIONS OF MEDICAL ASSISTANTS

Medical assistants usually work under the direct supervision of a physician, and they must adhere to the requirements of state statutes. As a general rule, medical assistants are allowed to perform injections, skin tests, or blood withdrawal in a physician's office only if the physician is *physically* present at the time of the treatment. This rule is frequently abused, and many medical assistants perform functions that are not included in the legal scope of allowable activity. The misconception is that they are working under the license and authority of the physician. This assumption is not true. *No one* may practice any form of healing art unless they *personally* possess the license to do so. Performance of a duty that is not within the scope of one's training or license is a criminal offense.

LEGAL DEFINITIONS

Supervisors may find themselves dealing with legal questions frequently in the day-to-day activities of leading others. The supervisor must be well versed in the law and understand the common legal terms. You, as a supervisor, may be called upon frequently to interpret the law as it applies to the health care industry. Each particular health care agency sets its own policies and procedures based on state and federal laws. It is important for you to have a basic knowledge of the law's terminology to assist your staff with any legal questions.

It is equally important to distinguish law from custom or policy. *Law* is defined as the standard of conduct established and enforced by an authority. In the United States, authority rests with the federal and state governments. *Criminal law* governs the actions and activities that may injure society as a whole. *Civil law* concerns the rights and duties of a private citizen. *Custom* is an action that is continued because of tradition or habit. This is not a law or official rule that demands adherance, and there is no legal punishment for failure to adhere to custom.

Sometimes custom is so strong and has been carried on for so long that everyone believes it to be law. *Policy* is not a form of law either. Policy is set by the organization or agency, and it differs from agency to agency. The specific agency decides on the provisions and also on the punishments for failure to comply with established policy. Many times custom or policy is followed so frequently that nurses feel that it must be a law. Nurses who move from one hospital to another and who are asked to do a procedure that is against established policy in the former hospital may feel that they are "breaking the law" by doing the task. They are only confusing law with policy.

The study of law is a fascinating one that demands much time and careful study. We do not need to go into a detailed study of the law to learn supervision, but a few important legal terms should be explained and defined as they apply to supervision. A knowledge of these terms helps you in the supervision of health care personnel.

License   A license is a legal document that permits a person to offer to the public skills and knowledge in a jurisdiction where such practice would be unlawful without a license. The state's licensing requirement is designed to protect the public from unskilled persons performing functions for which they are not trained.

Tort   A tort is a civil wrong—a wrong or injury done to someone that violates his or her rights. An example of a civil right is the right of privacy, which would be violated by divulging unauthorized information about a patient or by exposing a patient needlessly. Both of these situations are considered torts.

Assault   The legal definition of assault is the unlawful touching of another person without that person's consent. In the health care setting, a patient gives implied permission for certain routine procedures when he or she enters the hospital and signs the conditions of admission. Even so, the patient retains the right to refuse treatment or to leave the hospital. Performing surgery on a patient without consent, cutting a patient's hair without permission or putting restraints on a competent adult, are all examples of assault.

Battery   This is the unlawful touching of a person with the intent of bodily injury.

False Imprisonment   This legal term does not seem to apply in a health care agency, but forcing patients to remain in the hospital against their expressed desire is false imprisonment. The nurse has a legal responsibility to protect and restrain the confused patient or minor, but to detain a competent adult against his or her will is an infringement of that person's rights as a citizen.

177

LIBEL AND SLANDER

Libel is defined as the use of the *written word* to subject someone to ridicule or embarrassment. Using medical charts that may contain damaging or embarrassing information in a therapeutic manner does not constitute libel. Yet using those same charts in an unprofessional way, such as printing them in a newspaper story, would be considered libel. The person responsible for releasing the information would be subject to a civil suit if damage to the patient's reputation results.

Slander is using the *spoken word* to subject someone to ridicule or embarrassment. In the case of slander, a third party must hear the slanderous remark. If the remark is heard by no one but the speaker and the listener, there is no slander. For example, a patient is admitted to a gynecological ward with a diagnosis of pelvic inflammatory disease. The doctor is unsure about the possible organism causing the infection. The nurse calls the doctor outside the room and tells him that this same patient was admitted previously with a venereal disease and that this previous condition could possibly be contributing to her present condition. This is not slander. This is the professional exchange of information in a therapeutic way, with no possible ridicule to the patient. If the nurse phones a friend of the patient and tells the same story, this is slander and the rights of the patient have been violated.

Remember, slander is a defamatory statement that is spoken. The four legal categories of slanderous remarks are:

1. a false statement made that damages a person's job standing or professional reputation;
2. falsely accusing someone of a serious crime;
3. falsely circulating gossip that a woman is unchaste;
4. falsely stating that someone has a loathesome disease.

Although the language of the law is stilted and seems old-fashioned, the intent remains the same. Making any of these types of statements is a violation of a person's civil rights.

Libel applies to any damaging statements of the same nature as slanderous statements that are put into permanent form. This written word includes newspapers, television, radio, postcards, letters, or graffiti. Anything that is written and placed in a spot where someone else could possibly read it is considered libel if it damages someone's reputation.

Duties of the Supervisor

In the health care setting, the supervisor must be constantly aware of the possible damage of the written or spoken word. In the hospital, for example, many diagnoses are of a sensitive nature and may cause the patient great mental anguish if made public. Due to the nature of our profession, we are privy to information that could be damaging to patients, to other nurses, and to doctors. In the health care industry we deal with professional people whose licenses are involved, and great harm can come from the unguarded tongue.

"I can't believe it, she/he has made another error!"—These can be the most expensive words that a supervisor can utter. If such a statement is overheard by other personnel or patients, it can cause a problem. Any nurse who can prove in court that his or her reputation and professional standing was affected by that statement can sue the supervisor in a court of law. If the court action does take place, the supervisor must prove that the remark was true, that this particular nurse had, in fact, made several errors. If the remark can be validated, the supervisor is justified in making the remark, and no slander will be charged. But the nurse who can prove that the statement hurt him or her professionally—whether the statement was true or false—may receive monetary damages for defamation of character, another tort. For instance, the nurse was about to get another position and the prospective employer heard the remark and refused to hire her, then defamation of character will be declared, and the nurse may receive monetary damages in court. This decision holds true whether the statement was true or false.

The supervisor must be aware of the dangers of slander and libel and must guard against them at all costs. The ways to avoid slander and libel are simple, and they require nothing more than common sense and a professional attitude. Never discuss doctors with anyone. This caution applies to members of your staff, as well as to your personal acquaintances.

A statement that seems perfectly innocent to you, may be misunderstood by a lay person and cause damage to a doctor's reputation. A case in point is of a very skilled obstetrician working in a large city hospital. He was very adept at taking difficult deliveries, saving the mother and child by the use of emergency caesarian sections. The other doctors in the hospital frequently asked this doctor to consult on their complicated cases, and the surgeon frequently participated in deliveries. At a social gathering, a nurse in the department made the comment, "He does more caesarian sections than any other doctor on staff"— a seemingly innocent, true statement when heard by professionals in the field. Yet this particular statement was overheard by a woman in the community with no knowledge of medicine, much less the doctor or the situation. She interpreted the statement to mean that the physician did needless surgeries. She proceeded to spread the word among her friends that Dr. X was "knife happy." Eventually, the doctor heard the gossip and traced it to its source. The nurse was charged with slander and sued in a court of law. The court found that the doctor's reputation was, indeed, damaged. The court awarded damages to the physician in the form of monetary compensation.

Do not discuss a patient's condition with the family without the permission and knowledge of the patient and the doctor. A safe method of dealing with this problem is to make it a rule *never* to discuss the patient's condition with the family. If the family comes to you with questions, you can answer the questions using the amount of information that they provide as a guideline to how much to say. Never offer information about a diagnosis or condition. There may be a reason that the patient or the physician wants information withheld, and you may be breaking a confidence.

If you see an obvious error, you are bound by medical ethics to speak up. Yet before you say or do anything, be sure of your facts. Make sure that you *personally* know the facts surrounding the situation and are able to document them. Report this error to your immediate supervisor and to *no one* else. The alleged error will then be investigated and a resolution reached. Handled in this professional manner, there can be no charge of slander. As the supervisor, you may be the last in the chain of command, and you are responsible for dealing with the accusation. Once you are sure of the facts and have witnesses or documentation to prove the facts, you are ready to take the appropriate action.

If a situation involves testifying in a court of law under direct testimony to a question directly asked, your response is considered privileged information, and is not subject to a charge of slander. Be careful to answer only the question asked. Do not volunteer additional information. For example, you may be asked, "Did you see Miss Jones illegally take a medication on February 14?" Answer only "yes" or "no." If you say, "No, but on another day I saw her administering medication to herself," you may be guilty of slander or defamation of character.

Discussing employees with another professional in the interest of their jobs is not considered slander. For instance, if two head nurses discuss an employee in relation to some negative items on his or her evaluation form, that is not slander. If the discussion takes place in the coffee room, in front of others, it may be a violation of the person's civil rights.

Many situations can cause defamation, and they may leave the supervisor open to a charge of slander or libel. Be aware of how easy it is to fall into a difficult situation by giving too much information. Be very careful of every word you speak and write. In regard to slander and libel, you cannot be too careful. Your professional reputation, and those of your staff, are at stake and may be damaged permanently by one thoughtless remark by you or a staff member.

NEGLIGENCE   In the legally conscious society that we live in, the health care industry is constantly accused of serious crimes of negligence and malpractice. Most of these claims prove to be unfounded, but the mere accusation causes health professionals to be very frightened of the legal process. The fact is, 90 percent of the cases filed never go to trial. This is because most of the cases do not have sufficient evidence to warrant a court investigation. True, you hear stories every day of huge settlements being awarded to patients in cases of malpractice. These settlements are the exceptions to the rule, and nurses should be aware of this fact. The profession cannot live in a constant state of fear that their every action may cause a law suit. Many nurses cause damage to a patient because they are afraid to act, because of a possible legal action.

As a supervisor, you must stress to your st aff that, as long as they are following the policies and procedures of the health care agency, they are working within the legal limits. Negligence and malpractice can be eliminated by following the rules and regulations set out by the organization.

There are three classifications of errors in nursing:

1. a mistake or error that causes no injury to the patient;
2. negligence, defined as failure to act as the average nurse with similar skills would act, and,
3. gross negligence—the failure to use *any* caution or thought.

The most common forms of negligence seen in the nursing profession are:

1. *Failure to use adequate precautions to prevent injury:* This is a case of filling a hot water bottle too hot and burning a patient, or failing to use sterile technique. These cases involve a breakdown in approved technique and can be eliminated by simple knowledge and supervision.

2. *Failure to recognize and report untoward symptoms:* Nurses are obligated by the nature of their profession to be alert and watchful to the patient's condition. If nurses notice a change in the condition of a patient, their responsibility is to report this change and document it on the patient's record. Discharging this duty is simply a matter of using good nursing judgment. When in doubt, report any unusual condition.

3. *Failure to respond to a patient's summons:* This is probably one of the situations that each and every nurse can relate to easily. The simple act of neglecting to answer a patient's call light can be proven to be negligent if some damage occurs.

4. *Failure to carry out medication and treatment orders:* This action can also be interpreted to mean failure to record medications and treatments. The patient's chart is a legal record, and, if a medication or treatment is not listed, the law assumes that the medication was not administered or that the treatment was not performed.

5. *Failure to protect a patient's valuables:* Every health care agency has a policy concerning locking up a patient's valuables in a safe. As a supervisor, you must stress the importance of following this procedure. Not only rings and watches are involved, though. The dropping of a patient's dentures down the laundry chute can also be considered negligence.

6. *Failure to report one's own illness or fatigue:* The law requires that any persons too ill or too tired to adequately carry out their tasks should be relieved of duty. If you remain on duty and cause an error through your fatigue, or spread a communicable disease that you were aware of having contracted, you are guilty of negligence.

7. *Failure to have faulty equipment repaired:* Many times staff members continue to use equipment that is faulty because of the time and inconvenience necessary to repair it. If damage to the patient occurs, the nurse who knowingly used the equipment is guilty of negligence.

Although these are the most common forms of nursing negligence and the ones frequently seen in court cases against medical personnel, they should not cause you to become afraid of your legal standing. You must be aware that these cases of negligence are not all actionable. A legal case exists only if the patient can prove that injury occurred because of the negligence. In other words, these situations would be considered simple errors if no damage or injury to the patient occurred. This damage or the negligence act, must be proved by the patient. The statement by a fellow staff member that the error occurred, for example, does not constitute negligence in a court of law. The patient must show that an injury occurred. Nurses can feel secure against action in a court of law if they always carry out procedures as taught, never try to do an unfamiliar procedure, and never assume responsibility for tasks for which they are unprepared.

If an act of negligence has occurred and if the patient claims that damage has been done, the law steps in to make the final determination. The law defines two types of negligence:

1. *Simple negligence:* Failure to exercise ordinary care and caution.
2. *Gross negligence:* An act committed, not as negligent behavior, but as a criminal act. An act that is so bad as to cause death would be considered gross negligence. For example, if a nurse deliberately does harm to a patient, the act is gross negligence. This is a criminal act punishable by imprisonment and/or fine.

Negligence is the failure of a nurse to possess and exercise that degree of skills, care, and knowledge normally possessed by the nurses in that community. The law takes into consideration the abilities of the peer group of a particular nurse, and expects him or her to act in the same manner. The plaintiff, or patient, must prove that damage occurred because of the nurse's action.

RE IPSA LOQUITUR   This latin term means literally, "the thing is spoken for by itself." This is a legal claim made by the patient in a court of law. In other words, the negligent act was so clear-cut and easily seen by the average person that no defense is possible. The conditions necessary for this claim are:

1. an accident that does not ordinarily happen without negligence;
2. an accident that had to be caused by an agent or instrumentality under the control of the defendant, (the nurse); and,
3. there must be no contribution on the part of the plaintiff. The classic example of *re ipsa loquitur* in malpractice is the amputation of the wrong leg in surgery. If the patient can show that the average person can go into the hospital for a surgical amputation and expect that the correct limb will be removed, that alone is enough to cause the court to award the plaintiff financial damages for the pain and suffering resulting from the negligence.

NEGLIGENCE PER SE   If a nurse is sued by a patient who suffered damages because of his or her illegal activity (perhaps practicing medicine without a license) , the nurse would also be presumed negligent under the doctrine of law called *negligence per se.*

RESPONDENT SUPERIOR   This principle states that employers are responsible for the acts of their employees. The law defines the employer not as the person or institution who pays the salary, but as the one who directs and controls the activities of the employee. For instance, if a supervisor assigns a task to a nurse knowing full well that he or she is unable to do the task and if a negligent act causes damage to the patient, the supervisor is responsible for the financial damages, not the hospital.

WILLS

Many times supervisors are placed in the position of dealing with a patient who wishes to write a will—a written declaration for disposition of possessions after death. Never write a will for a patient. If the patient wishes to write a will without the assistance of a lawyer, the will must be written in the handwriting of the patient. If patients ask you to write for them, suggest that a family member be called to assist the patient to find legal council. If you are asked to witness a will that has been written in your presence, you should refuse to do so. A handwritten will, drafted by the patient, needs no witness to be legal.

If an attorney is present in the patient's room and is writing a will, he or she may ask you to witness the document. To do so is a mistake, and you should refuse to do so. In the unusual event that you or your health care institution is mentioned in the will, the document could be declared null and void because of undue influence on your part. The law states that it is a fraud to influence individuals to part with their possessions. Try to stay out of legal dealings involving your patient, and council your staff to do the same.

ADMINISTRATION OF DRUGS

One of the major causes of actionable negligence is a medication error. These cases could be completely eliminated if only the staff are reminded and supervised in the technique of never giving a medication unless they know:

1. the nature of the drug,
2. the average dose,
3. the therapeutic use of the drug,
4. the untoward effects of the drug, and,
5. the method of administration of the drug.

THE PATIENT'S RECORD

The primary purpose of the patient's chart is to record problems and solutions, that is, the care of the patient. The chart should show the complete picture of the patient's care: What was wrong initially, what was done for the patient, and, if anything went wrong, what was done about it.

The patient's chart is considered a legal document, and, as such, it may be entered as evidence in a court of law. The basic rules of charting must be reviewed so that all staff members are as careful of their charting as they are of their care. The chart must:

1. be written neatly and clearly,
2. avoid hospital slang that is not clearly understood by everyone,
3. use only standard abbreviations,
4. avoid monotonous or meaningless entries,
5. must contain no erasures, and,
6. must be signed.

As a supervisor, your responsibility is to make sure that the charting of your agency reflects adequately the level of care performed. Auditing the charts is a major responsibility that cannot be ignored.

Alice H. Kerr, R.N., an authority on the legal aspects of nursing, feels that nurses' notes are where the "goodies" are. In other words, lawyers can find more information about the actual care, or lack of care, of a patient in these notes than on any other part of the chart. The nurse's notes list the care of the patient in chronological order, with times and dates entered. Doctors list notes also, but their information is not as detailed and does not give as accurate a picture of the overall condition of the patient.

RECORDING INCIDENT REPORTS   A question frequently asked of supervisors is how to record on the patient's chart the writing of an incident report. If something untoward happens in the routine care of a patient, and if the hospital requires that an incident report be filed, the problem is how to note this on the nurse's notes. Usually the hospital's insurance carrier requires:

1. that the incident report be filed in the Nursing Office,
2. the information about the accident or error be placed in the nurse's notes, and
3. that *no* statement to the effect that an incident report was filed be written in the nurse's notes.

Insurance companies feel that if the care was faulty, the chart should report only the care given, not the existence of an incident report. Insurance companies usually say *not* to write the words, "Incident report filed." Their reason is obvious. Writing these words makes it very simple for an ambitious attorney to skim the charts and pick out an error with no effort whatsoever.

This argument makes sense as far as the insurance company is concerned, but it does not help the staff member. If an accident occurs, and if the hospital policy is to fill out an incident report, then that fact *should* be noted on the chart to protect the nurse in question. As far as the law is concerned, any procedure not listed on the chart is assumed not to have been done. If no note is written stating *specifically* that an incident report was filed, nurses have no proof of their actions.

The chart must record every aspect of a patient's care, both positive and negative. If something was done in error, it should never be omitted from the chart. If the patient charges damages because of the error, and if there is nothing listed on the chart concerning the situation, the court assumes that something is being covered up. Supervisors are expected to protect their employers, but they must also remember that they are the advocates for their staffs and, as such, expected to protect them.

The nurse's notes should show continuity. If there is an entry stating, "The bruise on left buttocks is slightly larger today," there had better be a notation concerning the original observation of the bruise.

Try to avoid unsolved mysteries in charting. If an abnormal skin eruption is noted on a patient, did it disappear? Was it treated or ignored? The solution must be included.

Some of the common mistakes in charting are caused by carelessness, ignorance, or habit. If the staff fall into a pattern of sloppy charting, this pattern continues until the supervisor takes steps to train all staff members in the correct method of charting. Basically, the nurse's notes should reflect, in as descriptive terms as possible, the true picture of the patient. Nurses should chart what they see, hear, smell, and feel, as well as the patient's complaints.

When making entries in the nurse's notes, try to avoid meaningless terms such as: "good condition . . . good night . . . usual day." These phrases tell nothing about the patient unless you are personally aware of the patient's status. For a critically ill patient, a "good night" might mean a half-hour of uninterrupted pain-free sleep. For the ambulatory patient about to be discharged, this notation would have a completely different meaning. "Usual day" means nothing unless the reader looks back over the previous notes to find out what a "usual day" entails.

In charting, there should be no conclusions. If you are charting what you see, hear, taste, smell, and feel, then no assumptions about possible causes for these observations are necessary. Terms that need definition or interpretation should be eliminated from the charts. "Better" is a value judgment, and needs the perspective of the charting nurse to be understood. Better than what? "Restless" is another example of a term that needs definition. Is the restless patient tossing and turning? Or is he or she bored and ready to go home?

Some additional factors to keep in mind:

1. *Avoid biased charting:* Don't let your opinion of a patient's diagnosis affect the way you chart. Sometimes your wording can be colored to emphasize certain symptoms that support your feelings about the patient's diagnosis.

2. *Don't let routine charting become careless or sloppy:* Don't let fairly routine charting become careless or sloppy due to the similarity of care given to all patients in the department. In postpartum care, for example, the care of most patients is fairly consistent. The charting can easily become too mechanical and may fail to accurately portray the patient's condition.

3. *Do not let your emotions show in your charting:* If a patient has tried you to the limits of your patience, do not let this appear in your notes. "Seems to enjoy putting on call light," is an example of emotional charting.

4. *Use common sense in your charting:* If the doctor's order reads, "Observe color and temperature of extremities q one hour," it only makes sense to chart the observations every hour.

5. *Write what you mean, and watch your spelling:* If nurses cannot spell terms that are used every day in their work situation, an observer may wonder about the level of their expertise. An ICU nurse who misspells common cardiac terms does not give the impression of competence.

KNOW THE LAW

Although the legal aspects of nursing get a great deal of publicity, there is little more to this subject than good common sense. The supervisor who is aware of the legal implications of various actions, and who is well versed on the policies of the organization, should have no problems concerning the law. Trying to instill in your staff the caution necessary to be careful, without creating an atmosphere of fear, is the task of the supervisor. Nurses must feel secure in the knowledge that if they follow the rules of the organization and practice the skills of the profession at the accepted levels, they have no cause to worry about the law.

DISCUSSION QUESTIONS

1. Discuss the Nurse Practice Acts and their impact on nursing.

2. Find out the provisions in your state's Good Samaritan Law.

3. Discuss the differences between law, policy, and custom.

4. How can the legal term "false imprisonment" be applied to health care?

5. What is the difference between slander and libel? Give an example of each.

6. Discuss the most common forms of negligence? How can each be avoided?

7. Why is accurate charting such an important part of the nurse's responsibility?

APPLICATIONS

The following application situations are examples of frequently encountered legal problems. Assume that you are the supervisor, and make the appropriate decision in each case. Try to answer all the questions before you turn to the answers on the following page.

Questions

1. When doing the change-of-shift rounds in the form of "walking rounds," could information heard by the other patient in the room be considered an invasion of privacy?

2. A hospital does not employ assistant head nurses to replace the head nurses on their days off. The staff nurse with the most seniority acts as the head nurse, with no additional pay. This responsibility is not included in the job description of a staff nurse. Can the hospital legally do this? Is the nurse within his or her rights to refuse to accept this additional responsibility?

3. Are nurses automatically covered by the Good Samaritan Law if they give aid at the scene of an accident?

4. A psychiatric patient is admitted to an acute hospital. Is the nurse liable if the patient hurts himself? Can the nurse legally refuse to care for such patients?

5. Can a nurse refuse to participate in a situation that he or she feels is unnecessary, such as preparing a very elderly, debilitated patient for tests unrelated to her illness?

6. If a physician orders a medication for pain (for example, Meperidine 100mb. IV q4h), may the nurse legally assess the patient's needs and decide on that basis to give a smaller amount?

7. Are nurses justified in confiscating medications a patient brings to the hospital and refusing to return them at discharge without a doctor's order?

8. If a private duty nurse makes an error in practice or in caring for a patient in a hospital, what is the liability of the charge nurse as the hospital's delegate?

9. Can a nurse legally set up a booth at a fair or public gathering and charge for services, such as taking blood pressures?

10. Can ward clerks *legally* make up medication cards from a doctor's orders?

11. Can non-nursing personnel, such as receptionists, office clerks, medical assistants, and the like, transmit a doctor's orders?

Answers

1. Yes. Your statements could be considered slander if they defame the character of the patient in question. The way to avoid this charge is never to discuss anything that could be legally or morally damaging in front of a nonprofessional. If the patient is unconscious, discuss only his or her physical condition. Include the patient who is conscious in the discussion. Talk about superficial things only; save the other discussion for outside the room.

2. No. The hospital cannot compel the staff nurses to perform the task of head nurse. The Nurse Practice Act states that nurses may perform only those duties for which they are trained, tested, and found competent. If you feel unprepared, you have not only the right to object, but also a legal responsibility to say so. The hospital cannot continue to demand this work from you.

3. It depends on where the accident took place. Some states offer the protection of the Good Samaritan Law only to the nurses licensed to practice in that state. You should check the restrictions of your particular state. Other states restrict the protection of the Good Samaritan Act to areas away from the nurse's place of employment.

4. Yes. The nurse, the doctor, and the hospital would all be liable if a likelihood that the patient would hurt himself and failed to take proper care.

No. You can't refuse to care for these patients. Your only recourse is to ask for a transfer to another area. Nurses are not legally allowed to pick and choose the patients that they wish to care for on a particular ward.

5. No. Unless this procedure violates personal moral or religious beliefs. Nurses may refuse to participate in a procedure that is contrary to their moral or religious belief, such as abortion, but they cannot refuse simply because they feel that a procedure is unnecessary. Follow the doctor's orders unless you have proof that the test is unnecessary.

6. Yes. This type of drug order generally implies that a smaller dose may be given. The doctor should be notified as soon as possible of the change in dosage.

7. Yes. The nurse may confiscate the patient's medications unless the doctor has written an order permitting self-medication. Once the medications are taken away from the patient, they cannot be returned without a doctor's order.

8. The charge nurse is responsible for all facets of patient care, including surveillance of private duty nurses. So if the charge nurse knew or should have known that the private nurse made an error, he or she and the hospital would share the liability.

9. Yes. There is no statute against nurses' setting up private practice to do routine "nursing" procedures.

10. Yes. They may transpose medical information from charts to cards, provided that they are not required to summarize, interpret, or reconstruct the information.

11. Yes. Legally a doctor can appoint anyone to transmit orders. A hospital can rule that only its RNs may receive doctor's orders, but this rule is *policy*, not *law*.

REFERENCES

GARLAND, J. V., *Discussion Methods*. New York: H. W. Wilson Co., 1951.

HUNT, DERALD D., *Teacher Training Supplemental Material No. 27*. California State Department of Education: Peace Officers' Training Program, 1960.

LONEY, GLENN M., *Briefing and Conference Techniques*. New York: Mc-Graw-Hill Book Company, 1959.

SUTHERLAND, SIDNEY S., *When You Preside*. Danville, Ill.: Interstate Printers and Publishers, 1952.

TAYLOR, H. W. AND MEARS, A. G., *The Right Way to Conduct Meetings, Conferences, and Discussions*. London: Morrison and Gibb, Ltd., 1964.

10

The supervisor as management

The concept of a nurse/leader functioning as a manager is a new concept that a great many nurses feel uncomfortable accepting. Health care is an industry, just like any other major industry. Supervisors in the health care industry are required to manage personnel and materials as an integral part of their jobs. The study of management as a science helps supervisors to understand the activities necessary to function as members of the management team.

Understanding organizational principles is the foundation or framework of supervision. Without a clear conception of how and why the organization is structured, the supervisor is unable to function as a member of the team. Too many supervisors feel that management is an area that belongs to business, not to nursing, and they fail to see the important fact that supervisors must be good managers as well as good leaders and good nurses.

All organizations, whether large or small, have the common need for a systematic plan of accomplishing work. This plan is referred to as *organization*, which is an arrangement of individuals with a common goal working in a systematic manner, enabling the efficient achievement of these goals. Without the plan, or organization, of the health care agency, work would not be accomplished and the goals of patient care would not be met.

Those responsible for maintaining this organization are called *managers*. The study of management is not a strange and mystifying

191

science. The myriad approaches to managing the activities of subordinates present a difficulty in studying management. Each management specialist or theorist proposes a new and somewhat different approach to management and organization, and, with the new theory, comes a new vocabulary of management terms. Since the basis of this textbook is supervision for nurses, and not the study of administration and management, we will look only at the principles of management as they apply to the health care setting.

Since management is not a strict science—because it does not have set rules and formulas that apply in every case—we must study management in terms of trends. Also, to understand your role in management, you must develop a sense of the progression of management as a science. Studying management from a historical perspective is therefore important. From the classical period of management theory right up to present day management science, much can be learned from each school of thought.

You will see the periods of thought as they developed and then, through an active learning process, apply each successive principle of organization. In this way, you become responsible for the extent of your learning experience. Guidelines to assist you are provided, but the burden is on you to read and evaluate each of the management styles. You should understand that each of these styles is still practiced, to some extent, in health care agencies today. At the end of this chapter you will understand the principles well enough to see the advantages and disadvantages of each, and you will be able to apply them to your own work situation.

Working through the learning application on "management as a science" gives you a better grasp of the framework of management. This section provides the foundation for further study of the subject. Read each essay on management style, then try to fill out the application sheet that follows. Spend as much time as necessary on each topic so that you feel comfortable with the ideas presented. A short summary is offered after each essay to help you organize your thinking. At the end of the exercise, you will be able to identify the three periods of management theory, and you will see the basic similarities and differences between the theories. The completion of this application gives you the tools necessary to understand organization and its evolution, as well as to give a logical plan for the accomplishment of goals in the health care industry.

Try to think of each of these principles as "name-calling." In other words, you are giving names and terms to ideas that you may have been vaguely aware of, but have never studied. Calling something by name or clearly understanding a concept does not solve all management problems, but it helps you to see the reasons behind behavior and some reasons why certain management tactics work and some do not.

APPLICATION: PRINCIPLES
OF ORGANIZATION

Objective

- To enable the student to learn the historical principles of organization by reading and then outlining them.

Procedure

1. There are three periods in organizational theory:
   a. the Classical Period—
      (1) rationality (Weber),
      (2) management as a true science (Taylor), and
      (3) principles (Gulick, Urwick).
   b. the Neo-Classical Period—
      (1) Hawthorne studies,
      (2) Human Relations Era, and
      (3) organization as overlays.
   c. the Modern Period—
      (1) systems approach,
      (2) open social systems (subsystems),
      (3) project organization, and
      (4) matrix organization.
2. Each student is expected to learn the basic facts of each period.
3. Read the essays, and fill out the principle sheet for each one.
4. The student then reviews each period in terms of general trends.

WEBER (RATIONALITY)

Max Weber was one of the leading scholars of the early twentieth century. Significantly, he was a founder of modern sociology as well as a pioneer in administrative thought. The major theme underlying most of Weber's work is the derivation and development of *rationality*. This concept led him to study different kinds of organizations in terms of their interactions with society as a whole.

Weber probed bureaucracy, which here is essentially synonymous with "large organization," to uncover the rational relationship of bureaucratic structure to its goals. His analysis led him to conclude that there are three types of organizational power centers:

1. *traditional*—The way things have always been done,
2. *charismatic*—subordinates accept orders because of an emotional response to the leader, and

3. *rational–legal*—subordinates accept order because they agree with the legality of such a situation.

Of the three types of authority, Weber recommended that rational–legal was the best way to obtain systematic relationships. Still, Weber was aware of the weaknesses of this structure. Not only do external forces exert constant pressures on the supervisor to follow norms other than those of the organization, but, in time, an individual's adherence to bureaucratic rules declines. His primary motive, therefore, was to build into the bureaucratic structure safeguards against external and internal pressures so that the bureaucracy could at all times sustain its autonomy.

According to Weber, a bureaucratic structure, to be rational, must contain these elements:[1]

1. Rulification and routinization— "an organization bound by rules."
2. Division of labor—"A specific sphere of competence."
3. Hierarchy of authority—"Each lower office should be under the control and supervision of a higher one."
4. Expertise—"Only a person who demonstrates adequate technical training should be allowed to perform tasks requiring that skill."
5. Written rules—"Administrative acts, decisions and rules are formulated and recorded in writing."
6. Separation of ownership—"Those in control or management of an organization should have no private financial interest in that organization."

This is Weber's ideal model: According to Weber, as these elements increase in their number and intensity, an organization becomes more rational and efficient.

Weber's theory contains two other essential aspects. First, he stressed the universality of bureaucracy. Since bureaucracy is the best known means for achieving rationality in human behavior, it is equally applicable in both the private and the public sectors of society. Second, for bureaucracy to work, man has to be a free agent. The relationship between man and bureaucracy has to be contractual rather than master–slave.

Most frequently, the critics take exception to his ideal type of bureaucracy and to the sharp distinctions he makes among the three types of authority. The latter objection is expressed because he does not take into consideration the fact that all three methods may be present in mixed forms.

[1] Max Weber, *The Theory of Social and Economic Organization* (a summary), ed. Talcott Parson, trans., A. M. Henderson and Talcott Parsons (New York: Oxford University Press, Inc., 1947), pp. 329–30.

Despite criticisms, Weber's vast contribution to organizational theory is becoming more recognized and is still present in management literature.

PRINCIPLES OF ORGANIZATION

Organization theory:

Period (Classical, Neo-Classical, or Modern):

Principal theorist:

Major theme summarized:

Major points in theory with definitions:

Strengths of theory:

Weaknesses of theory:

Examples of how this theory is used in health care at the present time:

Summary

Max Weber is the original theorist of organization thought and structure. At the time of his writing, little had been written about the actual process of organization. Workers were expected to perform for the employer with no understanding or conception of *why* the worker was carrying out tasks. Max Weber was the first to realize that if the relationship between employer and employee were an organized contract, both the organization and the employee would benefit. Although at first glance

195

Weber's ideas seem to be very simplistic, in reality, his treatise was a great breakthrough in management thought. He rejected the idea of master–slave and recommended the use of contractual methods to improve management.

The major theme of Max Weber's work is rationality, and his goal in organization was to achieve "rationality." In other words, workers should follow the norms of the organization because "legally" they are under contract to do so, and "rationally" because it makes sense to have a central leader responsible for the activities of subordinates. To obtain rationality, he outlined the ways in which an organization achieves its power. The goal of the organization should be systematic relationships, and Weber found these relationships develop in the use of the methods of authority—traditional, charismatic, and rational–legal.

Although the theory is very dogmatic and authoritarian, it is widely used in health care agencies to accomplish work:

1. All health care agencies function with rules and regulations.
2. Labor is divided according to type,
3. There is a chain of command,
4. All staff members possess the necessary expertise to function in the agency,
5. The policies and procedures of an agency are written,
6. In some agencies, ownership and management are separate.

DISCUSSION QUESTIONS

1. Why is Weber's work so important to management study?
2. What is the relationship of bureaucracy to health care?
3. In which situations would you choose to use Weber's theories?
4. In which situations would you want to avoid using these theories?

TAYLORISM (SCIENTIFIC MANAGEMENT)

Frederick Taylor, an early production specialist, applied the scientific method to the solution of factory problems. From this study he built orderly sets of principles that could be substituted for the trial-and-error methods then in use. The advent of Taylor's thinking opened a new era, that of "scientific management." His enormous contribution lay first in his large-scale application of the analytical, scientific approach to improving production methods. Second, while he did not feel that management could ever become an exact science, he believed that management could be an organized body of knowledge and that it could be taught and learned. Third, he originated the term "functional supervision." He felt that the job of supervision was too difficult for only one person, and that it should be delegated to many supervisors, each governing a single function.

Based on this analysis, he recommended that managers use scientific research to discover the "one best way" for doing a job. This approach would enable management to evaluate how much work should be accomplished in a set period of time. When this foundation had been established, it would be possible to make use of incentives for higher individual output. Furthermore, Taylor firmly believed that management, and management alone, was responsible for putting these techniques into effect.

Taylor prescribed five methods for scientifically managing an organization:

1. Management must discover the one best way to do a job.
2. It must standardize its equipment to do the best job.
3. It must train each worker for the job he or she will do.
4. It must use only "functional supervision."
5. Management must pay the worker in accordance with individual output.[2]

Taylor's ideas were opposed by management and unions. Also, job specialization had not reached such a point as to force attention to his theory.

Ironically, Taylor's general approach to management is widely accepted today in production-oriented business organizations. Scientific management became a movement that still has a tremendous influence on industry today. Numerous managers firmly believe that, if material rewards are directly related to work efforts, the worker consistently responds with maximum performance.

PRINCIPLES OF ORGANIZATION

Organization theory:

Period:

Major theme summarized:

---

[2] Frederick W. Taylor, *Shop Management* (a summary) (New York: Harper & Row, Publishers, Inc., 1911).

Major points in theory with definitions:

Strengths of theory:

Weaknesses of theory:

Examples of how this theory is used in health care at the present time:

Summary

Frederick Taylor followed Max Weber in the progession of management thinking. While Taylor agreed with many of the basic ideas of Max Weber, he disagreed on the simplicity of management. Where Weber felt that everything could be accomplished through rational thinking and organization, Taylor felt that the principles of science should be applied to organization.

Frederick Taylor felt that if the scientific method were used in management, the plan would be more logical, and the results would be greater efficiency and production.

The concept of "pyramid structure" or decentralization of authority can be attributed to Taylor, for he was the first to advocate functional supervision.

The five methods of scientifically managing an organization, as outlined by Taylor, are used almost daily in health care agencies. Basically, he says to find the one best way to do a job, train everyone to do the job that way, standardize the equipment to do the job, and teach all supervisors to direct the activities of these workers. In the hospital setting, this approach is used for all basic patient treatments. For example, if the patient is to have an enema, the equipment is standardized, the procedure manual tells how to do the procedure, the staff is taught the correct method of administering the treatment, and the supervisor is present to guide and direct the operation.

Many nurses feel that this theory is fine for the assembly line, but it has no place in health care. One of the problems we face in health care is the idea of production. As nurses, we resent the concept of patients being considered "production goals." In fact, they must be considered in these harsh terms if one is to understand the principle of goal achievement. We stress quality, not quantity, but even in a humanistic profession such as nursing, quantity is important. The successful manager realizes that the organization depends on task-centered goal accomplishment to achieve the stated objectives.

The one area that Taylor points out—that Weber ignored completely—is motivation. Taylor sees the workers' motivation as monetary, and he stresses the importance of paying the worker for his or her individual output. Again, we face the moral problem of putting the care and comfort of human beings on such a materialistic level. The supervisor must be aware of the basic facts of economics; the employee is working to earn a living. Granted, people have many other reasons for choosing nursing as a profession, but, if there were no monetary rewards to the job, few people would continue to nurse. The satisfaction of serving others and working in a helping, healing vocation is very important to the dedicated nurse, but earning enough money to meet the basic needs is more important. Today, we realize that Taylor saw only *one* of the reasons that employees work, and he failed to take into consideration all the other factors that motivate workers.

His suggestion that workers be paid for individual output, is still practiced in health care today. We do not pay the individual worker a set rate per task, as is practiced in the assembly line or in piece work, but we do promote staff on the basis of their individual output—which is essentially paying for output. In a few hospitals, Taylor's plan is practiced literally. In other words, nurses are paid per patient based on quality and quantity. This is an experimental program to improve efficiency and to lower costs. Each nurse is paid on a schedule of difficulty of care, for each client served. The idea is to increase individual motivation using money as the reward. The results of this experiment have not been analyzed for a long enough period to reach any conclusions, but it is an excellent example of Taylorism in health care. Other examples of monetary rewards are in staff profit sharing plans and yearly bonus checks.

In health care, Taylor's theories do work and are practiced in every area. Any functionally oriented organization can benefit from the study of Taylor's scientific management.

DISCUSSION QUESTIONS

1. In which ways does Taylor improve on Weber's basic ideas?
2. To whom does Taylor give the responsibility for a smoothly running organization?
3. In which medical situations would you choose to use Taylor's theories?
4. In which medical situations would you avoid using Taylor's theories?

GULICK AND URWICK (THE PRINCIPLES)

Luther Gulick and Lyndall Urwick were leaders in formulating principles of formal organization. Not only did they develop such activities, but Gulick went even further and defined administration as comprising seven activities:[3]

1. planning,
2. organizing,
3. staffing,
4. directing,
5. coordination,
6. reporting, and
7. budgeting.

These principles continue to serve as a starting point for anyone interested in dealing with different administrative processes.

The Gulick–Urwick principles deal primarily with the *structure* of the organization. Underlying all their principles was the need for an organizational division of labor. In other words, their approach rests firmly on the assumption that the more a specific function can be divided into simple parts, the more specialized the job becomes, thus workers become all the more skilled in carrying out their parts of the job. As the workers become more skilled in their particular jobs, the whole organization becomes more efficient. According to Gulick and Urwick, any division of work should be by:

1. purpose,
2. process,
3. persons or things dealt with, and
4. place where he renders his service.[4]

This four-determinant approach has been subject to much criticism. These determinants are difficult to apply to a specific organization since they often overlap, are incompatible with one another, and are quite vague. Planning the division of labor in a given organization is affected by many considerations not covered by the four principles. The division of tasks may be determined by the culture in which the organization is situated, by the environment of the organization, by the availability and

---

[3] Gulick's seven elements of administration are drawn from Henri Fayol's list of five: planning, organization, command, coordination, and control. See Henry Fayol, *General and Industrial Management*, trans. Constance Storrs (London: Sir Isaac Pitman and Sons Ltd., 1949), pp. 43–110.

[4] Gulick, *Notes on Organization*, p. 13.

type of personnel, and by political factors. In the final analysis, organizations are made up of a combination of various layers that differ in their type of division.

In addition to their labor-division principle, seven other related principles merit our attention:[5]

1. Unity of command—"nor man can serve two masters."[6]
2. Fitting people to the structure—"People should be assigned to their organizational positions" in a cold-blooded, detached spirit, "like the preparation of an engineering design, regardless of the needs of that particular individual or of those individuals who may now be in the organization."[7]
3. One top executive—no committees or boards to govern.
4. Staff assistance.
5. Delegation of authority—"In large organizations you must delegate the right to delegate."[8]
6. Matching responsibility with authority.
7. Span of control—"No supervisor can adequately supervise more than five or six subordinates."[9]

While Gulick and Urwick accepted the need for principles of supervision, along with a single center of authority and control in the organization, they differed on how these principles should be implemented. Besides failing to provide a workable guide to the division of labor, all these principles are *prescriptive* and fail to allow for the numerous differences in real, as compared with ideal, organizations.

PRINCIPLES OF ORGANIZATION

Organization theory:

Period:

---

[5] This list is suggested in part by Gross. See Bertram M. Gross, *The Managing of Organizations* (New York: The Free Press of Glencoe, 1964), pp. 145–48.

[6] Gulick, "Notes," p. 9.

[7] L. Urwick, *Elements of Administration* (New York: Harper & Row, Publishers, Inc., 1943), pp. 34–39.

[8] *Ibid.*, pp. 51–52.

[9] *Ibid.*, pp. 45–46, 125.

Major theme summarized:

Major points in theory with definitions:

Strengths of theory:

Weaknesses of theory:

Examples of how this theory is used in health care at the present time:

Summary

Luther Gulick and Lyndall Urwick improved and expanded the ideas of Frederick Taylor. Taylor proposed the scientific division of labor, and Gulick and Urwick continued this approach by expanding the division. The main thrust of their thinking was to develop an organizational structure based on the division of labor, but the areas of division were more specialized. Where Taylor wanted each worker to do one task and only one task, Gulick and Urwick felt that the division should be by function rather than by specific tasks.

Their categories—purpose, process, persons or things dealt with, and place where service is rendered—are difficult to conform to and lead to much confusion. People do not fit into little boxes, and they cannot be categorized so easily. Team leaders can identify with the overlapping that occurs if they remember the difficulty of assigning patients to the staff. It would be simple to divide patient assignment by "place where the service is rendered." Simple and sensible, yes, but nearly impossible. If, for instance, you wanted to assign nurse X to all the patients on one corridor and nurse Y to those on the other corridor, you would have to make sure that all the patients needed about the same number of nursing care hours. Also, the skill of the staff member has to be taken into consideration, as well as the availability of staff. The theory must have all aspects equal in order to work, and this condition seldom happens in the health care industry.

The divisions of administration into seven activities are used in all areas of management and remain the basis for the study of management. These areas are important, and dividing them in this manner makes the study of administration easier. Yet in actual practice, these divisions are as artificial and difficult to maintain as the four-stage approach. As often happens in trying to explain an idea, the idea becomes so complicated that it is destroyed.

DISCUSSION QUESTIONS

1. Why are the divisions of planning, organizing, staffing, directing, coordinating, reporting, and budgeting seen so often in management literature?
2. Compare and contract the theories of Max Weber, Frederick Taylor, and Gulick and Urwick.
3. In which medical situations would you choose to use the principles of Gulick and Urwick?
4. In which medical situations would you avoid the principles of Gulick and Urwick?

THE CLASSICAL PERIOD OF MANAGEMENT—AN OVERVIEW

1. Give some key words that describe the general feeling of the Classical Period.

2. What element did Taylor include that the other Classical theorists ignored?

3. What was completely forgotten in the Classical Period?

THE CLASSICAL PERIOD OF MANAGEMENT: A SUMMARY

The Classical approach to management is a set of theories developed over a period of many years beginning in 1890 and then summarized and classified in the 1930s. The main theorists studied in the Classical Period were Max Weber, Frederick Taylor, Luther Gulick, and Lyndall Urwick.

The main thrust of the classical theorists was formal organizational structure. Classical organization theory focused on the total organization and attempted to provide general truths or guidelines that would direct the manager in the accomplishment of work. The Classical Period was one of a "descriptive" process. All its theories revolve around the goals of economy, efficiency, and strong central control. These basic goals can be achieved by creating an organization on four basic tenets:

1. division of labor,
2. hierarchy of authority,
3. structure, and
4. span of control.

Through the study and writing of the Classical theorists, the pyramid structure of organizational planning has evolved. This structure is the basis of our modern health care organizational charts.

THE HAWTHORNE STUDIES

This series of studies, done during the late 1920s and throughout the mid-1930s, produced some very important, unexpected findings. To begin, a group of girls who assembled telephone equipment was selected for a series designed to determine the effect of their working conditions on their productivity.[10]

As the researchers varied working conditions, they found each major change was accompanied by a substantial increase in production. When the test was completed, the researchers decided to return the girls to their original conditions to see the effect on their work. To the astonishment of the researchers, output rose again, to an even higher level than it had been under the best of conditions. The hypothesis was that motivation to work, productivity, and the quality of work are all related to the nature of the social relations among the workers and between the workers and their boss. The findings are summarized as follows:[11]

1. The productivity of individual workers is determined more by their social "capacity" than by their physical capacity.
2. Noneconomic rewards play a prominent part in motivating and satisfying employees.
3. Maximum specialization is not the most efficient form of division of labor.
4. Employees do not react to management and to its norms and rewards as individuals, but as members of groups.

The tendency of experimentally chosen groups to show increased productivity and job satisfaction is now termed the "Hawthorne

[10] Edgar H. Schein, *Organizational Psychology* (Englewood Cliffs, N.J.: Prentice-Hall, Inc., 1963), p. 27.

[11] Schein, p. 29–40.

effect." The findings from this study have come to be misused in the literature to refer to any favorable effect on the performance of a group. In this experiment *treatment* was the significant factor. The girls were given the best supervisor, special privileges, and made into a cohesive group. The group did not hold previously established norms on what its level of production should be. The workers' cohesion around their own norms was too strong to change if a new group was not established. The primary lesson taught in the original experiment was that the level of production is set by social norms, not by physiological capacities. What this finding brought home was the importance of the social factor—that is, the degree to which work performance depends not on individuals alone, but on the network of social relationships within which they operate.[12]

PRINCIPLES OF ORGANIZATION

Organization theory:

Period (Classical, Neo-Classical, or Modern):

Principal theorist:

Major theme summarized:

Major points in theory with definitions:

Strengths of theory:

Weaknesses of theory:

Examples of how this theory is used in health care at the present time:

[12] A more comprehensive description of these researchers can be found in F. J. Locthlisberger and W. J. Dickson, *Management and the Worker* (Cambridge: Harvard University Press, 1939).

Summary

In the Classical Period, the individual was completely ignored. With the exception of Taylor and his monetary motivation, the Classical theorists were task-oriented and failed to see the needs of the worker.

The Hawthorne studies explored for the first time the idea of workers as *individuals*. These studies point up dramatically the error in this thinking. The work level improved not only when the conditions were improved for the girls, but also when they returned to the original work situation. Even more significant was the fact that when this same group of girls was given poor working situations—worse than those of the average worker—they continued to increase their output. This reaction was taken as proof that the nature of the work situation and the resultant group feeling are more important to the worker than some other aspects of the job. The study shows the importance of "groups" in the work situation and the need for developing a group spirit.

This so-called Hawthorne effect can be seen quite easily in a small, tight-knit unit in the hospital setting. The emergency room personnel present a classic example. They feel united, able to work together well because of their feeling of group unity and loyalty. Even when the work situation is less than ideal, such as when a major accident doubles the number of patients in the ward, the staff is able to cope and cope quite well. You may even hear the comment, "We can handle it, we are good and can handle anything."

This study is important because it points up so vividly the importance of *treatment* to the staff. As a supervisor, you must be aware of the Hawthorne effect and use it to your advantage.

DISCUSSION QUESTIONS

1. Can you, as a supervisor, initiate the Hawthorne effect?
2. If personnel are functioning as members of a group and a new staff person is added, what is the effect?
3. Where does the supervisor stand in relation to discipline with a group that functions as a tight-knit unit?
4. What is the difference between a group and a clique?
5. How can the Hawthorne effect aid you as a supervisor?
6. How can the Hawthorne effect hinder you as a supervisor?

THE HUMAN RELATIONS ERA

The human relations approach to managing and supervising is still widely accepted in administrative circles. A long line of research has added to the evidence that group solidarity and loyalty is associated with productivity and job satisfaction. Moreover, these experiments have provided a better understanding of organizational leadership, decision making, and communication. In regard to leadership, it was observed that the leader is able to set and enforce group norms through a particular style of leading a group.

Also, considerable time was spent analyzing the difference between formal and informal groups,[13] thus setting the stage for identifying and understanding the informal organization. After the social capacity of human beings was discovered, others began to notice that the social scientists were directing their attention to how certain factors—such as power, expertise, and the like—operated in a nonformal or informal sense. Thus the human relations approach to organization carved out a Neo-Classical theory, which devoted most of its study to an improved knowledge of the informal organization.

The assumption is that employees who are made happier through satisfaction of their social needs, become more cooperative and efficient. It refuses to regard individuals as economic entities and defines them as a social animals. Accordingly, once a worker's social problems are solved, management is able to make the worker's organizational existence a happy one.

PRINCIPLES OF ORGANIZATION

Organization theory:

Period (Classical, Neo-Classical, or Modern):

Principal theorist:

Major theme summarized:

Major points in theory with definitions:

Strengths of theory:

---

[13] R. Lippitt and R. K. White, "An Experimental Study of Leadership and Group Life," in *Readings in Social Psychology*, ed. G. E. Swanson, T. M. Newcomb, and E. L. Hartley (New York: Holt, Rinehart & Winston, Inc., 1952), pp. 340–55.

Weaknesses of theory:

Examples of how this theory is used in health care at the present time:

Summary

The Human Relations Era can be summarized by the statement, "the happier the worker, the more productive." The conclusion can then be seen that, as a supervisor, your task could be made much easier by simply making all your employees happy. You can easily see the major flaw in this kind of thinking: the simple fact that no matter what you do, you cannot make all people happy.

Although delving into this approach is a major endeavor, a certain amount of this thinking is necessary in any health care agency. Employee Christmas parties, bowling leagues, days off for birthdays—these are all examples of Human Relations Era thinking. The health care agency does these things simply to make the employee happy. They serve no direct benefit to the health care agency except to make happy, contented workers.

DISCUSSION QUESTIONS

1. Show how the Human Relations Era tried to form a theory around the Hawthorne studies.
2. How can you as the supervisor use human relations to your benefit?
3. How can human relations hinder the effectiveness of your organization?

ORGANIZATION AS OVERLAYS

The formal structure of an organization represents as closely as possible the framer's intended processes of interaction among its members. In the typical work organization, this structure involves definitions of task specialties and their arrangement in levels of authority, with clearly defined lines of communication from one level to the next. (See Figure 10–1.) However, the actual processes of interaction among the individuals represented in the formal plan cannot adequately be described

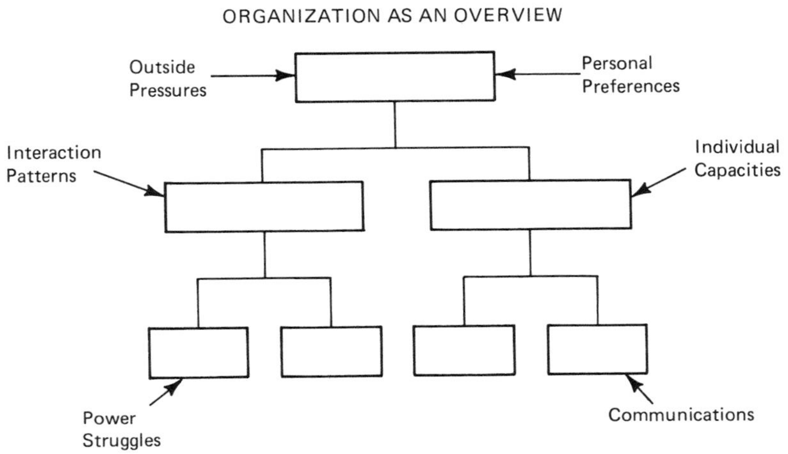

ORGANIZATION AS AN OVERVIEW

Figure 10–1. The typical job pyramid of authority and some of its interacting processes. *Adapted from John M. Pfiffner and Frank M. Sherwood,* Administrative Organization *(Englewood Cliffs, N.J.: Prentice-Hall, Inc., 1960), pp. 18–27.*

solely in terms of its planned lines of interaction. Coexisting with the formal structure are myriad other possibilities for interaction among persons in the organization, which can be analyzed according to various theories of group behavior. Further, these other interactions never function very distinctively, and all are intermixed in an organization that also follows its formal structure to a large extent. These modified processes must be studied one at a time.

A good way to do so without forgetting their "togetherness" is to consider each as a transparent overlay superimposed on the basic formal organizational pattern. The overlay approach aims to be realistic by recognizing that an organization also consists of a wide variety of contacts that involve communication, sociometry, goal-centered functionalism, decision making, and personal power.[14] Let us consider this complex of processes one at a time.

THE JOB-TASK PYRAMID   This pyramid constitutes the basis from which all departures are measured—the official version of the organization. Without this organization chart, the other networks (overlays) would not exist.[15]

[14] For much of the conceptual underpinnings of this essay, we are indebted to John R. Dorsey, Jr., "A Communication Model for Administration," *Administrative Science Quarterly*, 2: 307–324 (December 1957).

[15] Reprinted with permission of the author and publisher from *Administrative Organization* (Englewood Cliffs, N.J.: Prentice-Hall, Inc., 1960), pp. 18–27. Footnotes renumbered.

William Brownrigg deals with the job-task hierarchy in *The Human Enterprise Process and Its Administration* (University of Alabama: University Press, 1954).

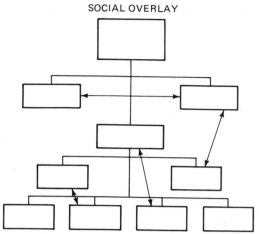

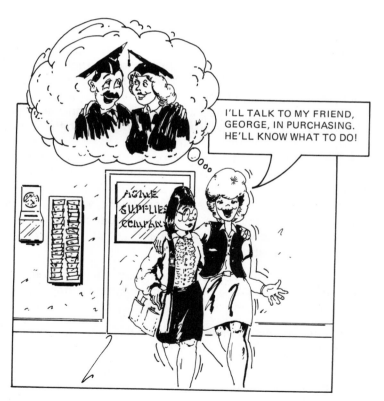

Figure 10–2. The social overlay. *Adapted from John M. Pfiffner and Frank M. Sherwood,* Administrative Organization *(Englewood Cliffs, N.J.: Prentice-Hall, Inc., 1960), pp. 18–27.*

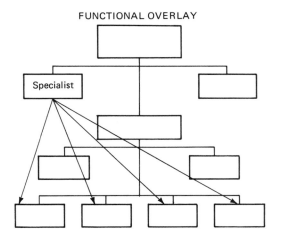

FUNCTIONAL OVERLAY

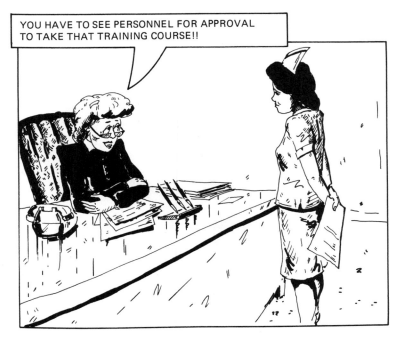

Figure 10–3. The functional overlay. *Adapted from John M. Pfiffner and Frank M. Sherwood,* Administrative Organization *(Englewood Cliffs, N.J.: Prentice-Hall, Inc., 1960), pp. 18–27.*

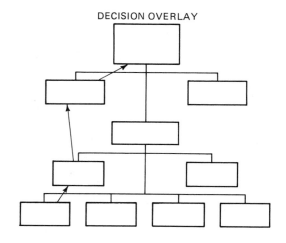

DECISION OVERLAY

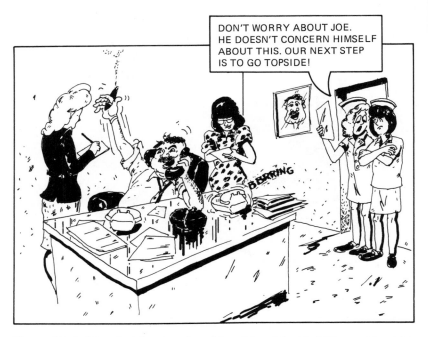

Figure 10–4. The decision overlay. *Adapted from John M. Pfiffner and Frank M. Sherwood,* Administrative Organization *(Englewood Cliffs, N.J.: Prentice-Hall, Inc., 1960), pp. 18–27.*

POWER OVERLAY

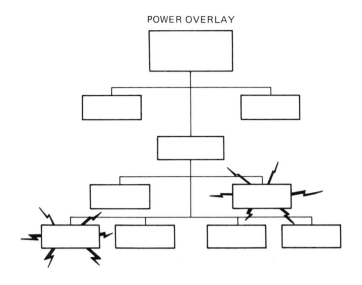

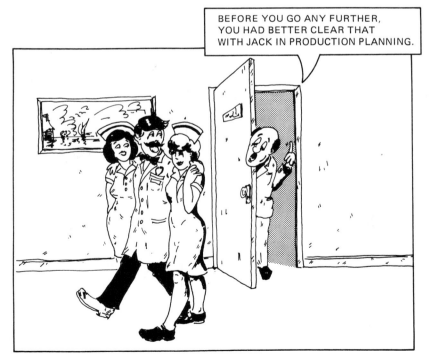

Figure 10–5. The power overlay. *Adapted from John M. Pfiffner and Frank M. Sherwood,* Administrative Organization *(Englewood Cliffs, N.J.: Prentice-Hall, Inc., 1960), pp. 18–27.*

THE COMMUNICATION OVERLAY

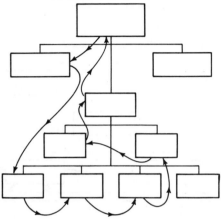

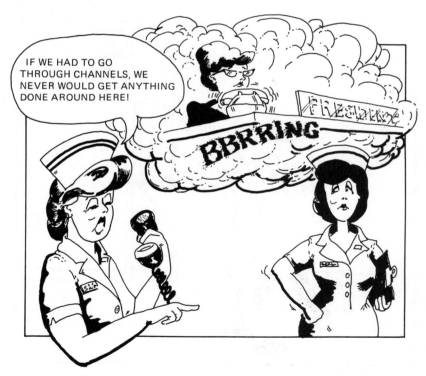

Figure 10–6. The communication overlay. *Adapted from John M. Pfiffner and Frank M. Sherwood,* Administrative Organization *(Englewood Cliffs, N.J.: Prentice-Hall, Inc., 1960), pp. 18–27.*

The Sociometric Overlay: "In any organization there is a set of relation-ships among people which is purely social; it exists because of feelings of attraction or rejection. It is the special friendships in the organiza-tion."[16] (See Figure 10–2, p. 210.)

The Functional Overlay: Functional contacts occur most typically where specialized information is needed; through them the staff or the intel-lectual "leader," exerts influence on operations without direct respon-sibility for the work itself. (See Figure 10–3, p. 211.)

The Decision Overlay: "Normally in an organization the decision pattern follows the structure of the formal hierarchy, that is, the job-task pyramid. However, the power and authority network, together with the functional network, may cut across hierarchical channels. The flow of significant decisions in the organization may not follow the hierarchical structure at all."[17] (See Figure 10–4, p. 212.)

The Power Overlay: "Power exists when one has the ability to influence someone to behave in a particular way or to make decisions. As a result, the mapping of power centers would seldom follow the pattern of a typical hierarchy."[18] (See Figure 10–5, p. 213.)

The Communication Overlay: "The information process is central to or-ganization system. It affects control and decision making to name just a few. Real patterns of communication are often very different from the prescribed channels of communication."[19] (See Figure 10–6.)

PRINCIPLES OF ORGANIZATION

Organization theory:

Period (Classical, Neo-Classical, or Modern):

Principal theorist:

[16] Fred Massarik, Robert Tannenbaum, Murray Kahane, and Irving Weochler, "Sociometric Choice and Organizational Effectiveness: a Multi-relational Ap-proach," *Sociometry* 16: 211–238 (August 1953).

[17] Herbert A. Simon, *Administrative Behavior*, 2nd ed. (New York: The Macmillan Company, 1947), p. xix. Simon's decision model is discussed in detail in Chap-ter 21.

[18] Henry C. Metcalf and L. Urwick, eds., *Dynamic Administration: The Collected Papers of Mary Parker Follett* (New York: Harper and Brothers, 1940), p. 49. Discussed in detail in Chapter 5.

[19] Robert Dubin, *Human Relations in Administration: The Sociology of Organization* (Englewood Cliffs, N.J.: Prentice-Hall, Inc., 1951), p. 173.

Major theme summarized:

Major points in theory with definitions:

Strengths of theory:

Weaknesses of theory:

Examples of how this theory is used in health care at the present time:

Summary

This approach is not so much a theory as it is an explanation of reality—the best laid plans of mice and men, so to speak. It is a way for you to explain the problems that confront you each and every day in the running of an organization.

Again, we see the benefit of name-calling. Knowing the overlays—being aware of their existence—is not automatically going to solve your problems. Yet knowing the mechanisms at work in any large organization can give you the direction to follow for solutions. If, for instance, you have a power overlay in a department, you are able to see it for what it is. You know that the power center is there and that it must be dealt with. If you were not aware of the power center, you might be tempted to think that all the other staff members are ineffectual, and in need of dismissal. Alleviating the power center probably solves the problem with less trouble than dealing with the entire staff.

The functional overlay, as another example, can serve a very useful purpose. If a disaster team is working in your hospital, you see the use of a functional overlay. For the time that the disaster team is in operation, the person in charge of that team is the head of the pyramid. Questions and orders come not from the administrator, but from the head of the functional unit at work. When the work of the special unit is over, the pyramid shifts back into its normal position.

DISCUSSION QUESTION

1. For each overlay listed on page 215, give solutions to eliminate its presence.

THE NEO-CLASSICAL PERIOD OF MANAGEMENT: AN OVERVIEW

1. Give some key words that describe the general feeling of the Neo-Classical Period.

2. What are the advantages of this period as compared with Classical thinking?

3. What are the disadvantages of this period as compared with Classical thinking?

4. Which elements of Classical and Neo-Classical thinking could be combined to make a more workable management model?

NEO-CLASSICAL ORGANIZATION THEORY: A SUMMARY

In the 1920s, there was a strong movement away from the Classical theories and toward a newer, more humanistic management theory. This trend gave rise to the Neo-Classical organizational thought or the more "informal" structure in organization. Neo-Classical theorists objected to the classical "mechanistic prescriptions" for management. These theories developed out of the knowledge that, within every formal organization, there develops a system of informal organization or of social groups. The Neo-Classical Period was therefore one of psychological study and research. The formal structure of organization was discarded in favor of one more social or informal. All this study led to the conclusion that group solidarity and loyalty are associated with productivity, effectiveness, and job satisfaction.

The Neo-Classical Period stressed communication, the sharing of decision making, decentralization, and leadership rather than command. The most important statements made in the Neo-Classical Period were:

1. the most satisfying organization is the most efficient;
2. organizations are more satisfying if the needs of the worker are met; and
3. organizational goals and objectives must meet the goals and objectives of the individual worker, as well as those of the social groups formed within the organization.

The Classical theorists assumed that the most efficient organization is also the most satisfying one, because it maximizes both productivity and the employee's salary. The Neo-Classical theorists assumed that, as employees were made happier through the satisfaction of their social needs, their cooperation and efficiency would be all the greater. The basic contrast in the two theories is that Classical theory views people as economic entities and Neo-Classical theory views them as social entities.

MODERN ORGANIZATIONAL PRINCIPLES

The modern period of organizational thought is one of constant change. Every few years, a new theory comes into fashion, and its proponents claim another solution to all organizational problems. However, the one element that modern theories have in common is action. In the current thinking, management is thought of as a process, a flow, a flux. Administration is a moving, action-oriented set of behaviors.

The following management strategies are presented with the idea of giving you a feeling for the modern approach to management. This subject is so vast and requires such a great deal of study that you are asked only to learn the *basic* philosophy of each of the modern theories. The basic understanding of these modern theories enables you to picture the newest ways of accomplishing work through systematic organizational structures. Study the diagrams to see the movement of the organization toward goal achievement.

Although each organizational theory is presented and studied as an independent entity, you must be aware that all modern organizational theory is a blending of many concepts. For the supervisor studying management theory, modern principles must be viewed in this manner. Rather than learn and discuss each theory individually, try to see the modern period as an amalgamation of general concepts and processes. Worksheets are provided to help you organize your thinking, but your goal is to see the modern period as the sum of its parts, not as individual theories.

The Systems Approach

Every system is a part of a larger system, and each is itself made up of a hierarchy of subsystems, sub-subsystems, sub-sub-subsystems, and so on—each of which is a system in its own right. The molecule, the cell, the organ, the individual, the group, and the society are all examples of systems. Increasingly, organizations are viewed from a systems perspective. Accordingly, the modern organization is dominated by the systems approach, which, in turn, is itself a set of theories, analytical methods, and plans.[20]

The primary difference between an organization and a system is that the former has a goal or goals to accomplish. A nursing organization is a system since it relates both men and materials, as well as integrates them in a dynamic fashion in order to conduct the work of the system, goal attainment. Consequently our idea of an organization is changing from one of structure to one of process.

The systems approach offers five significant benefits to a health care organization:

1. a vehicle for permeating the organizational boundaries of an agency;
2. a way to deal with complexity;
3. a new perspective on organization;
4. a conceptual underpinning for an empirical tool (systems analysis and design); and
5. a potential fund of scientifically pragmatic information.[21]

Why should we consider organizations as systems? The first reason is the increasingly complex and frequent change in our society, which is evident in both our social relations and technological innovations. Further, such complex change is equally prevalent within the organization itself. The second reason is the limitation of the previously discussed organizational theories: That is, you cannot view an organization as a closed static system. An organization is continually dependent on its environment for the inflow of materials and human energy. Yet we often find supervisors coping with organizational problems as if they were independent of changes in the environment.

[20] Daniel Katz and Robert L. Kahn, *The Social Psychology of Organizations* (New York: John Wiley & Sons, Inc., 1966).
[21] Stanley Young, *Management: A Systems Approach* (Glenview, Ill.: Scott, Foresman & Company, 1967).

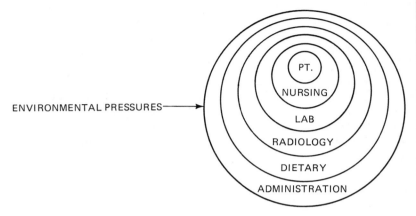

Figure 10–7. Systems approach to organization.

Second, the systems approach effectively helps us to cross boundaries to identify, establish, and make use of meaningful interrelationships between various organizations. Many health care agencies are becoming aware of the limitations of simplistic research. Problems in the sphere of health care, as in other fields, are seen more and more to exist within a broader system. In essence, it is an attempt to synthesize the research contributions of relevant fields into a single approach for the solving of a given problem. In terms of organization theory, therefore, the systems approach attempts to gather the necessary research information to construct a better organization.

Third, a systems approach provides us with a new perspective on the internal operations and environmental relationships of health care agencies, and it can result in a highly creative process. Its outcome is predominantly dependent on its users and on the resources on which they draw. Lastly, this approach is intended to be action-oriented.[22] (See Figure 10–7.)

PRINCIPLES OF ORGANIZATION

Organization theory:

Period:

[22] Paul M. Whisenand and R. Fred Ferguson, *The Managing of Police Organizations*, 2nd ed. (Englewood Cliffs, N.J.: Prentice-Hall, Inc., 1978), pp. 71–72.

Major theme summarized:

Major points in theory with definitions:

Strengths of theory:

Weaknesses of theory:

Examples of how this theory is used in health care at the present time:

OPEN SOCIAL SYSTEMS

The open social systems approach is a model that stimulates intuition and judgment. In contrast to a single scientific method, it extracts everything possible from existing scientific methods, and its virtues are therefore the virtues of those methods.

In the biological sciences, a systems theory is applied frequently in the study of plant and animal life at a variety of levels. In anthropology, the key element of analysis is cultural systems. In sociology, the concept of social systems is of crucial importance.

Research efforts, to date, offer considerable support for the use of an open social systems approach in analyzing health care agencies. A system is created wherever people or equipment perform a sequence of operations in a regular or predetermined order.

The open social system theory forms the distinctive qualities of modern organizational theory—its conceptual-analytical base, its devotion to empirical research data, its process orientation, and, most significantly, its integrating nature.

Social systems are contrived systems. Made by men, they are anchored in the needs, perceptions, attitudes, and motivations of human beings. Further, they form patterns of internal relationships for processing inputs into outputs. All open systems possess the following nine characteristics:[23]

[23] Katz and Kahn, *Social Psychology*, pp. 19–26.

1. *input*—takes material and ideas (input) from the environment;
2. *processing*—processes this information;
3. *output*—interprets and implements the information;
4. *cyclic character*—the product or service output furnishes the source of energy for an input and thus the repetition of cycle;
5. halting disorganization—open social systems process and store information to combat disorganization;
6. *information gathering*—to support feedback;
7. *stability*—a balance between organized structure and creative thought;
8. *specialization*—to achieve more accurate input; and
9. *equifinality*—they can reach the same final state from differing initial conditions and by a variety of paths.[24] (See Figure 10–8.)

In summary, the open social system's main focus is to view the organization as a system of interdependent relationships. The organization is viewed as a *process* that seeks to take an input and transform it into desirable results. All modern open social systems are comprised of five subsystems to accomplish work (Figure 10–9):

1. *operations*—to get work done;
2. *maintenance*—to train people and service machines;
3. *support*—to achieve good relationships;
4. *adaptation*—to achieve change; and
5. *management*—to control, direct, and coordinate the other systems.[25]

Figure 10–8. Equifinity: There is more than one way to reach a goal. The route doesn't matter; the goal is all that counts.

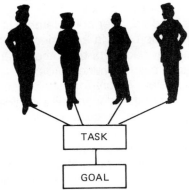

TASK

GOAL

[24] Katz and Kahn, pp. 19–26.
[25] *Ibid.*, pp. 39–44.

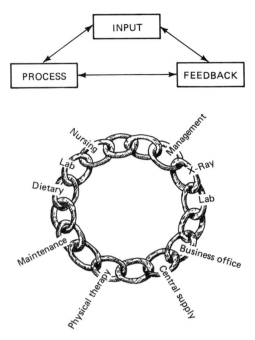

```
        ┌─────────┐
   ┌───▶│  INPUT  │◀───┐
   │    └─────────┘    │
   ▼                   ▼
┌─────────┐      ┌──────────┐
│ PROCESS │◀────▶│ FEEDBACK │
└─────────┘      └──────────┘
```

Figure 10–9. Open social systems. Each department in health care is one unit in a chain, joined for the organizational objective of providing patient care.

PRINCIPLES OF ORGANIZATION

Organization theory:

Period:

Major theme summarized:

Major points in theme with definitions:

223

Strengths of theory:

Weakness of theory:

Examples of how this theory is used in health care at the present time:

PROJECT ORGANIZATION

Highly technical industries have begun to utilize project organization when management decides to focus a great amount of talent and resources for a given period of time on a specific project goal. A project "team" of various specialists is put together under the direction of a project manager. In contrast to classical organization structures, there is a strong emphasis on direct horizontal relations between specialists: communication rarely goes up a scaler chain and back down.[26] (See Figure 10–10.)

Project organization offers greater flexibility and responsiveness to innovative ideas than the classical functional organization structure. There are some problems associated with its use, primarily role ambiguity for members of the team and the fact that the project manager must adopt a new approach to her job.[27]

Cleland and King point out that:

1. The project manager must become reoriented away from the purely functional approach to the management of human and nonhuman resources.

2. He or she must understand that a purposeful conflict may very well be a necessary way of life as the project is managed across many vertical organizational lines.

3. He or she must recognize that project management is a dynamic activity where major changes are almost the order of the day.[28]

These considerations make it clear that the project concept is not only a form of structural organization, but also a philosophy of management.[29]

[26] Beaufort Longest, Jr., *Management Practices for the Health Care Professional* (Reston, Va.: Reston Publishing Co., 1976), p. 116–119.

[27] Longest, p. 119.

[28] David I. Cleland and William R. King, *Systems Analysis and Project Management*, (New York: McGraw-Hill Book Company, 1968), p. 152.

224   [29] Longest, p. 119.

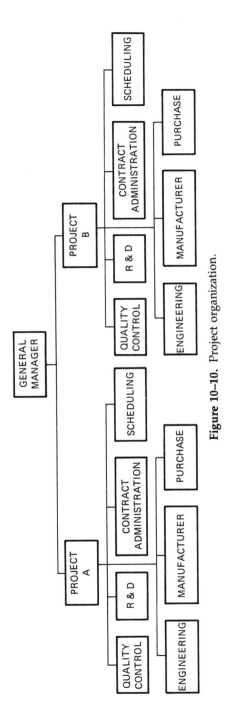

Figure 10–10. Project organization.

PRINCIPLES OF ORGANIZATION

Organization theory:

Period:

Major theme summarized:

Major points in theory with definitions:

Strengths of theory:

Weaknesses of theory:

Examples of how this theory is used in health care at the present time:

MATRIX ORGANIZATION

Superimposing project organization over the existing functional organization in most health care facilities results in *matrix organization*. It provides a horizontal, lateral dimension to the traditional vertical orientation of the functional organization.

Duncan Neuhauser has suggested that "hospitals can do this very easily (in fact, some already have). They do it by establishing patient care teams under the leadership of individual physicians for individual patients."[30] See Figure 10–11.

[30] Duncan Newhauser, "The Hospital as a Matrix Organization," *Hospital Administration* (Fall 1972), p. 19.

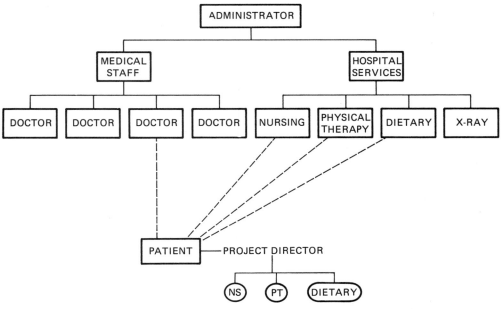

Figure 10–11. The hospital as a matrix organization. Several specialists join under a project director to provide their expertise for a specific patient. When the need for their services is no longer necessary for that patient, they return to the traditional pyramid structure. In this way, there is both vertical and horizontal organization.

Matrix organization incorporates some of the best aspects of project organization and functional organization. Its advantages may be summarized as follows:

1. The project (the care of a particular patient, for example) is emphasized by designating one individual as the focal point for all matters pertaining to that patient.

2. Utilization of manpower can be flexible because a reservoir of specialists is maintained in functional organizations.

3. Specialized knowledge is available to all programs on an equal basis; knowledge and experience can be transferred from one project to another.

4. Project people have a functional home when they are no longer needed on a given project.

5. Responsiveness to project needs (and patient needs) is generally faster because lines of communication are established and decision points are centralized.

227

6. Management consistency between projects can be maintained through the deliberate conflict operating in the project and the functional organizations.

7. A better balance among time, cost, and performance can be obtained through the built-in checks and balances and the continuous negotiations carried on between the project and the functional organizations.[31]

Note that the matrix organization concept does not do away with the classical organization structure—it simply builds and improves on it.

PRINCIPLES OF ORGANIZATION

Organization theory:

Period:

Major theme summarized:

Major points in theory with definitions:

Strengths of theory:

Weaknesses of theory:

Examples of how this theory is used in health care at the present time:

[31] Cleland and King, *Systems Analysis*, p. 172.

THE MODERN PERIOD
OF MANAGEMENT: AN OVERVIEW

1. Give some key words that describe the general feeling of the modern period.

2. Using the diagrams provided, try to fit your own health care agency into each of the four modes of organization.

3. For your particular health care setting, which of these models would be the most workable?

4. From outside sources, find out the basic definitions and ideas of at least two other modern management theories. Possible sources:

MODERN ORGANIZATIONAL
THEORY: A SUMMARY

Modern organization theory is concerned with developing an intentional structure of roles and relationships capable of carrying out the objectives of the organization. The goal is to relate all people and things within an organization to the goals of the organization. The modern period of organizational thought grew out of a human need for cooperation. It is essentially a blending of the Classical and Neo-Classical schools of thought to produce goal attainment through efficiency and employee satisfaction.

Studying the modern period of organizational design is difficult for several reasons:

1. The present intensified study of organizational design has produced many new and abstract concepts.
2. There is no valid statistical data to objectively compare the benefits of each design as they apply to health care.
3. The solution to the problem of organizational design has been sought by so many diversified groups that each has developed a language that is unique to that school of thought. At times, each group does not even agree on what constitutes "organizational design." March and Simon said it best: "The literature

leaves one with the impression that after all not a great deal has been said about organization, but it has been said over and over in a variety of languages."[32]

Modern organizational thought does not discard Classical and Neo-Classical thinking; it simply builds and improves on it. No set pattern of organization applies to every health care agency. Final goal achievement can be reached in a variety of ways. You, as a supervisor, can use a variety of ways to achieve organizational goals. The management process is not one of rigid solutions to problems, but rather one of a variety of satisfactory solutions to management problems.

REFERENCES

BERNSTEIN, P., "Workplace Democratization: Its Internal Dynamics," *Organization and Administration Sciences,* 7 (1976).

BRADFORD, L. AND D. MIAL, "When Is a Group?" *Educational Leadership,* 21 (1963).

CARTWRIGHT, D., AND A. ZANDER, *Group Dynamics: Research and Theory* New York: Harper and Row, Publishers, Inc., 1968.

HOMANS, GEORGE C., *The Human Group.* New York: Harcourt, Brace and Jovanovich, 1950.

MILLER, G., "Living Systems: The Group," *Behavioral Science,* 16 (1971).

MILLS, M., *The Sociology of Small Groups.* Englewood Cliffs, N.J.: Prentice-Hall, Inc., 1967.

REEVES, ELTON T., *The Dynamics of Group Behavior.* New York: American Management Association, Inc., 1970.

SCHEIN, E., *Organization Psychology,* 2nd ed. Englewood Cliffs, N.J.: Prentice-Hall, Inc., 1970.

SCHUTZ, W., "Interpersonal Underworld," *Harvard Business Review,* 36 1958.

---

[32] James G. March and Herbert A. Simon, *Organizations* (New York: John Wiley & Sons., Inc., 1958), p. 5.

11

The supervisor and group relations

THE STUDY OF GROUPS

Within any health care agency, the supervisor functions as a group leader and a coordinator of group behavior. Formal groups are established within an organization for a realistic division of labor and for a more organized work force. These formal groups are specifically formed by the management for the express purpose of accomplishing work. Usually these groups are well-established and their existence is known to all employees. The major function of a supervisor is to control these groups and to assist them in the accomplishment of work.

The supervisor must therefore understand group behavior because it has a major impact on the inner workings of the agency—that is, no goal can be reached without the cooperation of the individual members of the formal groups. This group behavior, a scientific phenomenon, can be studied as a consistent response to certain stimuli. With the increased complexity in health care delivery systems, health care agencies have become increasingly aware of the need to further divide the work force into more specialized groups. These groups are divided by function, the type of work done, the type of client served, and the actual function served. Without such division, the organization could not function as a smoothly running system to achieve the goal of patient care delivery. We are aware of the group's existence to provide for a subdivision of tasks, but we must completely understand the inner workings and activities occurring within the group. These activities are so consistent that they can be studied as a psychological basis for supervisory functions.

DEFINITION OF GROUPS

A *group* consists of a number of people who interact, who are aware of each other, who have common goals, and who perceive themselves as a group. The gathering of several people does not necessarily constitute a group. For example, a crowd sitting in a stadium watching a football game is not necessarily a group. Although this crowd has a common goal (watching a football game), they do not perceive themselves as a group, and they have limited interaction. They are not a group. Yet suppose a member of the crowd suddenly suffers a heart attack in the stands. As the members of the crowd gather around this person and begin to administer first aid and to seek help for the stricken person, they would become a group. They are now interacting, they are aware of each other, they have the common goal of helping the person, and they perceive themselves as a group working together to achieve a goal. This immediate formation of a group causes the group members to become mutually aware, and the cohesiveness of the group begins to form.

This cohesiveness would be seen if, for example, the paramedics asked the group members to leave the area. The group would respond, not as individuals, but as members of a group, and they may be hesitant to leave the victim. What might be considered to be morbid curiosity is really a response to the threat of breaking up the group. Long after the patient has been transferred to the hospital, the group members cling to the ties that originally bound them and continue to discuss the situation. They may even go as a unit to the hospital to visit the victim. This is "group" behavior.

The size of a group varies with the purpose of the group. A group may be two people, or it may be one hundred people. The size is determined by the amount of mutual interaction and by the level of awareness of each other as members of the group.

In the health care setting all members of the organization or agency as a whole may not be considered a group. They have a common goal, but, in a large agency, they are not mutually aware of each other and do not all communicate. In the individual units, the formal groups are formed.

There are two main classifications of groups: (1) formal and (2) informal.

Formal Groups

Formal groups are established by the organization and exist for a specific purpose. The characteristics of a formal group are as follows:

1. The group has a leader.
2. It has followers.

3. Rules and regulations govern group behavior.
4. The group has assigned tasks.
5. The group is aware of the specific duties to be performed by the group.
6. The organization expects a standard of performance.
7. There are rewards and punishments for adherence or for the lack of adherence to group rules. These are tangible, and they are known to all members of the group.

As a supervisor, you are concerned with these groups, but their functions are well established and well-known. The task of supervising these groups is simply one of coordination and direction. Keeping the lines of communication open and firmly following the organizational structure assure smooth operation of these formal groups.

Informal Groups

Within the formal groups, smaller and less structured groups form. These "informal" groups exist not to meet the organizational goals, but to meet the needs of the individuals within the organization. The health care agency is not responsible for the creation of these groups, and it has no formal control over their activities. The informal group has these characteristics:

1. The group has a leader.
2. It has followers.
3. Informal or unwritten rules regulate the conduct of group members.
4. The group exists for a purpose, and group members have specific tasks to perform. These tasks may not be firmly established, or written, but they are important to the group, and they are followed.
5. Members expect a certain level of group behavior. Again, this expectation is not written, but it is well-known.
6. There are rewards for following group norms in the form of group approval.
7. There are punishments for not following these norms in the form of peer pressure, and possible exclusion from the group.
8. The norms for the group are usually more strictly followed than the norms for a formal group because they are set up by the group.

In health care, these groups exist, and they must be handled and understood as an integral part of the organization. Supervisors have no control over their formation, but they do have some control

233

over their behavior. The groups are usually formed to fill a specific need in the staff, and these groups are very powerful. Most work that is accomplished in the organization is because of the work of these formal and informal groups. The supervisor who is knowledgable and informed on group behavior is better able to relate to these groups and to coordinate the efforts of both formal and informal groups in accomplishing work.

Since we are familiar with the formal groups and their function and activity in health care, we will limit our discussion to the informal groups formed within the organizational structure.

The Functions of Informal Groups

Informal groups are formed to fill a need that is not met by the organization. For example, they may be formed to meet the social needs of the staff; the group that meets for coffee break, lunch, and after-work social activities is meeting for the express purpose of interaction and pleasure. This is a very cohesive group, and a threat to one member becomes a threat to the entire group. There are many other names for "groups," including some that carry a negative connotation. Groups may be referred to as clubs, teams, subunits, and cliques—whatever their name, the effects are the same. Groups always exist; they are inevitable. There is no way to stop their formation. The groups are mobilizing forces. Work is accomplished by the social or informal group. Groups produce both good and bad consequences. If you, the supervisor, know the groups and their behavior, you can enhance the good behaviors and decrease the negative consequences.

Informal groups serve the function of giving the individual a social identification. In a large organization, the individual worker may be lost in the shuffle. Becoming a member of an informal group assures the staff member that he or she is important and belongs to the group. The social group bridges the gap between the individual worker and the organization. The social group gives the worker a greater sense of identity and greater control over working conditions. One person can do little to change the organization's structure or rules and regulations. A group, on the other hand, can unite and accomplish much more. This unification gives the worker strength and an improved self-image.

How Groups Are Formed

Formal groups are formed by the organization to achieve the organizational objectives. The organization divides the work and establishes formal work groups to accomplish the tasks. In a sense, they establish who works with whom. The assignment of a staff member to a unit or department is a simple example of a formal group formation.

Group assignment by the organization sets the framework for the formation of informal groups. Once the formal work groups are established, the social units develop to fulfill the unmet needs of the individual. No one works in a vacuum, and no person wants to feel that they are a "work unit" in an organization. Because human beings want to derive more than financial rewards from working, they make friends and have a certain level of social interaction to make their professional duties more enjoyable. The relationships that develop may enhance the organizational goals, or they may detract from them. A smoothly functioning, cohesive work group that enjoys working together because of the social interactions present generally assumes greater responsibilities and is more efficient. A social group that is more concerned with their personal needs than the needs of the organization is nonproductive. As a supervisor, you are aware of the inefficiency of a group that enjoys "coffee breaks" more than the tasks of the agency.

In any organization, individuals may belong to more than one group at a time. The formal groups—of permanent shift assignment, of department assignment, and the like—are groups to which every member of the organization belongs. At times the organization may also form temporary formal groups such as committees, task forces, study groups, and classes. Individual staff members may belong to one of these temporary work groups in addition to their basic assigned work group. In addition to belonging to the formal work groups, the members may belong to one or more informal groups. They may have friendships, club memberships, or just relationships formed because of similiar work situations or assignments.

When persons belong to both formal and informal groups and to numerous groups in each division, they are subject to many stresses. The norms of one group may be in direct conflict to the expectations of another. Members may feel torn in their loyalties between groups. Usually, individuals adhere to the norms and wishes of the informal group if it is in conflict with the norms of the organization. Since each informal group sets its own goals and norms of expected behaviors, the group may act differently from the way the organization wishes. The peer pressure is so strong that the organization has trouble changing the goals of the informal group.

If you control the informal groups, you will succeed. Informal groups formed for social relationships form with or without approval from the agency itself. The goals of the supervisor are to control the informal groups and to try to merge their goals with those of the organization.

Types of Informal Groups

There are three basic types of informal groups:

1. horizontal groups,
2. vertical groups, and
3. random or outside groups.

HORIZONTAL GROUPS These groups are composed of members who have the same work area, the same job level, and basically the same work assignments. They are usually formed just because of the physical makeup of the organization. People who consistently work together and who do the same tasks eventually make social relationships that are independent of the formal structure.

VERTICAL GROUPS These groups are composed of members who are on different hierarchal levels. They may consist of the special friendships or relationships between a superior and a subordinate. They have little to do with the formal chain of command. They fulfill the social needs of both staff and supervision. The communication between these groups is more informal and does not follow the established communication system.

RANDOM GROUPS These groups are formed to serve functions not served by the organization. They may be composed of members of the organization, or they may be outside groups. These are social groups, clubs, or units within the health care agency, or they may be church, social, community, or political groups outside the agency. These groups influence the behavior of their members more than any other type of group, because the members *choose* to belong to these groups and because their membership is contingent on conditions set by the social group. Commonly, the members of a social group feel conflict between their group commitments and the organizational requirements. A staff member request for a specific day off or for special consideration to meet family or social commitments is an example of conflicting values between formal and informal group membership.

The supervisor must be aware of the pressures and of the influence that informal groups exert on people. Allowing flexibility in the work situation to assist groups members to fill all their needs means greater job satisfaction and increased efficiency. Simply discounting any outside activities only serves to strengthen the ties to the informal group and builds up a hostile feeling in the employee. You must recognize the importance of these social relationships, and encourage staff members to have a satisfying social life, while still carrying out their professional responsibilities. You, too, are engaged in this conflict between your professional and your social needs, and you should be able to feel empathy toward your staff.

Informal Group Dynamics

The individual group members bring to the group their personal needs and desires. These needs are integrated into the goals of the group and become the overall group objectives. Each of the members receives personal satisfaction from belonging to the group, which meets many personal needs such as: the need to belong, the need for self-determination or self-esteem, the need for self-expression, the need for value expression, and the need to demonstrate and assert one's own personality. These are very important to the development of a well-rounded and totally integrated person, and allowing the social group to meet these needs enhances the individual's contribution to the organization.

The informal group can integrate the individual's personal and organizational goals through the use of group discussion of problems, feedback on decision-making situations, support and reinforcement, and the sharing of rewards and punishments. To work most efficiently with groups, the supervisor must decrease the organizational power and authority and give more power and influence to the informal groups.

The informal group fills a need for conformity function in the individual. The informal group exerts great pressure on its individual members to conform to the group's norms. No matter how "independent" a person is, he or she conforms in some way to one informal group or another. It may just be the family group or friends who also believe in nonconformity, but, whatever the group, the individual conforms. As a general rule, groups that require more-than-average conformity are more attractive. The club that is costly, that has strong rules and regulations, that has strict requirements for membership, and that limits its membership is more highly sought than the group that has little conformity or group identity. If the membership in the group is very desirable, the members change their goals and behaviors to conform to the group norms. Hence the pressure of the group can be enough to change the views of one of its members. This conformity function is not necessarily bad; it sometimes performs the function of keeping staff members united toward a common desirable goal.

The informal group also provides the occasion for motivation. Allowing the group to accomplish organizational goals through the use of participatory supervision encourages them to use creativity and innovation in the accomplishment of these goals. This group motivation increases job commitment and job satisfaction. Workers no longer work because the organization expects them to do so; they work because it fulfills their needs and increases their sense of belonging to a group. Supervisors do not erode their authority by allowing group influence; they enhance it.

Group Problems

As a supervisor dealing with groups, you should be aware of the common problems associated with groups. These occur frequently, and the alert leader recognizes them as "group" problems, not as individual problems. The solution comes only in dealing with the group as a whole, not one individual.

MISGUIDED GROUP LOYALTY   Many times members of the group do not admit the existence of problems or errors because they feel a sense of loyalty not to the organization, but to their informal group. The group's objectives and the organization's objectives are not the same, and the individuals feel that they should protect the autonomy of the group.

The solution to this problem can be achieved only by understanding the motivation of the group and by attempting to reach some compromise in the value systems of the group and of the organization. However, no members of any group should be allowed to compromise the goals of the organization because of their informal relationships. The group members must be counseled so they realize that the organizational goals are paramount, and that you may allow no deviation from the primary purpose of the health care agency. If a change in procedure or a modification of policy is possible and if it does not change the basic position of the agency, a compromise may be possible. Trying to discipline the group member who is in error or who refuses to reveal an error, only results in stronger group unity and further covering up of situations. At the first indication of this misguided loyalty, the entire group must be approached to reach a solution.

GROUP SELF-CENTEREDNESS   If the group is a very cohesive one and if it is able to accomplish much work, the members may feel that their interests are the only ones necessary to consider. At organizational meetings these people may be only concerned with satisfying their own needs, at the expense of other areas in the agency. Self-centeredness— where one department is concerned only with obtaining funding and equipment for itself—is a common occurrence in the hospital setting. The department's members see no need to share resources or staff with other areas of the hospital. This group has lost sight of the overall objectives of the organization.

The structure of the agency must be explained in detail, and this group must be made to see that they are only a part of the team that provides patient care services. Allowing this group to participate in budgeting and planning operations makes them feel more accountable to the organization as a whole, and it may take away some of the self-centered feeling. In this situation, dealing only with the leader of the group does not satisfy the group's needs. The leader might be convinced of the agency's general plan and of the need for sharing of resources, but he or she may not convey this to the group. The group then feels cheated and may refuse to participate. You should take the time to go to the group members and explain the policy of the agency. Never let this responsibility be delegated to the group leader. In routine matters, this step may not be necessary, but for critical or important decisions the group must be told of the agency position by the supervisor.

AGGRESSIVE GROUP BEHAVIOR   A group may consist of many members with very militant feelings about the organization or other groups. If these feelings become the tone of the group, there can be many problems. The group may begin an attack on the agency and undermine the organizational structure. Constantly degrading, belittling, or criticizing the management can result only in hostility. With this aggressive behavior, no work can be accomplished, and the group destroys the organization. The supervisor should be alert for the signs of an aggressive group: backbiting, criticism, gossip, stealing, and lying. If these symptoms are detected, the supervisor must go to the group and try to ascertain the reason for these behaviors.

One reason for this aggression is frustration. If the health care agency is not responding to the needs of the group, or if it is unwilling to accept any suggestions from the group, they respond with aggression. Being open and approachable does much to eliminate this problem. If changes can be made, they should be made quickly before the aggression gets out of hand.

Another reason for aggressive behavior is fear. If the group feels that it is in danger of losing its identity, it responds with hostility. Changing the working areas of many of the group members or scheduling the group on different shifts makes the group feel threatened, and they respond with aggression. Giving the established group a new leader or a new procedure without allowing them to prepare for the change also increases their level of fear. Try to institute any change in the group behavior slowly, with respect for the feelings of the group. If you detect any resistance, discuss the situation with the group members and attempt to resolve differences before they become major problems.

GROUP RUMOR SPREADING   One of the major problems in group behavior is the spreading of gossip or rumors. This is not necessarily hostile or aggressive behavior. The main reason that group members spread unfounded rumors is that they are, in fact, uninformed on an issue.

239

Each group within the organization wants to feel important. The group feels important when it possesses "inside" information of the workings of the organization. If they do not actually know what is going on, they fabricate a story to gain the attention and approval of other groups. Every person wants to know what is going on in the organization at all times. The group is then the primary transmitter of information.

The elimination of all gossip or rumor is impossible. The only solution to the situation is to make sure that the information that is passed is accurate. Keeping all members of all groups informed on the changes and decisions made by the agency management helps to prevent the circulation of false or inaccurate information. If you hear some rumor or gossip that is untrue, immediately trace the source of the information and deal with the group responsible for the initiation of the gossip. Discuss the situation with the group, and see if the rumor was started because they did not possess the accurate reports. If so, clear up the inaccuracy, and caution the group against spreading false rumors. Impress the group with the danger of spreading inaccurate information, and enlist their support in curtailing the spread of gossip.

INTRA-GROUP COMPETITION AND CONFLICT   In some instances, intra-group competition can stimulate the overall effectiveness of the organization. Healthy competition between groups may motivate them to achieve their maximum effectiveness. An example may be setting a goal for contributions to the United Fund or hospital building fund and allowing the groups to compete for a prize given to the unit that donates the most money. This sort of competition can be done in a spirit of fun, and the groups may become very enthusiastic about such projects.

In most cases, though, intra-group competition should be avoided. The groups usually view competition as a threat to the autonomy; because they resent the competition, conflict results. You should try to keep intra-group competition to a minimum by allowing each group to maintain its own identity and by separating each group's functions so that none are ever in direct competition. Increasing the contact between the groups and maintaining free communication in the agency also helps to avoid competition. If each group feels that its contributions are important and necessary to the overall effectiveness of the organization, competition is minimized. Never compare one group to another by words or actions. Set standards of behavior and performance for each unit or group individually, and have the group try to achieve their own goals, without comparison to other groups.

If intra-group competition and conflict have reached a point that they are interfering with work accomplishment, the only solution is to separate the group by rotating its members. This solution causes some emotional reaction, but it is easier to deal with than the anger and hostility caused by competition.

INTER-GROUP COMPETITION   With competition within the group usually comes a power struggle for leadership. If factions with conflicting goals develop within a group, the group begins to divide. In a social group, usually the solution is to let the group members work out these problems for themselves. If the problem is a major one, the group dissolves or divides. Thus the problem is eliminated, because a social group exists only if it serves a purpose for *all* its members, and individuals do not remain in a group if it does not meet their needs. The peer pressure is so strong that the group polices its own internal conflict.

When formal work units are in conflict, you must do something to resolve the conflict. As the group begins to divide, perceptions become distorted, and communications decrease. The members feel a real threat, and the work of the agency is affected. If a solution cannot be reached through mediation and discussion, you must dissolve the group by transfer or by the threat of discipline. There is no room in the health care industry for internal conflict, and small problems must be curtailed before they develop into open warfare. If two members are engaged in a power struggle, you may have to be the one to decide who should retain control of the group. Remember, the goal of supervision is to guide and direct the activities of others to achieve organizational goals. You cannot let the feelings or emotions of a group situation affect your handling of the problem. Step in as soon as you see that the group is unable to solve the problem, and make use of your authority. Impress on the group that you will not tolerate conflict and that, if they cannot solve their own problems, you will take action. If the group feels that it will lose its identity if you use your authority to transfer or discipline group members, they may take steps to resolve their differences without your help.

WORKING WITH GROUPS

The supervisor who understands group formation and behavior is better able to deal with the behavior of groups. The goal of working with groups is to achieve the degree of control necessary to allow the groups to exist and serve the needs of the individual, while accomplishing work toward the organizational objectives. As the level of cooperation between groups increases, the agency becomes more unified. Encouraging communication within and between groups eliminates most problems. The participation of group members in the planning of agency policy and procedure also fosters a feeling of worth and belonging, and it enables you to work with the groups, not against them. You must be aware of the 'groups', of their members, and of their leaders (formal and informal). Knowing the usual pattern of behavior for any particular group aids you in providing tasks that are consistent with the image that the group has of itself. Try not to deviate from the established group patterns, and allow the group members the freedom to control and direct the activities within their own group.

The existence of groups is inevitable. The best supervisors know how to function within the group system, and they are able to identify and correct problems before they affect the health care agency.

GROUP DECISION MAKING

In the health care industry most decision making is done as a group procedure. Rarely is a decision left to one individual without the need for group consultation. As a supervisor, you know the many meetings that you are expected to attend, as well as the many groups within which you interact. Since so much time is spent in the process of group decision making, understanding the interactions within these groups is very important.

Some people believe that working in groups is frustrating. This belief is not necessarily justified. Real creativity and cooperation can emerge if the group is given the freedom to act independently. Group decision making does not breed conformity. In actual practice, groups tend to make riskier decisions because they have the moral support of an entire group. Since no one individual has to take the blame for an error in the decision-making process, the group can "take" a change. We all participate in groups every day, and each day decisions are made in these groups. Rarely do we take the time to analyze why we behave the way we do or why group members behave as they do. Only through the thorough study of issues and personalities at work in groups can we make generalizations about group decision making. Understanding the dynamics of decision making in groups helps you to make better decisions and aids you in knowing yourself and your staff.

Observation of Group Decision Making

If you stood back and watched a group attempting to make a decision, you would consistently see two issues at work in the groups:

1. *Task Issues:* These statements and comments are directly concerned with accomplishing the work of the group. Also called "content issues," they are the reason for the group meetings. Statements such as, "Well, we could change to a flexible schedule," or, "If she replaced the staff nurse for her lunch break, . . ." are task or content statements. They refer directly to the subject at hand.
2. *Process Issues:* These issues relate to how the group is going to work to achieve the task goal. Process issues consist of the action or the movement of the group to initiate or to continue the

decision-making process. Process statements would be: "Should we vote on it?" . . . "I think that everyone should say what he thinks, and then we will discuss all the ideas," or the like.

Observing the task and process issues in a group gives a supervisor valuable clues to the group's personalities. Sitting back and quietly observing teaches you more about your staff than any number of one-to-one conferences. The alert supervisor can judge the prospects of successful completion of the decision-making task merely by watching the interaction of the group. One subtle clue, for example, is the interjection of a comment such as, "The last group we had was wonderful." This remark may be a person's way of expressing unhappiness with the way the process is going and disagreement with the decision being made. It is less threatening to talk about what happened before (past history) than it is to discuss what is happening at the present meeting.

Some other areas to observe in group activity are the communication patterns and the method of reaching consensus.

The communication pattern is easy to watch. Who talks to whom? Who controls the conversation? Who is the unofficial leader? Who constantly interrupts? Who is silent and contributes nothing? Who do people look at when they talk? All these questions are important if you are to understand the behavior of your group in action. Each one is an important clue to the relationships in the group. Understanding these relationships assists you in leading the group.

The method of actually making the decision or of reaching a consensus is also important. Did one person "railroad" the decision? Did the group vote? Did one faction coerce another faction? Observe and record this information to better understand your group. Remember that once the group decision is made, it is very hard to undo. It is now a group project, and more than one person is emotionally committed to the decision. If the decision is to be changed, you have to deal with the feelings and emotions of each and every member of the group.

Behaviors in the Group

A group can be observed according to the behaviors that it consistently demonstrates in its activity. Three such behaviors are always present in any group activity. Ideally they should balance out for successful group decisions. The behaviors are:

1. task behavior,
2. maintenance behavior, and
3. self-oriented behavior.

TASK BEHAVIOR   Persons who demonstrate task behavior are displaying behavior directly concerned with accomplishing the task. They are con-

243

cerned with getting the job done. They may be initiating discussion, seeking opinions, clarifying issues, summarizing, or taking consensus.

MAINTENANCE BEHAVIOR   These persons are concerned with the relationships in the group. They are the "oil" in the group. Their activity is usually directed toward improving or patching up a relationship, harmonizing, encouraging, or compromising.

SELF-ORIENTED BEHAVIOR   Whereas task and maintenance behaviors are concerned with getting the job done, self-oriented behavior is directed toward impeding or changing the process of the group. Persons who display self-oriented behaviors disturb the work of the group and cannot be ignored. For some personal reason, these individuals must engage in an activity that calls attention to themselves, and this need usually disrupts the work of the group. A leader must understand the reasons behind this behavior and attempt to channel this energy into the work of the group.

Some examples of self-oriented behavior are: talking or laughing with a neighbor, telling long and boring stories, making smart remarks, blowing smoke rings at the ceiling, doodling, clearing of throats, asking for statements to be constantly repeated, and nodding or silently making some indication of agreement or disagreement.

When self-oriented behavior is demonstrated in a group situation, the leader's responsibilities are to evaluate the reasons behind the behavior and to eliminate the need for the protective self-oriented behavior. Causes of self-oriented behavior are usually problems having to do with:

1. identity,
2. control and power,
3. goals, and
4. acceptance.

IDENTITY   Certain members of the group may wish to call attention to themselves because they feel that they have no identity in the group. These members are unsure of their role in the group situation or of their expected behavior in the group. Because of this identity problem, they use self-oriented behavior to call attention to themselves; in effect, they say, "Look at me. I'm here."

CONTROL   If a group member feels that he or she is losing control of the group or does not have the desired power in the group, that person may try to obtain control or power through the use of self-oriented behavior.

GOALS   If the goals of the group are not the same as the goals of an individual member, the discrepancy sometimes causes self-oriented behavior. The group member may either disagree with the group goals or lose all interest in the project. Rather than leave the group or ignore its working, such individuals may choose to try steering the group away from the original goals and toward that member's desired objectives. The member's objectives may be simply to meet for a social chat, and so he or she may use humor or other distracting behaviors to control the group.

ACCEPTANCE   A member of the group who is unsure of his or her acceptance in the group may try various ways to gain the group's approval. It may be through monopolizing the conversation or by telling jokes to "make everyone like him".

Ways to Eliminate Self-Oriented Behavior

The best way to eliminate self-oriented behavior is to understand and to eliminate its cause. Dealing with the specific behavior itself does not accomplish your goals because, even if the person conforms to the group standards, the underlying cause of the self-oriented behavior is still present. The needs of the individual are not being met.

THE PROBLEM OF IDENTITY   If a member of the group demonstrates self-oriented behavior because of an identity problem, assure the person that he or she does indeed belong to the group. The first approach is to use the person's name and ask for an opinion or statement: "Bill, do you have something to offer?" This is a perfect way to stop the self-oriented behavior and get the group working together. Usually the member stops the behavior and may even offer something of value to the group's operation. The most important thing to remember is to use the person's name: Bill's problem is identity, and sometimes just acknowledging that you know his name and that you will call on him is enough to eliminate the self-oriented behavior.

THE PROBLEM OF CONTROL AND POWER   If one member of the group feels threatened by your power as the leader and wishes to take control of the group, that person can cause serious problems. The best way to handle the situation is to analyze why the person wants the control. Is the group headed in a direction opposed to that person's point of view? Is your control too directed and structured to suit the member's needs? Is there a personality conflict between you and that member? Whatever the reason, you must know why there is a power struggle, and then eliminate it. One way to decrease this power conflict is to allow active

245

participation in the group process, while decreasing your own control of the group. If the group feels that everyone's ideas and opinions are important and that you are the moderator rather than the leader, the power struggles are lessened.

THE PROBLEM OF GOALS   Before the start of the group meeting, you have likely established mutual goals for the group. If not, the individual members will be unsure about why they are meeting and may not focus on the purpose of the meeting and accomplish work. If only one member has conflicting goals, you must deal with that person. If an attendee is bored and not interested in the task, and if you cannot stimulate interest in the group project, the best solution is to eliminate that member: "Jane, obviously you are not interested in working on this project, perhaps you should go back to the unit." Most of the time, this tactic is not necessary. A simple reminder of the reason for the meeting usually stops the self-oriented behavior: "Betty, the recipe sounds delicious, but we are here to decide a departmental policy. Perhaps, you could discuss that on your own time."

THE PROBLEM OF ACCEPTANCE   For members new to the group, taking the time to introduce each and every member to the new persons usually gives the needed acceptance and group intimacy. If you are introducing new members, take the time to tell something special about them. This technique makes them feel that they are important and that you value their contribution to the group: "Bill is here from Boston Memorial where he set up a primary care unit. He is very knowledgeable on the subject, and we look forward to his input."

If regular staff members suddenly feel that they do not belong or that the group does not like or accept them, you must look to the past history of the group and see if that feeling is indeed justified. Are all the members' ideas discounted? Do they have difficulty gaining the floor? These are questions that help you to assess the validity of their feelings and to deal with their feelings. Praise and genuine emotional support do much to give group members a feeling of belonging.

If you, as the leader, are able to analyze the reasons behind the self-oriented behavior, you will be ready to deal with these behaviors and eliminate them. The exhibition of self-oriented behavior impedes group work, and you must take immediate steps to keep the group working together toward the common goal.

Types of Group Behavior

Whatever the reason for self-oriented behavior, it represents a person's way of dealing with an increased level of tension or anxiety. Each person has a different way of dealing with these emotions, and the astute leader can identify the basic ways of displaying them. Three types of emotional behavior result from tension and from the attempt to resolve the underlying problems:

1. *Tough emotions*: This reaction involves the display of anger, hostility, self-assertiveness. The group member may fight with the others, try to control the others, use a loud and demanding voice, or argue every minute detail to death.
2. *Tender emotions:* This behavior is demonstrated by a desire to agree, to help to make friends with the others, to side with one group or another, to be overtly friendly to the group members.
3. *Denying any emotions:* Members may withdraw from the group and refuse to participate, or they may use "logic" or "reason" to explain every action. In effect, they are saying, "I don't have to become emotionally involved in this, because I can logically show the reasons behind my opinions." They hide behind the knowledge or logic that they possess to cover their own feelings.

Corresponding to their types of reactions, individuals have different styles of reducing tension and of expressing emotion. Three "pure types" have been identified:

1. *The "sturdy battler" orientation:* Acceptance of tough emotions and denial of tender emotions—the "Let's-fight-it-out" type of person. The sturdy battler can deal with hostility, but not with love, support, and affiliation.
2. *The "friendly helper":* Acceptance of tender emotions and denial of tough emotions. This "let's-not-fight-let's-help-each-other" type person can give and receive affection, but cannot tolerate hostility and fighting.
3. *The "logical thinker":* Denial of all emotions—"Let's reason this thing out." Cannot deal with tender or tough emotions, shuts eyes and ears to things going on.

These are the "pure types." No one is completely one way or another, but each has a blend of all types. As a leader, you must understand which "person" is speaking and respond to that stress personality. You must understand that friendly helpers achieve their desired world of warmth and intimacy only by allowing conflicts and differences to be raised and resolved. They find that they can become close with people only if they can accept what is dissimilar as well as what is similar in their behavior. Tough battlers achieve their world of toughness, conflict, and free expression only if they can create a climate of warmth and trust in which these are allowed to develop. Logical thinkers achieve their world of understanding and logic only if they can accept that their feelings and the feelings of others are also facts, and that they make an

247

TABLE 11–1
Three bests of all possible worlds

FRIENDLY HELPERS	STURDY BATTLERS	LOGICAL THINKERS
Love	Conflict	Logic
	Task Maintenance Behavior	
Harmonizing	Initiating	Gathering information
Compromising	Coordinating	Systematizing
Encouraging	Pressing for results	Evaluating
	Methods of Influence	
Appeasing	Giving orders	Rules and regulations
Appealing to pity	Offering challenges	Logic
	Threatening	Facts
	Personal Threats	
They will not be loved.	Lose power	The world is not orderly.
They will be overwhelmed by hostility.	Become "soft"	They will be overwhelmed by love or hostility.

important contribution toward their ability to understand interpersonal situations. (See Table 11–1.) Ideally, the three styles can be shown as corners of a triangle, with the well-balanced person fitting right in the middle. (See Figure 11–1.)

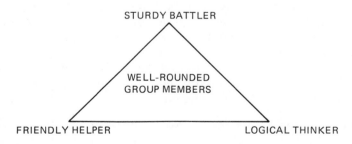

Figure 11–1. The "well-rounded" triangle.

CONCLUSIONS

The successful supervisor understands the importance of groups and of understanding group behavior. You cannot "wish" away personal conflicts. These conflicts must be met and dealt with for a smoothly running organization. Understanding the reasons behind behavior is more important than merely keeping the group on the right track. You must know why the group is not on the right track. In the well-functioning group, no one person should take responsibility for maintenance of the group. The entire group should actively participate in the group's objectives. Groups that ignore the individual emotions and feelings of the members may meet several times for the same issue, and they may still be unable to make a decision. Good group function ensures sound decisions and committed members. Teamwork needs practice, but the results are worth the effort.

DISCUSSION QUESTIONS

1. What is the difference between "formal groups" and "informal groups"?
2. How do "informal groups" develop?
3. Why is it so important for a supervisor to learn group behavior?
4. In a conflict between the member's "formal group" membership and "informal group" membership, which wins? Why?
5. Why do people become members of groups? What functions do the groups serve?
6. Make a list of all the "formal" and "informal" groups to which you belong. Include both professional and private groups.

APPLICATION: GROUP DECISION-MAKING EXERCISE

Objectives

- To introduce the supervisor to the group processes
- To practice the techniques of group observation
- To learn to control detrimental group or individual behaviors.

Directions

1. Divide into pairs.
2. Make concentric rings.
3. One partner sits in the ring; the other sits behind the first to observe his or her behavior.
4. The partner who is participating in the group does either task A or task B.
5. Observers rate the group and especially the partner's behavior. (See Table 11–2.)
6. Observers do not talk.
7. Be especially alert for task-, maintenance-, or self-oriented behavior. (See Table 11–3 for a summary guide of these behaviors.)
8. When task A is completed, partners switch and do task B.

249

TABLE 11–2
Observer rating form

DIMENSION	OBSERVATIONS (BEHAVIORS THAT LED YOU TO MAKE THE OBSERVATIONS YOU DID)*	IMPACT ON GROUP OR INDIVIDUAL
Communication pattern		
Decision-making procedures		
Task behavior		
Maintenance behavior		
Self-oriented behavior		
Types of emotional styles (sturdy battler, friendly helper, logical thinker)		
Content versus process issues		

* It is extremely important when giving another person feedback (sharing observations) that you be able to point to *specific behaviors* that led you to make your observations.

TABLE 11–3
Application: Group decision making

I. Group Decision making
  A. Issues at work
    1. Task or content issues—the reason the group is meeting.
    2. Process issues—how the group works to achieve the task.
II. Task, maintenance, and self-oriented behavior
  A. Task-oriented behavior
    1. Person concerned with getting the job done. Seeks opinions, initiates, clarifies, summarizes, takes concensus.
  B. Maintenance behavior
    1. Person trying to improve or patch up some relationship.
    2. Constantly tries to harmonize, encourage, compromise.
  C. Self-oriented behavior
    1. The person is trying to meet some personal need or goal without regard to the group's problem.
    2. May try to be humorous, silly, angry, and so on.
III. Three pure types
  A. Sturdy battler—acceptance of tough emotions and denial of tender emotions. "Let's fight it out." Can deal with hostility, but not with love.
  B. Friendly helper—acceptance of tender emotions. "Let's not fight, let's help each other." Cannot tolerate fighting.
  C. Logical thinker—denial of emotion. "Let's reason this thing out." Shuts eyes and ears to much that is going on.

Task A

Rank the following items in terms of their importance for improving the effectiveness of organizations. Place number 1 by the most important item, number 2 by the next most important item, and so on down to 10, which represents the least important consideration. Make your rankings in terms of organizations in general. You must come up with one set of rankings that reflects the group's consensus.

_____ Create conditions so that employees can participate in making decisions that vitally affect them.

_____ Develop early retirement programs to weed out people in the older-age categories who are nonproductive.

_____ Give craft, technical, or social skill training to improve skills at all levels.

_____ Expand personal contact between top management and the rest of the organization.

_____ Fill jobs on qualifications rather than by seniority.

_____ Improve the incentive system for nonsupervisory personnel.

_____ Institute a regular replacement hiring program.

_____ Discharge all poor performance personnel, including supervisors.

_____ Stress feedback in communication programs.

_____ Put key categories of employees on merit salary.

Task B

Rank the following items in terms of their importance in selecting a middle manager, such as department head, who is effective in making and carrying out decisions. Place number 1 by the most important item, number 2 by the next most important item, and so on down to 10, which represents the least important consideration. You must come up with one set of rankings that reflects the group's consensus.

_____ Able to grasp the structure of the organization quickly and to use it effectively.

_____ Able to give clear-cut instructions.

_____ Keeps all parties who are concerned with a decision fully informed on progress and final actions.

_____ Able to change own conclusions when they prove to be wrong.

_____ Goes about decision making by developing a range of alternatives before coming to a final verdict.

_____ Able to grasp instructions and to act appropriately in terms of them.

_____ Capable of making fast decisions under time and other pressures.

_____ Able to delegate effectively.

_____ Capable of seeing appropriate relations among a variety of items.

_____ Able to resist shaping an opinion before all the facts are in.

DISCUSSION QUESTIONS

1. What kinds of things seemed to help each group perform the task? What inhibited?
2. Did either group talk about how they were going to do the task (process)?
3. How did it feel to be in each role?
4. What observations did you make?
5. Were there any self-oriented behaviors? How did the group react?
6. How did the friendly helper affect—or was he or she affected by—the tough battler or logical thinker?
7. Were any power factors noted?
8. As we have done this discussion, we have functioned as a group. Did you notice any specific types of behaviors?

REFERENCES

HERZBERG, F., B. MAUSNER AND B. SNYDERMAN, *The Motivation to Work.* New York: John Wiley & Sons, Inc., 1959.

MASLOW, A., *Motivation and Personality*, 2nd ed. New York: Harper & Row, Publishers, Inc., 1970.

STEERS, R. AND L. PORTER, *Motivation and Work Behavior.* New York: McGraw-Hill, Book Company, 1975.

WAHBA, M. AND L. BRIDWELL, "Maslow Reconsidered: A Review of Research on the Need Hierarchy Theory," *Organizational Behavior and Human Performance*, 15 (1976), pp. 212–240.

12

Training and educational functions of a supervisor

THE DIFFERENCE BETWEEN EDUCATION AND TRAINING

One of the most important functions of the supervisor is the training and education responsibility. Every supervisor is faced daily with the need to teach. The supervisor's responsibility is to assist in the training of new staff members, to provide advanced training for experienced staff members, and to serve as a counselor on training and education for all who need assistance. Even though many health care agencies employ "in-service" individuals to coordinate the training and educational needs of the organization, the supervisor is still frequently called upon to assist in the planning of training programs.

The training or teaching function may be formal or informal, but, whatever form it takes, the supervisor must use the best techniques and most recent material. You must show by your example that the constant study of new procedures and scientific developments is necessary to assure competent health care delivery. A part of this vital function is to know which educational opportunities are available to staff members, both in and out of the organizational setting. You must be an effective teacher and an able planner of educational programs. Most important of all, you must encourage staff members to actively seek educational opportunities in and out of the agency, in order to better themselves professionally.

You must also realize that the words "education" and "training" are not synonymous. *Education* is learning for the learner's sake.

253

In other words, it is the opportunity for self-improvement in the specific area selected by the student. Education often deals with concepts and ideas rather than technical skills. *Training* is learning for the job's sake. It is the study of specific skills and information necessary to improve performance on the job. Training improves performance because it gives information that can be immediately put to use in the health care setting. Pre-service training and education prepare staff members to engage in the basic pursuit of their profession. In-service development improves the skills and knowledge of staff members or teaches a specific skill to learn a new assignment. In-service may take the form of a review to refresh the established learning, or it may be the teaching of a new idea or procedure. Some educational offerings may result in both education and training, depending on the type of study.

DETERMINING EDUCATIONAL AND TRAINING NEEDS

The supervisor uses many methods to determine the need for a specific educational or training need, some of which are:

1. conferences with other supervisors,
2. surveys,
3. questionnaries,
4. observation of major changes in departmental or organizational policy or activity,
5. requests from staff members, and
6. input from administration, physicians, and the community.

Planning the Program

In order for an educational program to be successful, there must be careful planning before its initiation. All too often such programs are started without consideration for the basic feasibility of the planned program. These guidelines include:

1. Does the learner have the mental and physical potential to learn?
2. Does the learner have the mental and physical desire to learn?
3. Can the desired changes in behavior take place?
4. If so, how can this change best be accomplished? By:
   a. increased self-awareness?
   b. additional information?
   c. additional skills?
   d. additional choices or alternatives?

e. changes in habit?

f. encouragement, feedback, reinforcement?

Once the need for a program has been established and the best method of presentation selected, the supervisor is ready to start the planning of the program. Any training or educational program must include these four elements:

1. selection.
2. competence,
3. functional subject matter, and
4. consideration of the working conditions.

SELECTION   The selection of "what" is to be taught—the subject matter or skills is the most important part of the training function. The supervisor must use any means available to choose topics that are necessary and that best meet the needs of the organization and of the individuals in that organization.

The selection of "who" should take part in the program is also important. Experienced nurses should have different classes and subjects from new employees. Nurses' aides usually require different programs from other staff members. Generally, the training group should all have the same basic knowledge and skill level.

COMPETENCE   Competence refers to the skill and educational level of the person selected to teach the class. Teachers must not only possess a high level of knowledge and understanding of the subject matter, but they must also be able to impart this information in a professional way. The task of the supervisor is to choose the most skilled person to teach the educational of training program.

FUNCTIONAL SUBJECT MATTER   When instituting an educational program, the supervisor must be sure that the subject matter is pertinent and serves some useful purpose. General interest subjects are not functional unless they serve to improve the level of performance or education of the members of the organization.

WORKING CONDITIONS   Since many of the educational and training programs in health care are conducted on duty time, the supervisor must be aware of the working conditions and the educational setting. Asking a staff member to leave a busy working situation to come to a class may cause frustration and hostility. Students must come to the class with a real desire to learn, and this attitude cannot be accomplished if their minds are on the tasks that remain unfinished on the ward.

Setting a comfortable environment for learning is also important. Quiet, calm surroundings lend themselves to the learning process better than a busy setting. The use of a closed classroom makes the student feel more receptive to the presentation. In any type of educational program, the student must feel relaxed and unhurried. The teacher must make sure that the student is as receptive as possible through the use of a proper environment.

TYPES OF EDUCATION AND TRAINING

Orientation

THE INITIAL INTERVIEW   The first opportunity for education and training comes at the initial interview. Frequently, as the supervisor, you are in the position to conduct this interview, and you must be aware of the numerous opportunities for teaching in this situation.

The initial interview is a perfect place to build a supportive attitude with new employees. In this first meeting, you can do much to instill a feeling of belonging and concern in staff members. By setting an example of interest and knowledge, you make new persons feel as though the organization cares about them as individuals. Listening quietly to everything that employees have to say and being genuinely interested set the tone for furure dealings with them.

During this initial interview, you should give new staff members some idea of the work of the department or health care agency, the backgrounds of fellow employees, and the basic organizational rules and policies. Giving this information in a supportive and knowledgeable way conveys to employees that everyone in the organization is committed to achieving the goals of the organization.

THE FORMAL ORIENTATION   In the formal orientation, employees receive more detailed information about the job that they are expected to do and about the organization itself. This orientation may take a few days to several weeks of classroom instruction, followed by on-the-job training. Whatever form the orientation takes, employees should be told:

1. the salaries of their jobs,
2. the duties and responsibilities expected (job description),
3. working hours, shifts, benefits, and sick time,
4. the organizational rules and regulations,
5. organizational policy,
6. the expected ethical conduct,

7. the opportunities for advancement,
8. their places in the organization (where they fit on the organizational chart, their subordinates and supervisors),
9. the general objectives of the health care agency and the specific goals of their areas of responsibility,
10. the methods of discipline and the procedure for grievance,
11. any necessary community information,
12. the health care agency's evaluation procedure, including a blank copy of the organization's evaluation form, and
13. the basic information necessary to begin her tasks, such as layout of the agency and the like.

Much additional information can be taught in an orientation program, but this is the basic information needed by the new employee in order to begin working.

Advanced or In-Service Education

Experienced staff members are taught new procedures and information through the use of in-service education. This education is the responsibility of the in-service director or of the supervisor. Whoever is responsible for this training must be interested in the welfare of the patient and of the staff members, realize the importance of the teaching function, and have excellent teaching skills. The basic goal of any supervisor in the training function is to instill a desire to learn in the staff. Staff members learn because they are taught the importance of acquiring the information. If they see the need and the benefits, they will be motivated to learn.

The advanced or in-service education of staff members may be accomplished in many ways, but basically it is divided into: (1) informal education and (2) formal education.

INFORMAL EDUCATION The informal education consists of information given to staff members in a setting other than a formal classroom. It may be anything from a word of advice in the corridor, to a patient care conference on the wards. Supervisors must remember that anytime they give information to a staff member, they are teaching.

The same rules apply to you, as an on-the-job teacher, that apply to the teacher in a formal classroom. You must be informed on the subject, willing to take the time to share the information, interested in the participation of the staff member, and skilled in the techniques of teaching. What seems to you to be a simple comment on an employee's behavior may really be an important lesson for that employee. What seems simple to you may very well be unclear to the staff member,

257

and taking the time to point out a simple solution to a problem may be very meaningful to that person.

Clear, concise instructions delivered in a patient tone of voice do much to educate your staff, both to new methods and to your supportive attitude. Try to seek out opportunities to give information and education to your staff. This suggestion does not mean that you must carry a blackboard on your back. It simply means taking those extra few minutes to correct a procedure and to give a few ways to improve the situation. With any form of criticism you should furnish ways to change the behavior. This is teaching. In the long run, the time spent on this task saves you much time in discipline and in repairing the damage done by mistakes or misunderstandings.

Many times just explaining "why" *you* do certain things is an excellent way of teaching your staff. The staff may look to you as a role model, and they may try to pattern themselves after you if they see that you are capable and efficient. Explaining the reasons behind decisions or actions can reduce misunderstanding and also help the staff understand the organizational objectives. Most adults respond best to this form of informal teaching. Try to be open to new ideal from the staff, and assure them that you too are willing to learn. Ask the staff members why they are interested in learning. If the employees feel that they are contributing to the educational experiences in the health care agency, they will be more enthusiastic and willing to participate.

Any written or verbal memo distributed to the staff is another form of informal teaching. If you are writing a memo, make sure that the information is clear and correct. If the material is difficult or involved, have someone else read your message before you send it to the staff. That way, you are sure that your intended message is understood. Sometimes, when you are writing a message, it seems perfectly clear to you, but another person can detect areas that are not understandable or that are vague. Don't hesitate to have another person critique your work if it is very important. A few minutes spent rewriting a message can save you hours of explaining later on.

If your goal is to change policy or procedure, make sure that your attitude conveys support of the new procedure. The staff is unsure of change. Never, by word or attitude, express negative feelings about the proposed change.

The education of staff members always carries with it a certain amount of anxiety or tension on the part of staff members. They are unsure of new ideas because they are unfamiliar with them. Your task is to reduce the anxiety and tension and help the staff succeed in learning the new behaviors without fear or rebellion. Allowing the group to express their feelings and opinions aids you in initiating changes. If they feel that they have had a chance to vent their emotions, they become more open to your suggestions and to those of the health care agency.

258

FORMAL EDUCATION   The formal education of staff members takes the form of an organized class, usually in the structured setting of a meeting room or classroom. The continuing education programs, in-service education programs, and teaching lectures are examples of formal training carried on in the health care setting. These classes should be conducted by the most experienced and knowledgeable person available, and they should give information that is important and valuable to the growth of the staff. Education is to help persons reach their fullest potential, and this aim can be achieved only by a skilled teacher.

If, as a teacher, you seem unsure or frightened, the staff sees this immediately, and thus you reduce the effectiveness of the class. One way to reduce your fears is to plan carefully for the class and then present the material in a way that is interesting and informative. The only way to achieve consistent success in teaching is to practice. Use every opportunity to practice and to improve your teaching and public speaking skills.

Try to vary the speakers at in-service education programs. No matter how skilled the teacher is, the group grows tired of hearing the same voice at each meeting. Go into the community and find interesting and informative people who are skilled at teaching and who have some valuable material to share with your staff. The more creative types of educational planning yield great benefits for your staff.

As a supervisor, you must be aware of any and all educational programs offered to the members of your staff. You must read all literature about seminars, training sessions, lecture series, and college classes offered in your area. If you stress the importance of education to the staff, you must be ready to provide the resources for that education. Try to find out about as many programs as possible, so that you can offer a wide variety of choices to the staff. If possible, preview the seminars or college courses, to assess the value and the quality of instruction. It is frustrating to a staff member to attend a class that is poorly developed or outdated.

Encourage the staff members to seek education beyond that provided by the health care agency. Many states require mandatory continuing education for relicensure, and this requirement is a perfect opportunity for you to encourage the employees to take outside courses. If staff members are interested in obtaining education for higher degrees, help them find the programs that best suit their needs, and then offer support and guidance. If possible, arrange the working schedule to allow for the time needed to attend classes. The supervisor who encourages continuing education and then makes provision for the staff to obtain this information will be respected.

If your health care agency has a financial assistance or reimbursement program for continuing education, make sure that you understand the provisions and explain them to your staff. Offer to help the staff member obtain this financial assistance, and try to find alter-

259

native programs that offer additional help. Many times the financial help or the extra time off is all that stands between staff members and their educational goals. Better educated and trained staff means better care in your institution. Taking the time and effort to investigate the programs and courses available in your area can only help you and your organization.

One way to encourage educational involvement in the staff is to rotate the staff members, allowing different persons to attend different educational offerings. Try not to consistently send the same person to conferences or seminars. Allow every employee the opportunity, perhaps as a reward, so that everyone has the chance to grow professionally. Many times a staff member gains more from a conference than the department head who has been to the same conference many times before. Asking staff members to attend a conference, and then having them present the information received to the other staff members, is a good way to involve every person in the training function of the organization. A person involved in the planning and presentation of an informational topic learns as much, if not more than, the participants.

THE STUDENT/EMPLOYEE AS AN INDIVIDUAL

No matter which form the training takes, formal or informal, you must remember that each student is an individual and that your approach must meet the needs of that individual. The successful teacher is the one who responds to each student as a unique person, not as a member of a group. Assisting a student learning occupational concepts necessitates effective communication on an instructor–learner level. In order to facilitate this communication, the instructor should have an understanding of the "self" concept and its interrelation with the learning process.

The Nature of the Self

The *self* is the individual's interpretation of a continually changing world of experience. Most of these experiences are at a conscious level. The person can analyse past and present experiences and relate them to the current situation. A portion of the world, as the individual sees it, gradually becomes differentiated from the rest of it: This is the self. The way each individual perceives this changing world of experience is reality for him or her. The person sees and interprets this reality. The "self" is the portion of the world that is within the individual's control and that he or she consciously controls.

As individuals have more and more experiences, they begin to organize their reactions into a fluid pattern, changeable but organized and consistent with their self-concepts. The self-concept is their way of looking at themselves, and their way of meeting their needs as they see them. All thinking, feeling, and behaving are usually consistent with the self-concept.

The "Self" as It Tends to Interfere with Learning

The self tends not to accept new situations as new, but in terms of situations with which we are familiar. Individuals feel more comfortable with established, familiar situations. The self would like to believe that the new situation is the same as the old familiar one. Somewhat afraid of a new situation, individuals approach it with some degree of anxiety, which in turn tends to obscure those details that make it different from familiar situations. Individuals suddenly realize, usually too late, that this new situation is not a "truly new" situation but rather has some similarity with an older one. Identifying this similarity helps individuals to accept the change and to integrate it into their "selves."

Basic Assumptions Regarding Behavior Self

The supervisor/instructor must understand the complex emotional interactions in the student in order to change behavior. Behavior is anything done in response to a stimuli, either internal or external. In the teaching/learning situation, the instructor attempts to be the stimulus to change behavior or to educate the individual.

In order to change behavior (or persons' responses to "self"), the instructor must know the basic assumptions about behavior and self:

1. Behavior is caused by stimuli and is meaningful to the person. Good or bad, the behavior fills a need. Instructors must be aware of the underlying needs for the behavior if they are to change it.
2. The causes that underly behavior are always multiple. To change behavior, or to teach, the instructor must respond to more than one motivation in the student.
3. Each individual is an indivisible unit. One technique does not work for all students. The instructor must employ various strategies of instruction.
4. Every human individual is a dynamic energy system, not just a machine acted upon from without. You can never entirely separate the self-concept of a person from the professional en-

vironment. An educational program is only valuable to employees if they see the meaning or relevance in it.

5. Each individual is different from every other individual.

THE LEARNING PROCESS

Because learning and teaching are parts of one general process, superior teaching rests in part on a clear appreciation of learning. An awareness of the mechanism of this process helps both students and teachers in their joint undertaking. One approach subdivides the learning process into three steps:

1. comprehension.
2. recall, and
3. creative thinking.

Comprehension

Successful comprehension—the absorption—of a new idea generally requires a motivation and a desire to learn. Students usually wish to learn if they see that the material presented may be useful and if they feel that they are making visible progress. Comprehension of a new idea requires an adequate background of related knowledge or prerequisites to the subject. The new idea must be expressed in a vocabulary that is familiar to the student. If the new idea requires a technical jargon or the use of specialized, precise meanings of familiar words, then these vocabulary problems must be met first. They must not be permitted either to obscure the idea or to impair or prevent comprehension. True comprehension requires undivided attention.

Recall

Recall is the process of remembering, of which several levels or degrees are recognized. The lowest level is *recognition recall,* by which we remember an item only after someone else has jogged our memory. In fact, we do not "recall" it at all, but only "recognize" it as familiar after it has been recalled for us. Recognition recall is exhibited by those whose memories for anecdotes are only good enough to spoil the other fellow's jokes but who cannot contribute much themselves. *Volitional* or *spontaneous recall* is the process of successfully remembering something previously learned. Obvious examples of volitional recall include the successful repetition of the multiplication tables or of the names of students in a class.

In a restricted but useful educational sense, the word *knowledge* means only the power of volitional recall of comprehended material.

Knowledge is a two-step process: First comes comprehension or understanding of the item; later comes recall or remembering the item. In this sense the concept of knowledge does not necessarily extend to the next intellectual step, which involves creative thinking or, more simply, the new use of knowledge.

Creative Thinking

The ultimate aim of a teacher must be more than the mere acquisition and transmission of knowledge. These processes alone simply preserve knowledge, without contributing any intellectual progress. The society in which we live would not exist if the body of knowledge possessed by the early scientists had merely been passed along, generation after generation, without being enlarged.

Students are responsible for developing efficient and effective methods of study. Their so-called "learning aids" may include notes taken in class, notes made during private study of the textbook and of library reference materials, solutions of problems, and a textbook marked up by their own marginal notes, underscorings, and annotations. Yet only a few students give as much as 1 percent of their study time to the development of efficient study habits and techniques. Such self-investigation is very much worthwhile and can usually increase learning by 5 to 50 percent. Remembering that the nursing student's investment of time alone amounts to about 6,000 hours, an increase of a few percentage points in learning efficiency is significant.

Students' study aids and methods must aim not only at comprehension but especially at improvement in their powers of recall. Educational experiments have shown that great improvements can indeed be made by individuals in their ability to recall previously learned material. Study methods should involve aids to both comprehension and recall. Students whose systematic efforts to develop their powers of recall consist only of cram sessions before quizzes are missing a large share of their educational opportunity. Throughout the learning process, the powers of recall should be constantly stimulated and exercised. Creative thinking and recall can often be cultivated simultaneously.

CHARACTERISTICS
OF ADULT STUDENTS

Immediate Responsibilities of Adults

The immediate responsibilities of adults, and hence the education that is suitable for adults, differ from those of youth and children in at least four ways:

1. Adults have the responsibility for carrying on all the functions of government, including voting, holding office, and other functions of citizenship.
2. Adults have the responsibility of maintaining economic stability as it relates to themselves, their families, and their communities.
3. Adults have the responsibility of parenthood and of maintaining a well-adjusted home and family life.
4. Adults have the responsibility of providing the social, cultural, and spiritual environment for present and future generations.

How Adult Students Differ

Not only do adult students differ among themselves in age, occupation, physical condition, living standards, education, ambition, mental ability, aptitudes, and attitudes, but they differ from secondary school students in that adults come to classes solely because they want to. Hence they don't take their classes, their progress, or their teachers as a matter of course. Also, they have a richness of experience that younger students lack, and, as a result, they are able to lend to classes individual judgments that often shed a new light on old problems, theories, or facts. The teacher has a potential assistant in every adult member of the class.

As a rule, most adults who come to organized education classes are well-motivated, eager to learn, and very appreciative of good teaching. They are more sensitive to physical surroundings such as lighting, seating, ventilation, and heating. They like to be comfortable, they enjoy learning comparatively short units, and they usually want to cover ground as rapidly as possible.

Adult students appreciate systematic, business-like procedures, as well as tangible evidence from time to time that their needs are being met. They immediately stop coming to class if they feel their time is not being used to good advantage and if they feel their needs are not being satisfied. Adult students welcome variety and like informality. They like to be treated like adults with mature minds, successful backgrounds, and rich, varied experience. They welcome a chance to laugh and a chance to relax. They come for business, but they enjoy the followship and congenial atmosphere always found in a good class for adults.

Ability of Adults to Learn

The fact that adults can learn is by now so firmly established that it requires only brief mention here. Experiments show that the general ability to learn reaches its peak at about the age of 25. The ages

25 to 45 are superior to childhood, as well as equal or superior to early adolescence, in the ability to learn.[1]

Principles Essential to
Effective Learning

Adult learners must see some immediate benefit. The content of the course, whether it provides information, skills, or both, must be immediately useful to the adult. Unlike the adolescent student, the adult student does not study for some remote, uncertain future.

Adults must want the instruction; they must be motivated. Their presence in the class does not necessarily indicate that they want what they are getting. They may want part of it or expect to get what they want later in the course. If teachers are well acquainted with the needs and objectives of their students, they are in a position to make sure of their motivation. They do not take their interest for granted. Rather, as the occasion requires, they take time to develop in the minds of their students a realization of their need for the subject matter, or they present other subject matter. Interest and motivation naturally arise from the students' expectations of success. Thoughtful teachers create occasions to emphasize and to call attention to the student's progress, through comment, encouragement, praise, and expression of personal satisfaction with their work.

Adults want specific, concrete, practical lifelike situations. They question the abstract or theoretical approach. They require some knowledge of physics and mathematics, for example, to understand fully the concepts of pharmacology, but they will not study them until they first see the occasion for their use. Courses in skill development should duplicate practical, everyday functions. Dramatizing content, demonstrations, illustrations, and visual aids presented on the adult level make content more lifelike.

If the student activity is tangible, concrete, and evident, it enables adults to measure and realize the rate of their progress and growth. One of the great advantages of discussion methods in instruction is that students must take active parts.

Adults require participation in class activity. They do not come as spectators or as members of an audience. They want demonstration, illustration, and explanation, but they also want to work things out for themselves. If the particular situation can be presented to them as a problem to solve, their interest, satisfaction, and learning are all multiplied. While adults want participation in class activity, especially in

[1] Edward L. Thorndike, *Adult Learning* (New York: The Macmillan Co., 1928), p. 147.

the fields of their particular interests, many of them do not take the initiative in participating. As a teacher, your responsibility is to consciously and continually create situations that call for participation on the part of all students.

In general, adults are very ready to engage in class activity if given an opportunity. Some classes lend themselves to participation more easily than others. The project method, exercises, problems, conference, and informal discussions are based on active student participation. The benefit in general participation far exceeds that indicated by each individual act of participation. It builds up class unity. The class as a whole feels drawn into the instruction, becomes part of it, senses the instructor's awareness of its interests and personalities, and appreciates being called on to help carry along the instruction, realizing that the teacher values the experiences and opinions of class members.

Adults have experiences and interests to which new material should be related. Most adults have had experiences, contacts, or interests that have to do with the course subject and that may be utilized to advantage by the teacher. One of the major characteristics of a class for adults is its many different types of members. The students in an adult class usually have a wide range of differences in age, ability, interests, and occupational and cultural experience. These differences give rise to a great need for adaptation of subject content and methods of instruction. In order that each student may understand each step in the development of the course, individual instruction is frequently necessary.

Often adult students, because of their knowledge or experience, are able to make substantial contributions to the content of the course, even though some of the contributions or opinions may not be entirely sound. The teacher, wherever possible, should allow the students themselves to discover their own errors. Teachers may do so by stating the problem or issue, helping the students to assemble and study the data, classify the data, and in the process of arriving at a conclusion, emphasize the desirability of keeping judgment suspended until a logical conclusion is reached.

In return for their input, adults require subject matter adapted to their individual objectives, needs, and capabilities. Teachers many times fail to see that a carefully planned course may fit the needs of some adult students but may not contribute towards reaching the objectives of others. It is also likely that students may come into the class with an intense interest in the subject but without the required background or learning that enables them to profit by the course as planned. The successful teacher of adults must have ways and means of discovering the needs and capabilities of the students.

Adults must enjoy the instruction. The chief source of enjoyment to adults is found in the knowledge that they are progressing toward an understanding of the material presented and that it is useful to them. In order to make this progress, learning must take place in an atmosphere to their liking and adapted to their level. As adults and as responsible members of the community, they resent anything bordering on adolescent schoolroom discipline or restraint. You, as the teacher, can secure order and attention to instruction because these students want the instruction provided, not because you demand or require attention.

GENERAL PLAN FOR
AN EDUCATIONAL CLASS

No success in teaching can be achieved without careful planning and organization before the actual teaching process begins. Supervisors who are also able instructors see the need for these detailed plans, and they never omit this step. Using a step-by-step system to plan a lesson is essential to assure that the needs of the students are met.

No matter how informal the teaching is, five steps of instruction are always included (see Table 12–1). You may not have to write down the proposed steps for an informal or on-the-job teaching session, but these elements are present in any type of teaching encounter:

1. assessment,
2. objectives,
3. topic,
4. alternatives, and
5. evaluation.

Assessment

This initial step to any teaching situation begins with the observation of a need for some type of education. It may be as simple as noticing a problem with an employee and correcting it verbally, or it may take the form of planning for a formal course in a specific topic. The assessment stage consists of seeing a need or a problem, and then deciding to respond to that need. The method of response, the educational process, depends on the situation. In this stage, the supervisor develops an overview of the problem, how it started, how it became apparent, the extent of the problem, the present effects of the problem, and any examples of situations caused directly by the problem. This is essentially a process of seeing a need and documenting it.

Since adult students respond to an educational program better if they see the need for the program and can see the benefits to learning another or refined behavior, the teacher's assessment is quite important. Carefully considering all aspects of the assessment stage assures

267

TABLE 12–1
General plan or format for a training class

I. *Assessment* (problem):
   A. An overview of the problem, how it started.
   B. Present effects.
   C. Give example, if possible.

II. *Objectives:*
   A. Tell the group what you want them to do.
   B. Give the reason for the class.
   C. Define terms.

III. *Topic:*
   A. Ask yourself "What, exactly, do I want to get across to the group?"

IV. *Alternatives* (motivation):
   A. Redefine or re-explain in different terms.
   B. Make learning reasonable, meaningful.

V. *Feedback* (evaluation):
   A. Test to see if the students understand.

that the program will be necessary and meaningful. This process of assessment is not only part of the planning stage, but it should also be included in the presentation of the topic. It is not enough for *you* to see the need for the program; you must relate this need to the students. This requirement makes the assessment stage part of the actual introduction of the class. Making this assessment interesting by including examples does much to spark interest in the class, and it aids the teaching process.

Objectives

Once you have established a need for the class, you must decide on its future outcome. What do you expect to have happen at the conclusion of the educational process? This goal should be written in terms of behaviors. In what way will the behavior of the students be changed at the close of the class? As an example objective for a four-week training class, the student should be expected to:

1. see the need for oral hygiene in the bedridden patient.
2. understand the physiology and anatomy of the oral cavity,
3. understand the factors that contribute to poor oral hygiene, and
4. be able to perform the procedure for preventive oral hygiene.

Listing the possible outcomes and anticipated objectives enables the student to understand more completely the need for the class. Students become acquainted with the topics and terms to be covered, and they have an understanding of the benefits to themselves and to the organization. This step completes the introduction phase of the class, by preparing the student for the educational process.

Topic

In this stage, you present the subject to the class. In planning the presentation, you should ask yourself, "What, exactly, do I want to get across to the group?" The subject should be broad enough to interest the students, but it should not be so broad that adequate coverage is impossible. Try to narrow the class down to the essential material necessary to teach the subject or to relieve the problem. Most teachers make the mistake of trying to cover too much material in one session.

Students have only a limited attention span, and once the group's attention starts to wander, no learning takes place. Make sure that any new terms are completely defined and that all areas are clear and concise. Do not insult the intelligence of the group by covering topics that are very familiar and well-understood, but do not assume that the group knows more than they do. Listen to the questions asked by the class. These questions give you a good indication of the level of the group's knowledge. You must meet the needs of the group as a whole, and this necessity may mean slowing down the pace of the class to allow the slower students to catch up.

In a one-to-one teaching situation, this step can be accomplished by questioning the student as to his or her present level of knowledge on the subject. Once you have established a baseline, you are ready to start the introduction of the new subject matter.

No matter how skilled your group, everyone benefits from a review if it is handled correctly. Most topics should be introduced with a very brief review to help the students prepare for the new material. One good method of review is to give a pre-test to the group. Two or three questions reviewing the material serve as a beginning to the class, and they enable you to tailor the class to the needs of the group. If the class is a continuing one, perhaps meeting once each month, the review stage is essential to maintain continuity in the learning situation. Review is also a good way for you to assess the success of your teaching ability, and you can stress areas that seem to be weak.

In the presentation of the topic, use any methods that help the students achieve success: lecture, group discussion, skill demonstration, films, flip charts, slides, film strips, lectures from physicians or other skilled persons, self-instruction in the form of programmed lesson plans, peer demonstrations, or outside reading and research. (See Appendix A at the end of this chapter for a conference format.) The topic presentation can be in any form, but, whatever form you choose, make sure that it meets the needs of the student and accomplishes the goals of the instruction. As you vary your teaching techniques, your students receive more and more benefit from the class. Try new approaches, be creative and innovative. You may want to discuss with the class the methods of instruction that they feel would best meet their needs. The key to any teaching method is to make sure that the student is interested and is actively learning. Do not hesitate to change techniques if your method does not seem to be working. Watch the class, and you will be able to tell if their attention is wandering or if they are not comprehending the information.

Alternatives

The alternatives phase of the learning process is an extension of the topic presentation. In this stage, you redefine or re-explain the topic in different terms. For the student who understands the procedure or subject, this step serves as a review. For students who are still unclear about the subject, it may serve to clear up the puzzling points.

In the teaching a skill, this stage takes the form of allowing the student to practice the skill under supervision. A skill cannot be learned without actual practice. What seems clear in an explanation may be more difficult in actual practice. Allow the class to practice the skill as many times as necessary to assure that they are proficient in the task. Try not to control the group too closely in this stage. Allowing the group to proceed at their own pace, and to make mistakes gives you the opportunity to see errors and to give guidance. If you control them too closely, they are never able to see if they can actually do the procedure on their own. In a very difficult task or new procedure, the class should be able to practice their skills in a classroom situation first, and then be allowed to practice, with supervision, on a patient or in a real situation. Classroom practice is one thing; doing a procedure on a patient is completely different. Both types of application are necessary.

The alternatives stage of learning serves to motivate students to learn as much as possible because they know that they are not only expected to learn the subject, but also to demonstrate their skill.

Evaluation

This is the most important part of the learning process. At this stage, students demonstrate their ability to perform the behavior or skill without supervision. As an instructor, you have an opportunity to evaluate the success of your teaching, and students the chance to demonstrate their mastery of the behavior.

The preliminary part of evaluation may take the form of a question-and-answer session at the close of the class. Asking for questions from the group, or proposing questions yourself, enables you to see if your students understand the material. So-called "dumb" questions at the end of a session are not "dumb" at all. They are indicators that the class did not meet the educational objectives established at the start of the process. You may have set too high goals for the students, or you may not have presented the material in a way that resulted in learning. Whatever the reason for this lack of understanding, it gives valuable feedback concerning the future needs of the group. If one or two members of the group seem to be the only students who are unclear on the subject, you may want to work independently with these students and allow the remainder of the group to progress to additional subject matter.

The real process of evaluation takes place in the test procedure. Testing may take the form of an actual pencil-and-paper test or of simply observing behavior in the clinical situation. Whatever form you choose, the students should know that a testing procedure will take place, and they should be allowed to prepare for this step. Knowing that they will be tested sometimes increases the motivation to learn. Demonstrating that they can write the answers to questions or perform a skill proves to them that they have succeeded, and this accomplishment increases their confidence.

The last part of the evaluation stage is for you, the instructor, to take stock of the class and decide if the goals have been met. If your goal in the educational process was to teach a skill to eliminate a problem, you can now analyze the situation and observe the success or failure of the class. Is the problem reduced or eliminated? If so, the educational process was successful and resulted in goal attainment. If not, you can evaluate the level of success and change your techniques or review the subject to reinforce the learning. If the goals were not met because of too high a level of expectation, you can write new objectives for the group and begin the process of learning at a different level or by using another approach.

THE FOUR STEPS OF INSTRUCTION

Many successful teachers use a four-step procedure to present their material. This simple procedure can be adapted for teaching either information or skills. Incorporating many of the considerations about the learning process, about adult students, and about the five elements of planning a training program, the four steps in instruction provide teachers with a handy checklist when working up a lesson plan. The four steps are:

1. motivation,
2. presentation,
3. application, and
4. testing.

Tables 12–2 and 12–3 detail their applications in teaching information and skills.

TABLE 12–2
Four steps of instruction adapted to teaching technical information—Example: mathematical calculations

I. *Motivation:*
   A. Use attention-getting devices, such as approriate charts, photographs, blackboard drawings, or three-dimensional objects.
   B. Show how this math process fits into the future occupation of the student.
   C. Show how this process builds on previous math knowledge.

II. *Presentation:*
   A. Teacher works example on board labeling all elements of the problem.
   B. Explains plan of attack on this type of problem.
   C. Teacher uses questions and makes certain that students understand how this math process is applied.

III. *Application:*
   A. Teacher works another example, step by step, having the students follow each step by working the problem at their seats.
   B. If many students are having trouble understanding, then the teacher asks a capable student to go to the board and work an example explaining the process in his or her own words.
   C. Teacher sends a typical group of students to the board to work on the example while remainder of students do problems at their seats.
   D. Teacher observes students at the board to see if plan of attack is logical and to see if consistent errors are made by the students.
   E. Teacher reteaches if necessary.

IV. *Test:*
   A. Several typical problems are assigned to be done by the students under test conditions.
   B. Quiz questions are immediately corrected, and the students are given an opportunity to see their scores.
   C. Students needing special assistance after the quiz are given individual help by the teacher and/or by other students who thoroughly understand the process.

TABLE 12–3
Four steps of instruction adapted to teaching a skill

I. *Motivation:*
   A. Prepare the learner by stimulating interest. Cite examples and personal experiences to arouse curiosity.
   B. Show how this skill fits into the future occupational needs of the student—objectives.
   C. Show how this skill builds on previously learned skills.

TABLE 12–3 (*cont.*)

II. *Presentation:*
   A. Give demonstrations.
   B. Follow proper procedures.
   C. Explain procedures.
   D. Emphasize key and safety points.

III. *Application:*
   A. Have learners perform the job.
   B. Supervise performance closely.
   C. Check and correct errors.
   D. Develop correct habits.
   E. Check key and safety points.
   F. Have learner repeat operations if necessary.

IV. *Test:*
   A. Have learners perform the job.
   B. Ask prepared questions.
   C. Give written tests.
   D. Give performance tests.

WRITING A LESSON PLAN OR INSTRUCTIONAL ANALYSIS GUIDE

When you are doing informal teaching, a written guide is not necessary or even desirable. No one expects a supervisor to write down every aspect of a simple direction or critique. Yet in the formal educational setting, this lesson plan is necessary.

The best teachers are not just skilled public speakers; they are also skilled at planning and implementing an educational objective. They take the time to write down all the organizational plans for their classes. This plan also serves the purpose of organizing their thinking so that they can accomplish the objectives in the simplest and easiest way possible. If you are unsure or frightened about teaching, prepare a lesson plan to help you present the material well with as little nervousness as possible. Having everything written down assures that you will cover every necessary area and not forget to discuss an important issue. Even the most skilled teachers occasionally get nervous or distracted, and they need the guidance of a prepared plan for reference. You may feel that you know the subject so thoroughly that you do not need to refer to notes or to planned lessons, but going without them is a risky practice. Teaching a subject is much different from actually doing the procedure, and it requires a whole new set of skills. Writing down the plan insures that what you know and wish to convey is being expressed to the students. Appendix B to this chapter contains a step-by-

273

step guide to serve as an example for your own lesson plans. This guide can be adapted to meet the needs of any type of educational setting.

The careful planning of the lesson assures you maximum success and simplifies the process of teaching. Detailed preparation of these guides makes the teaching topics and techniques that you use available to anyone, and it encourages other members of your staff to teach the same subjects. If this guide is kept as a constant reference, the ongoing education of new employees becomes more and more efficient. Ideally, your lesson plan should be so well written that any person could use the same plan to achieve the same results.

QUALITIES OF A GOOD TEACHER

The teaching function of a supervisor is an essential one that demands much attention to detail and advance planning. Supervisors are expected to teach every day, so the importance of developing good teaching skills cannot be over-emphasized. Supervisors who are good teachers have easier jobs because their staffs are able to function independently with more efficiency and quality. Basically, which qualities make for a good teacher?

THE ABILITY TO GUIDE AND DIRECT BY STIMULATING INTEREST IN THE GROUP The group that is motivated to learn accomplishes more than the group that attends class because it is "mandatory."

PATIENCE To teach demands much patience, along with a calm, supportive attitude. Allow students enough time to learn a new behavior without belaboring the point.

GOOD PERSONAL HABITS OF SPEECH AND GROOMING The class spends most of its time looking directly at you. If your appearance is less than perfect, the class spends valuable time critiquing your appearance and not listening to what you have to say. The ability to use your speech effectively and efficiently is also a necessary skill. Such techniques as varying the tone of your voice, speaking slowly and clearly, and using correct grammar all assure that your group is listening to what you are saying and not focusing on how you say it.

THE ABILITY TO SET A GOOD EXAMPLE No matter how skillfully you teach a subject, if you do not practice what you preach, the staff notices and loses respect for your teaching ability. Make sure that you perform every task and behavior in the way that your class is taught to do it.

274 *ENTHUSIASM* If you are genuinely interested in what you are teaching and if that enthusiasm comes across to the class, they become infected

with the same enthusiasm and learn more. Convey by words and actions that you care about the subject and that you sincerely want the students to learn.

THE ABILITY TO CONTROL THE CLASS   The supervisor/teacher is not expected to rule the class with an iron fist, but you should exercise that degree of control necessary to keep the group on the subject and not allow the group's attention to wander. A member of the group who is not interested in the subject, or who wishes to take control from the leader, can do much to interfere with the objectives of the class. The group respects you more if you maintain control, and not allow one member to monopolize the discussion or gain the group's attention for a side topic. Always start and end the class on time.

THE ABILITY TO DISPLAY EXPERTISE   Successful teachers know their subjects and are able to express this knowledge to the group. You should not try to dazzle the group with your intelligence; showing off only frustrates them, increases the anxiety level in the group, and prevents learning. Being able to sense the level of the group and speak to that level is a necessary skill for the teacher.

THE ABILITY TO USE A VARIETY OF TEACHING AIDS AND TECHNIQUES   Variety in the methods of instruction assures the interest of the group. A method that does not interest one student might be perfect for another. The use of several methods in each session does much to meet the needs of *all* the students.

THE ABILITY TO SIMPLY EXPLAIN A SUBJECT   A good teacher is able to analyze a subject and explain as simply as possible the basic elements of the topic. Keep the vocabulary within the level of the group, and use as few words as possible to convey your message.

THE ABILITY TO KEEP THE CLASS THINKING   A group actively involved in the educational process is constantly challenged and learns more. The goal of any educational session is to provide the information necessary to motivate the students to practice the procedure or to further their education on the subject. In other words, you stimulate the group to *apply* the education.

DISCUSSION QUESTIONS

1. Why is the supervisor expected to be a teacher?
2. What is the difference between "education" and "training"?
3. How does the supervisor determine the educational needs of the staff?
4. What are the various levels of training in health care? How does the supervisor meet the needs of these levels of preparation?

5. How is the orientation interview used as an educational process?
6. How can the supervisor/teacher stimulate interest in learning in staff members?
7. Describe some methods of instruction. Explain when each type of instruction should be used.
8. Describe the steps in the instructional process.
9. What is the importance between formal and informal teaching?
10. What is the importance of a written lesson plan?
11. A student is being disruptive in a formal class setting. Describe the possible ways to control this individual, without decreasing the total class effectiveness.

APPLICATION: HELPING LEARNERS

Subject

What the instructor can do to help the learner.

Objective

- To learn six ways in which the instructor can make learning easier and/or more effective for the learner.

Introductory Information

Each of the six recommendations covered in this lesson is based on actual observations about the learning process made by capable instructors in training situations. Even though you could just memorize the list, you will probably use them more often and more intelligently if you know why each recommendation aids learning. This assignment helps you develop that understanding.

Some Observations About Learning

1. *Principle of Motivation:* We learn best when there is a need for learning.
2. *Principal of Readiness:* We learn new things best in terms of old.
3. *Principle of Practice:* We learn best by doing.
4. *Principle of Effect:* We learn best if we can expect and experience success.
5. *Principle of Experience:* The more we do a thing, the better we are able to do it, and the more we enjoy doing it.

Some Recommendations for Teaching

1. Have a long-range goal, in addition to the immediate aims.
2. Teach from the known to the unknown.
3. Tie knowledge and skill together.
4. Proceed from simple to complex, easy to difficult.
5. Reward success.
6. Provide for practice or drill.

Application: Preparing a Lesson Plan

Prepare a lesson plan for a nursing topic. Use the general format for teaching a skill or technical knowledge under the following headings:

1. Unit Title
2. Goal
3. References
4. Material Necessary
5. Motivation
6. Student Performance Goal
7. Presentation
8. Application
9. Evaluation

REFERENCES

ARGYRIS, CHRIS, *Executive Leadership: An Appraisal of a Manager in Action.* Hamden, Conn.: Shoe String Press, 1967.

FIEDLER, F. AND M. CHEMERS, *Leadership and Effective Management.* Glenview, Ill.: Scott, Foresman & Company, 1974.

PRATT, WILLIAM V., "Leadership," in *Selected Readings in Leadership,* 3rd ed., ed. Malcolm E. Wolfe and F. J. Mulholland. Annapolis, Md.: United States Naval Institute, 1965.

STOGDILL, R., *Handbook of Leadership: A Survey of Theory and Research.* New York: Free Press/Macmillan, 1974.

APPENDIX A: FORMAT FOR A CONFERENCE

Problem:

Write an overview of the problem, how it started, present effects of the problem. Give an example of the problem, if possible.

Objectives:

Tell the group what you want them to do, that is, the reason for holding the conference. Get the group interested. Be sure to define your terms, for example, problem, morale, policy, supervisor, and so on.

Topic:

Write a complete sentence in terms of "What . . . ." Ask yourself, "Exactly what is the question (or problem) I want the group to answer?" Writing the topic in terms of "what" brings out a concise statement.

Alternate Topic:

Try to ask the same question in a different way. Use it if the conference is slow to start; however, do not be too concerned if the group does not respond immediately.

Chart Headings:

Write down a few key words from the topic identifying each column (if 2 two-column chart): such as, "Advantages—Disadvantages" or "Cause—Solutions."

Facts or Chart Points:

List on your "hot sheet" the points you believe are important under the proper column. This is your analysis of the problem. Use them, throw them out if the discussion lags, but do not force them on the group.

Conclusions:

Write out your conclusions based on your analysis. Note: Do not be concerned if the group's conclusions are different from yours.

APPENDIX B: A SAMPLE OUTLINE FOR A LESSON PLAN

The lesson plan or unit guide is the teacher's road map for teaching a unit of instruction. It identifies:

1. the scope and task organization,
2. what the student sees and hears during the teacher's presentation.
3. what the student will be required to do during and after each lesson, and
4. how the teacher will determine whether the student has achieved the established goals.

Although the guide follows a step-by-step method of instruction, the presentation and application steps alternate continually throughout the unit.

Organizing the Instructional Guide

I. Selecting the Unit Topic: A unit is an entity that is identified by its content and not by time conditions. It is the part of the instruction that focuses on a central theme, such as the "Respiratory System" or the "Use of a Fetal Monitor." A unit normally consists of several segments formed through analysis of the needs of the subject and of the group. A good unit follows four steps of instruction:

A. The *motivation* or *introduction* step introduces new ideas and experiences to be taught. It is essential that this step be designed to focus the students' interest on the lesson to be learned and to provide them with a motive and enthusiasm for learning. This step must be related to known ideas and experiences.

B. The *presentation* step consists of the delivery of the subject matter.

C. The *application* step affords the learner the opportunity to put the subject matter to use.

D. The *evaluation* step helps the instructor to determine how well the student has learned.

II. Writing the Unit Title:

A. Write unit titles that are concise, complete and descriptive of the unit content. Remember, this is the students' first introduction to the subject and must spark their interest.

B. Skill-type unit titles should begin with, "How to . . . ."

C. Informational unit titles usually begin with:
 1. "Kinds of . . . ,"
 2. "Types of . . ," or
 3. other qualifying modifiers of a subject of study.

D. Supervision unit titles usually begin with chapter headings from the textbook, such as:
 1. "Interpreting Organizational Policies" or
 2. "Discovering and Adjusting Grievances."

E. Avoid titles that are too brief and consequently open to conjecture such as "Nursing," "Supervision," "Laws," and the like.

III. Writing the Unit Objectives:

A. The unit objectives should indicate the scope of the instruction and should be written in terms of the skills, knowledge, and attitudes that you expect the students to develop.

B. Objectives should encompass two specific areas:
 1. the desired learning accomplishments, and

2. general description of the conditions and limitations of what is being taught.

In descriptive form, the objectives reflect the purposes of the instruction and set the teaching parameters for organization and presentation. Unit objectives should be correctly written so that they are understandable to students as well as to other teachers.

C. For example, a unit on "How to Give an Enema" in an introductory class for nurses' aides might have the following objectives:

1. to teach the proper use and care of equipment;
2. to learn the kinds of enemas used and learn how to administer them, and so on.

Or a unit on "Essentials of Organization" might have the following objectives:

1. to discuss various types of organization in industry;
2. to establish the need for organization policies.

Or a unit on "Anatomy of the Eye" might have the following objectives:

1. to acquaint the student with the basic anatomy and physiology of the eye;
2. to explain the pathology and treatment of the eye.

Also, there might be indirect or hidden objectives:

1. to get the students to participate in open discussion;
2. to build confidence within the supervisor's or student members' group.

IV. Planning the Motivation Step:

A. The motivation step is easier to plan after the complete unit instructional analysis guide has been written. After considering the various teaching factors, you can develop the motivation step so that it is more applicable to what will be taught.

B. In writing the motivation step, list the techniques you will use to arouse interest and to prepare the student for the learning experience. Ideas that can be included:

1. relate personal experiences;
2. relate the lesson to previous lessons;
3. state future use of the skills and information covered;
4. use exhibits and displays; or
5. relate it to other interests of the students.

V. Identifying the Instructional Segments:

A. Instructional segments are major divisions of a unit. Through an analysis of the unit of instruction, segments of instruction are identified. Each segment is a bit of cohesive instructional activity, and the total instructional segments within a unit of instruction provide for sequential and coordinated learning experiences.

B. Factors that determine the number of instructional segments in a unit are:
1. the overall goals of the course;
2. the relationship of this unit to the course and instructional level;
3. educational and skill level of the students;
4. time allotted to the unit;
5. equipment, tools, and materials available;
6. ability of the students;
7. previous experience of the students;
8. judgement of the teacher;
9. sequence of the unit in the course;
10. any special licensing examination requirements.
C. Included in each instructional segment is the following:
1. student performance goals;
2. level of instruction;
3. the key points and feedback for the segment;
4. the activities and checkup items.

VI. Writing Student Performance Goals:

A. Each instructional segment has its own student performance goals. These goals are specific in content and describe what the student will know or be able to do after the instructional segment has been learned. Descriptive statements include the following:
1. what the student will be given to perform the instruction task;
2. description of the performance;
3. what is the minimum acceptable standard for doing the task.
B. Performance goals contained in the instructional segments are student-centered goals, while unit objectives are more general in scope and tend to be teacher-centered. Properly stated, student performance goals should contain the three following elements:
1. Given:. . .
2. Performance: . . .
3. Standard: . . .
C. An example of a student performance goal is:

PHYSICAL FACTORS EFFECTING QUALITY A.M. CARE
Student Performance Goal

Given:
Reference material and procedure manual information about procedure.
Lecture material and demonstration of the procedure.
Performance:
Students will answer ten questions dealing with morning care as it relates to medical/surgical patients, and demonstrate

281

their ability to perform the procedure.
Standard:
Correct answers for at least seven questions and demonstrated proficiency in the procedure.

VII. Planning Key Points and Activities:

    A. Use a brief step-by-step outline style for skills development.
       1. Start statements with action words such as "cut," "measure," "fasten," "adjust," and the like.
       2. Refer to available job or procedure sheets, and attach them to the instructional analysis guide.
    B. Use a topical outline form for technical instruction. (Supervision lessons are classed as informational.)
       1. Develop a foundation from which you can teach.
       2. Present concepts, principles, and required information.
    C. Plan the teaching techniques you will use in presenting the material. Include such items as:
       1. teaching aids to be used;
       2. drawings and terms to be written on the board;
       3. sample problems (include the solutions in the instructional guide).

VIII. Planning Feedback and Checkup Items:

    A. List the activities you expect the students to carry out as a means of applying (doing, using, practicing) the skills and information covered in the presentation step of the instructional segment. Include such items as:
       1. assignments;
       2. questions, question topics, and problems;
       3. projects;
       4. reports;
       5. experiments;
       6. jobs, operations, or procedures.
    B. Develop techniques and methods to provide feedback that indicate whether the students have learned what was presented in the instructional segment.
    C. Indicate the teacher's part in supervising, checking, and correcting the above activities.

IX. Completing Instructional Segments Presentation and Application Steps:

    A. Develop the student performance goals for each instructional segment.

B. Use the procedure outline for developing the presentation and application steps for an instructional segment as outlined in Parts VII and VIII.

C. Continue this procedure until all the instructional segments for a particular unit have been completed.

X. Plan the Evaluation Step:

A. List the techniques to be used to evaluate the students' performance and knowledge.

B. Include performance tests, along with written or oral tests, used in this step.

XI. Complete Additional Items of the Unit Instructional Analysis Guide:

A. references,

B. materials,

C. supplemental tests and instruction sheets should be attached when completing the instructional packages.

13

Evaluation

KEEPING UP THE QUALITY
OF CARE

The quality of nursing care depends on the performance level of each employee and the development of every individual's potential to the fullest. Consequently, in supervising other personnel, nurses find that staff evaluation becomes a necessary part of the supervisory task.

Staff evaluation has as its aim the development of personnel who are self-reliant and capable of helping themselves. Ideally, the evaluation should aid both the employee and the supervisor. For head nurses and supervisors, such evaluations take two forms: (1) on-the-job and (2) formal counseling sessions.

On-the-Job Evaluation

In this face-to-face situation, also referred to as "incidental counseling," there is little or no advance planning. It is uncomplicated, simple, and done so many times a day that the nurse may be slow to recognize it as evaluation at all. There are a number of purposes to incidental counseling. Some of these are: to give information or facts, to get information or facts, to interpret facts, to give advice or training, to help solve a problem or improve a situation, or to correct performance or action.

Formal Evaluation

In contrast, formal evaluation and counseling are concerned with the total picture of a person's performance on the job. Formal evaluation takes a broader view of performance and behavior with an eye to the overall development of employees and their roles in the health care organization. The formal evaluation session should be thought of as a periodic summary or counseling session, built on an accumulation of previous informal evaluation encounters and anecdotal notes. The annual evaluation of employees is the most common form of employee appraisal in nursing services across the nation.

You should recognize, however, that formal evaluation should, by no means, be restricted to a session once a year. Evaluation is an ongoing process that continues every minute of every working day. Formal evaluation is an integral part of the supervisor's duties and one that should be thought of as essential to the staff and to the employee. In actual fact, though, the task of evaluation is often looked upon as a difficult and thankless task. Most supervisors dread this part of their job more than any other.

Perhaps part of the problem is that formal evaluation techniques are often improperly used. The evaluation situation can never be a scientific tool, but it should be objective and valuable to everyone involved. Eliminating personal opinion and emotion is essential to writing personnel evaluations. However, no system of evaluation has been devised that is really adequate. The fault lies not in the system, but in the fact that the system must be administered by human beings. No one likes to be placed in the position of judging another individual, and that is precisely what the formal evaluation does. Staff members feel threatened at evaluation time, and this emotion interferes with their acceptance of the counseling session. An evaluation interview should be a time of growth for the employee, not one of disciplinary action.

WHY HAVE EVALUATION?

The purposes of formal evaluation are broader and more inclusive than those of on-the-job evaluation, but the basic goals remain the same for both:

1. *To help the employee to do a better job.* This goal includes making sure that the tasks and standards of the job are clearly understood by the individual employee.

2. *To give employees a clear picture of how they are currently performing.* Emphasis is placed on strengths as well as weaknesses. Supervisors or head nurses cannot be professionally helpful if they find nothing of value in a person, and if they find no strengths in that person's performance. Often, as one's strengths are identified, weaknesses come into focus. It is not easy to point out an employee's weaknesses, but this must be done.

3. *To develop an effective and strong relationship between the supervisor and the employee.* Strong relationships are needed to allow frank talk about the job, how it is being done, how improvement is possible, and how the task can be facilitated. Wise supervisors recognize that evaluation sessions provide opportunities to demonstrate interest and to inspire confidence.

4. *To reach an agreement on plans for improvement in the individual's overall performance.* Such agreement necessitates active participation on the part of the employee, and participation is predicated on acceptance and understanding. Acceptance and understanding by the employee make for the difference between the person who comes out of a counseling situation saying, "Whew, I'm glad that's over," and the one who exits saying, "Whew, looks like I've got a job to do."

5. *To provide a basis for development and training.* Often an analysis of the evaluation interviews for an entire department can isolate weaknesses and assist you in providing pertinent training programs.

6. *To aid in job placement, assignment, and promotion.* The evaluation can indicate strengths and weaknesses and help you to capitalize on them.

7. *To lay the groundwork for discipline.* Ideally, the evaluation interview should not be used for discipline, but, if certain areas of concern are outlined and documented, it can assist you in the decision to take punitive action.

8. *To encourage all supervisory personnel to take the time to coach employees.* It should come naturally to supervisory personnel to let their staff members know how they feel about their progress, but some supervisors need the requirement of an evaluation interview to take such action.

PROBLEMS IN EVALUATION

The major problem in evaluation programs is the lack of preparation of the evaluators. The usual method of training supervisors for this task is to hand out the evaluation forms and give a deadline for their return. Usually no more explanation is given than to "fill out the form." Because of such inadequate preparation, most supervisors go into the area of evaluation "blind," and they make several common errors.

Overly Generous Praise

The most common error is to be too generous in praise of an employee, while neglecting the opportunity to help staff members to see their weaknesses. The reasons for this error are easily seen. It is much easier to err on the side of generosity and to avoid antagonizing an employee. Nurses who are unfamiliar with the techniques of evaluation, or who are unsure of their roles as supervisors, take the easiest path to gain staff approval. Low ratings of an entire staff also reflect on the quality of the supervision in that area. It looks much better for supervisors if all of the ratings in the department are high, thereby raising their esteem as leaders. If raters have less experience than the person they are evaluating, they have difficulty being really critical of that person's behavior.

Leaving "Room to Grow"

Another mistake that evaluators frequently make is to start every new employee off with an average rating, then gradually raising the rating at each evaluation period. The thinking behind this approach is that you leave the new employee "room for growth." This method is a serious error that should be discouraged from the start. It is damaging to the organization and defeating to the employee. If staff members deserve to have the highest ratings in every area the first time they are formally evaluated, then they should receive those ratings. The rating scale is not the place to build in employee growth.

As the counseling session progresses, employees have an opportunity to set goals for the coming year. By learning more and more about the job and about the profession, employees show growth and improvement. If your rating form calls for such categories as poor, fair, average, good, and excellent, then employees should be rated on how their work fits into these categories. If all areas are excellent, then rate all areas excellent. When a first-grader, for example, deserves all As, he gets them. This rating does not mean that he does not have anything more to learn, it means only that, for the present time, he is meeting all the criteria for an excellent rating in every area. The following year, the criteria change, and so do the ratings, if necessary. It is the same in health care. Employees who do well in their work know that they have done well, and they deserve to be told. Nothing is as defeating to new employees as doing their best possible job and then receiving average ratings—"so they can grow." If excellent employees receive average ratings, they may be so discouraged that they will seek employment elsewhere, and you will lose a valuable asset.

Rating Specialty Units

Specialty units also cause concern for the evaluator. Since the staff is usually well trained and of above-average skills to work in such areas, the temptation is to rate them above-average just because of their additional preparation. These staff members should be rated on how well they do *their* job, no matter how critical in nature it is. They should be evaluated on how well they perform the tasks assigned to them, not on the nature of the tasks. Nurses working in specialty units should be compared with nurses doing similar work, not all nurses in general.

Prejudices and Biases

No matter what type of system you use for evaluation in your health care agency, it cannot be a useful tool unless everyone is using it in the prescribed manner. Inconsistent use of the system leads to confusion and useless data. Unless every evaluator understands the system and each item on the rating form, evaluation can never be objective. Each supervisor responsible for writing evaluations should be taught the organization's definition for each item. Without that definition, nurses rate each item with their own interpretations, and the evaluation is not valid.

Each and every nurse has personal prejudices and emotional biases. Occasionally, these show up on evaluations. If a supervisor is very appearance-conscious, for example, this factor shows on every rating form that he or she writes. As another example, a nurse who feels that bedside care should be performed only by female nurses is unable to write an objective evaluation of a male staff nurse. The way to eliminate this problem is to be aware of your own personal prejudices and to eliminate or overlook them, if possible.

If you are unable to overlook your prejudices, one solution is not to write an evaluation on any individuals who are affected. Another frequently offered solution to this problem is allowing two people to write an evaluation on a staff member. This is a viable alternative only if the evaluations are written independently and without consultation. Each supervisor should write his or her own evaluation, and, in the counseling session, the employee should see both forms. The discussion should include the employee and both evaluators. The reason for this requirement is to avoid a compromise evaluation. When two people with different viewpoints get together to reach consensus, the result is a blend of opinion, not a clear-cut definition of behavior. Employees deserve to see the highs and lows of their behavior, not an average of two opinions.

Seniority

Another problem in evaluations is allowing the seniority of an employee to affect the rating. Long-term staff members tend to receive higher ratings simply because of the length of time they have served the organization. Although loyalty is a good quality, it should not be used as a basis for judgment of behavior. A staff member is rated on behavior, not seniority.

"One-Time" Behavior

Rating on incidental, rather than pattern or consistent behavior, is another mistake often made. If a staff member makes an error, disciplinary action is usually taken at the time. If so, the entire evaluation should not be affected by this "one-time" problem. The way to avoid rating on the basis of incidental behavior is to keep anecdotal records of day-to-day activities. Then, at the time of the yearly interview, the evaluation reflects the entire year's performance, not just one or two incidents that stand out in the evaluator's mind. Remember, evaluations are continuous, not just yearly.

The "Halo Effect"

Try to avoid the "halo effect" in writing evaluations, which allows one highly favorable, or one highly unfavorable, attribute to color the entire evaluation. If a nurse is very dependable and can always be counted on to "pitch in" when things are busy, this characteristic tends to make the supervisor overlook the employee's quality of care. If appearance is important to you, a neat well-groomed nurse *seems* more efficient than a sloppy one. The way to eliminate the "halo effect" is to rate one item at a time, thinking only in terms of that item, not the overall evaluation.

Evaluation by Those Other Than Supervisors

The biggest problem in written evaluations is that they are often done by supervisors who do not know the employee. In some health care agencies, supervisors are expected to write evaluations on every person working on their shifts. The only way that they can do so is to interview the immediate superior of the staff member and try to assess behavior in this manner. This method should never be accepted. The evaluation process is effective only if it is done on a decentralized basis. Those closest in supervision to the employees should write the evaluation and no one else. This requirement means an increase in the number of persons writing evaluations, as well as an increase in the number of training hours necessary to adequately prepare the raters, but the results are worth the effort. More staff growth and motivation take place if the staff know that their evaluations were written and conducted by a person well aware of their strengths and weaknesses.

EVALUATIONS FORMS

Evaluation rating forms sometimes measure the wrong things. Some form items rate personality traits rather than accomplishments. The forms tend to rate persons, not the jobs they are doing. Personality rating does not work because traits don't necessarily accomplish the goals of the organization. Further, you cannot consistently or fairly evaluate the intangible personality traits listed on most forms. Although evaluations cannot be totally objective, they should be as objective as possible, and personality judgments cause emotional bias and subjectivity. Most nurses do not even agree on which traits are necessary to accomplish the goal of the organization. Basically, an evaluation should measure goal achievement. Goals can be reached only by improving individual performance. To do so, you need facts, not abstractions.

Standardized Forms

To simplify the process of writing evaluations, most health care agencies have gone to a printed form to be used on all employees. The purpose of the printed form is to standardize the format for all evaluations. If each person were asked to write an evaluation, using any method they thought appropriate (essentially an evaluation on a blank sheet of paper), there would be no consistency whatsoever. The content of each evaluation would depend entirely on each nurse's understanding of the job and its duties and responsibilities, as well as the evaluator's analytical ability and personal feelings. To avoid this problem, printed forms list specific behaviors and allow the evaluator to rate the employee on these behaviors. Standardized forms help the health care agency compare the performance of their staff on a similar scale.

Use of Judgmental Words

The simplest of these forms is the type that lists behaviors or personality traits and then asks the evaluator to rate the employee on these traits, using a scoring grid. (See Figure 13–1.) There are several problems with this type of form, most of them caused by the arrangement of the form itself.

Office Memorandum · UNITED STATES GOVERNMENT

TO   :   DATE:

FROM :   Chief, Personnel Division

SUBJECT: PROBATIONARY PERIOD REVIEW OF

Hospital and VA policy provide that a placement review must be made not later than the end of the 10th month following an employee's probational appointment. The purpose of this review is to determine whether the employee should be retained in his present position, assigned to other duties more in keeping with his abilities, or separated for failure to meet the requirements of Federal employment. This checklist will assist you in making the required review and certification.

Please complete and return this form to Personnel Division, in a sealed envelope, within 10 days.

PERFORMANCE FACTORS	EXC	VG	SAT	WEAK	UNSAT
Volume of work produced - speed in working					
Quality of work produced - freedom from error					
Dependability in meeting deadlines - keeping work current					
Knowledge of job techniques or work procedures					
Organization of work - does important things first					
Initiative - goes ahead without waiting to be told					

PERSONAL TRAITS

Cooperation with fellow workers and supervisors					
Attitude and job interest					
Reaction to constructive criticism					
Disposition and temperament					
Use of good judgment					
Learning ability - speed in grasping new ideas or work processes					
Oral expression - clearness of speech					
Appearance - neatness - grooming					

OTHER FACTORS CONSIDERED	YES	?	NO
Has prearrangement of annual leave & attendance been entirely satisfactory?			
Has conduct been satisfactory in every respect?			
Does employee accept work changes and emergency assignments willingly?			
Is this employee able to work closely with others without friction?			

OVERALL EVALUATION : ☐ EXCELLENT; ☐ VERY GOOD; ☐ SATISFACTORY;   ☐ UNSAT
IN PRESENT POSITION

<u>Please complete reverse side also</u>

I certify that this employee's performance, conduct and general traits have been found satisfactory/unsatisfactory. I recommend/do not recommend that he be retained in his present position beyond the 12 month probationary period.

_____   _____   _____   _____
Immediate Supervisor   Title   Ext.   Date

THIS EVALUATION HAS BEEN DISCUSSED WITH ME:

_____   _____   _____
Division/Service Chief   Employee's Signature   Date

Figure 13–1. Sample standardized evaluation form.

Evaluation

1. **Please explain** briefly any weak or unsatisfactory entries under the first two sections as well as any "no" or doubtful entries in the third section of the reverse side.

2. **What** action has been taken or is planned to overcome any deficiencies shown?

3. **Do** you feel that deficiencies shown are sufficiently compensated for by strong points, to warrant a satisfactory rating? **Please explain.**

4. **Do** you feel that this employee is reasonably well placed in his present position? If not, **what** type of work do you think would be more suitable?

5. **What** additional training would be desirable for this employee?

6. **What** assistance can the Personnel Division provide in counseling, training, or better utilizing this employee?

7. Other comments or recommendations.

_____   _____
Signature of Personnel Representative   Date

Figure 13–1 (*cont.*)

AMBIGUOUS TERMINOLOGY   With this form, the rater is asked to make a checkmark for each category on the scale. The terms used on the scale vary from form to form, but almost all the terms are open to free interpretation by the evaluator and by the staff person receiving the evaluation. Some examples are:

> Excellent—Very Good—Satisfactory—Weak—Unsatisfactory
>
> Above Average—Average—Below Average
>
> Excellent—Good—Average—Fair—Poor
>
> Competent—Improvement Needed—Unsatisfactory

Each of these examples leaves room for subjective judgment on the part of the rater. A choice must be made, usually not on a definite scale, but on the rater's opinion. People do not fit into boxes, and most supervisors run into the situation of giving a person a satisfactory plus or an average minus. Each of these rating words has an emotional tone. One person might consider "Average" equivalent to performing as most nurses with similar background and skill. This definition is positive. Someone else, however, might think that "Average" means "ordinary" or performing to the minimum degree necessary for success. This person sees "average" as a negative term. When these two opposing views are joined in the form of an evaluation and counseling session, there can be no growth or harmony, just a discussion of semantics.

If a scale must be used, it should not use the types of words that bring emotional feelings into play. One system is to use percentages: "75 percent" to "100 percent" rather than "Poor" to "Excellent." In other words, the staff person performs, say, as well as 85 percent of other staff members with similar duties and training. The sound of "85 percent" is less emotional than "Good." There are many numbers from 75 to 100, and this range gives the rater a wider choice and more of a chance to be specific.

Poor Layout

The second set of problems with this grid formation on a rating scale is human nature. We are human, and, try as we might, we cannot eliminate our human failings, or "quirks." When the form is set in a pattern like that of our first example, it is too easy for the rater to see the entire form all at once. The eye travels to what it wants to see, and only to that. For example, suppose the evaluator handed a form to a staff member with a pattern as shown in Table 13–1. Which item would the staff member look at first? Of course, the "Poor." This reaction starts the interview off on a negative note, one thing a supervisor tries to avoid.

The idea behind an evaluation is growth, and there can be no growth if a person is concerned only with areas of weakness. Most nurses who are evaluated with this type of form can immediately recall

293

TABLE 13–1

E	G	A	F	P
x				
x				
				x
x				
x				

their areas of weakness, but are hard-pressed to remember the areas in which they excelled.

Other errors that occur with this grid formation are on the part of the evaluator. To eliminate the "halo effect," the supervisor must evaluate one area at a time and think about each area individually. Suppose you have done just that—rated each item individually—and now that you are finished, you take a look at your form, shown in Table 13–2. You may be tempted to say to yourself, "That employee is not that good." You may, arbitrarily, lower one or more of the ratings just to more "accurately" portray the person's abilities. Not fair! The evaluation was designed to rate separate items, not the overall picture of how you see the employee. Once the rating is finished, leave it alone.

Other quirks show up in this system. Suppose you have to rate an employee very low in one area. You know that the person is going to see that area immediately. The tendency is to raise another area to "balance" the evaluation, thus aiding you in your interview. You are not raising the area because the employee deserves a higher rating, but just to balance your books.

The form illustrated in Figure 13–1 is very poor because of the grid formation, which causes the evaluator to make decisions based not

TABLE 13–2

E	G	A	F	P
x				
x				
x				
x				
x				

on fact, but on emotion. The sooner this pattern can be eliminated, the better.

Improper Emphasis on Nonmeasurable Behaviors

A problem on most evaluation forms is the categories themselves. Just removing the "colored" evaluation terms and the grid formation does not automatically improve the form. You must look to the traits and behaviors listed for evaluation, which are often not definable or measurable in a standardized way. Some common terms listed on evaluation forms are: professional competence, ability to get along, attitude toward patients. These are vague terms—terms that no two people see exactly the same way. Each item on an evaluation form should be measurable; that is, each person using the form should know what the behavior means and have a scale to rate the behavior.

Punctuality is an example of a measurable behavior. The supervisory staff can set aside the criteria and rate each person on them. For instance, using a "Good—Average—Poor" scale:

Tardy one to zero times in one year = Good

Tardy two to three times in one year = Average

Tardy three or more times in one year = Poor

Punctuality is thus rated the same way by every person using the form. Employees who receive poor ratings can be shown that they did not meet the criteria for receiving any higher rating. There is no room for discussion or argument.

Not all behaviors, however, can be made as measurable as punctuality or appearance. Yet each and every behavior can be discussed, and guidelines can be set by the staff concerning an accurate definition of each category of response for each behavior. The goal is to measure each person on the same scale and to eliminate personal opinion. This goal can be achieved only by using measurable behaviors.

Some items on an evaluation form are unnecessary, almost silly. Honesty is an example. Nurses are professionals and therefore considered honest. If they are not, they should not be employed at the health care agency. To rate nurses "Average" in honesty makes no sense. Does that mean that they lie and steal no more or no less than every other nurse? Silly, of course. Yet this item continues to appear on forms, serving no useful purpose. A nurse who rates a "Poor" in honesty or integrity should have been counseled much sooner than at a yearly evaluation interview.

If the items on the evaluation form are not measurable, staff members do not know specifically what they are doing right or which areas need improvement. Trying to define or explain why you rated an employee low in "Judgment" is a difficult task. Explaining why calling the doctor at 3:00 A.M. for a laxative order shows "Poor" judgment is much easier, and much more learning takes place. Make the items behavior-oriented, and the definitions will come much easier. Remember, rate the tasks, not the personality of the person.

If the grid formation, judgmental words, and nonmeasurable behaviors are eliminated, you are well on your way to a workable evaluation form. The only additional necessary items are: (1) a space for comments and (2) a space for goal setting.

Comments

Comments are essential on an evaluation form in order to make the tool personal and useful. Checkmarks in specific boxes do not mean as much to staff members as specific comments about their behavior.

Again, we have problems with the layout of the form. Given our nature, when we see comments on a form, our eyes immediately travel to the comment section. The value of the rest of the evaluation may be lost. So starting with a negative comment is bad psychology, but, if it is the only comment written on the form, the staff member sees it first.

To eliminate this problem, some health care agencies institute a policy requiring that a comment be written explaining any Above-Average or Below-Average rating. This idea is very sound. The purpose of the evaluation is learning, and in this way specific behaviors can be pointed out in comment form. The comment may even include specific ways that the problem can be eliminated or reduced. (The training program for those individuals using this system has to include the warning not to yield to the temptation of giving all average ratings.)

Goal Setting

For the evaluation form to be a tool for growth, it must contain an area for the setting of specific goals or objectives, perhaps the last page. One method of dealing with goal setting is to give the goals and objectives section of the form to employees several days prior to the evaluation interview. Have them fill out their objectives for the coming year and bring the form to the interview, which is a perfect opportunity for the staff member and the supervisor to discuss the goals and see how they fit into the goals and objectives of the health care organization. If a specific goal is set, there should also be a definite date for the completion of the behavior. At that time, the supervisor and the staff member would meet again to discuss the goal and assess its success or failure.

OTHER TYPES OF RATING SYSTEMS

Because of the problems in the existing printed forms, some health care agencies have gone to alternative rating systems. Some of these systems are quite good, but some have tried so hard to eliminate prejudice that thay are of little use to the organization or to the employee.

Job Description Evaluation Form

One method that is being used with success is the job description evaluation format. Copies of employees' job descriptions are used to evaluate their progress. The procedure is very simple: A scale of acceptable behavior levels is established, and, by this scale, employees are rated on every task that they are expected to do. The theory is that the persons are rated only on the tasks that they have been hired to do, not on personality traits or on vague nonmeasurable statements.

The problem is that the job descriptions do not always contain behaviors that the organization needs to evaluate. For example, with other types of evaluation forms, staff members occasionally complain that, although they were hired to give quality patient care, they are evaluated on their team spirit or loyalty to the organization. These traits are important to the goal attainment of the health care agency, and, while the job description evaluation eliminates this criticism, it does not allow the agency to evaluate them. The only way that this system can really work is to include in the job description not only task behaviors, but also attitude and personality traits that are necessary to perform well. If the job description is well written and complete, it is a very effective way of evaluating performance.

Health care agencies that do not use this specific format for evaluation, but that receive criticism about the rating of personality traits as well as task behavior, can improve their evaluation technique very easily. If, when employees are hired, they are given copies of the evaluation form, as well as copies of the job description, they have a clear idea of what the agency requires of them. Many times employees do not even realize that they are to be rated on attitude. This misunderstanding is easily corrected by showing them the evaluation form used by your agency and by explaining that not only will they be expected to perform the behaviors on the job description, they will also be expected to be loyal, prompt, honest, and so on.

Self-Evaluation

One of the most common of the newer methods of evaluation is allowing employees to rate themselves. Usually the rating done in

297

preparation for an evaluation interview with the supervisor. The supervisor also rates the employee on a separate form. At the interview, the two forms are compared to give a composite evaluation for the file.

There are many problems in this system. Usually, the really good people rate themselves too low on the scale, and their ratings must be raised during the interview. This sort of change feels good to staff members—boosting their egos—but it defeats the purpose of a self-evaluation. The purpose is to get an accurate picture of employees as they see themselves, not to spend the entire interview session patting them on the back. If employees really feel that their behavior is not as good as the supervisor sees it, then there has been a breakdown in communication, which should have been eliminated long before the yearly evaluation interview.

On the other hand, some employees may rate themselves very high for a variety of reasons. This tendency turns the interview into an exercise in tact for the supervisor, rather than a learning experience for the employee. The supervisor spends valuable time convincing employees why they are not really that high on the rating scale. In such cases, the interview may be a learning experience, but, more often than not, it is only an occasion for hard feelings and negative thoughts about evaluation.

The only time that self-evaluation really works is if the employee is carefully taught the purpose of the evaluation and the methods of preparation. If all members of the staff understand the purpose of self-evaluation and are willing to give a really accurate picture of themselves, the system is profitable to them and to the agency.

One area in which this is the system of choice is the evaluation of supervisory personnel. Those nurses on the management level are usually well aware of the evaluation technique and give an accurate rating of their current status. This approach can mean a valuable time of self-reflection and self-evaluation.

Peer Evaluation

Along the same lines as self-evaluation is the system of peer evaluation. This system is based on the premise that only those who work side-by-side with each other are in a position to really evaluate the quality of each other's work. This method works well if everyone is taught the procedure, is willing to be objective in their ratings, and is willing to invest the necessary time to participate.

The problems come when the evaluation is used as a weapon. Abusing this system is all too easy—patting friends on the back or stabbing enemies in the back. Although most staff members would not abuse this system, some individuals would. With any abuse, the value of the evaluation system is reduced, and staff members cannot respect its validity.

In supervisory roles this system works well, just as self-evaluation. The difference is in the training of the raters.

Goal Setting (Management by Objectives)

This excellent system of evaluation combines the best of the printed form with the attributes of self-evaluation. The basis of the method is a cooperative effort by the employee and the supervisor to list goals and objectives for the coming year. Usually, this goal setting is an addition to the usual printed evaluation form, which lists behaviors and rates them according to some scale, but it may also exist alone. The goals that the employee sets must be consistent with the expectations of the employer, they must be measurable, and they must be attainable within a certain time limit.

This method would seem to be the answer to all the problems of employee evaluation. It rates the employee on the quality of task behaviors expected by the health care agency. It also provides for the recording of employee growth. Employees do not feel threatened by this rating system because they are actively participating in the goal-setting process. This logical plan for action motivates employees to set goals that would otherwise seem unattainable, because they feel the cooperative spirit between management and staff. The built-in reward system is that employees see their own growth as each yearly review takes place.

Although this system seems nearly perfect, there are a few problems. First, the evaluation takes a great deal of time. Employees must take the time to write their goals. Supervisors must also write goals, and, at the interview, employee and supervisory goals must be compared and refined. Training the employees to write goals and objectives for themselves is a lengthy procedure. Most people are unable to immediately understand goal setting, and some people have never thought in terms of career goals. If an organization is willing to take the time and effort necessary to institute this procedure, the rewards may be increased in terms of employee motivation, morale, and productivity. Using management by objectives, supervisors must be aware of the fact that, although employee productivity increases at first, it tends to equal out in the long run. In other words, employees set very high standards for themselves at first and meet them, but, as time passes, the results are usually the same as in any other form of evaluation.

The Perfect Evaluation(?)

So what is the answer? Is there a perfect evaluation technique? No—no one system works for everyone in every health care setting. The individuals and the organization must be considered before any system can be selected. The best evaluation technique for your organization is the one that is the simplest and easiest to use and the one that meets the needs of the majority of the staff. Remember, no evaluation system is perfect, but many are better than others. The principle goal is to keep the evaluation process as objective as possible. Keeping in mind the fact that the major purpose of evaluation is employee growth will assist you in choosing the best system for your particular situation. Basically, the elements of a good evaluation system are:

1. The standards of the system must be well established and known to everyone. Explaining the plan and outlining the guidelines of the rating system eliminate many problems.
2. Subordinates should be rated on an established system, which is used by all persons in the evaluation role. It should be based on performance standards, not personality traits. If job description evaluations are used, the criteria should be: Was the duty performed satisfactorily to obtain the desired results?
3. All persons writing employee evaluations should be properly trained in the procedure. This training includes: instruction on what to rate and how to rate it, sharpening observation skills, resolving differences in values, being made aware of the fact that everyone makes errors, and improving counseling techniques.
4. The best evaluation systems include goals mutually set by the leader and the employee.
5. Any evaluation system must be a regular program, one that can be expected to be the same each time the evaluation takes place. If there are changes in format, the employee must know about these changes before the yearly interview.

IMPROVING YOUR EVALUATION TECHNIQUES

If you are in the position of writing evaluations, you may not have any control over the format used in your institution. This lack of control does not mean that the quality of your evaluation cannot improve. No matter which system you use, the principles are the same. Observe your employees constantly. Watch, listen, and record behaviors that are pertinent to an analysis of employee proficiency or deficiency.

Never write an evaluation on an employee you don't know. Take the time to seek out that employee's immediate supervisor, and train him or her to write the evaluation.

Know your evaluation forms, and know the agreed-upon rating scales. Try to keep your personal opinion out of any evaluation, and rate only on organizational objectives. Remember to avoid "personal prejudices" and "halo effect" items.

One good technique is to inform employees that their yearly evaluations are coming up. This forewarning gives them time to think about the previous year and to establish some tentative goals for performance. It also gives them time to formulate any questions that they may have.

During the interview, it is valuable to ask employees, "What are your most important jobs, as you see them?" If their answers are very different from how you see the job, you have a more complete picture of the employee's performance and job expectations. Another important question to ask is, "What changes would you like to make in your job?" This too assists you in helping the employee to reach the objectives of the agency. Employees seldom tell you specifically what jobs they cannot do, but certain questions give you this information. Asking, "What is the hardest part of your job?" helps you to see employee weaknesses, as well as needed training areas. This question could also help you to analyze the assignment of tasks. You may see an area in which you demand too much from an employee.

Since the purpose of the evaluation is to assist staff members, you should offer to help improve. "How can I help you more?" is a good query that enables employees to express their feelings about your supervision.

THE EVALUATION INTERVIEW

After you have written an evaluation of an employee, the presentation of the information to employees is as important as the content of the evaluation form. Plan for the evaluation interview carefully, and have all necessary materials available. You should review the form briefly before the staff member arrives so that all information is fresh in your mind.

For the meeting itself, select a suitable place. Privacy and freedom from interruptions are essential and conducive to frank discussion. Select a suitable time for the interview. Discussions and decisions are hampered if work pressures keep either of you from concentrating on the task at hand. Avoid scheduling an evaluation interview shortly after you have had to reprimand an employee.

Be sure that you know precisely what you want to accomplish during the interview. Make certain that you have a specific plan. Have all the facts, and be clear about the strengths and weaknesses that you are going to discuss with the staff member. Be prepared for disagreement. After all, we don't all have to agree on everything. With this in mind, you can face the fact that not every session will be totally pleasant.

Try to create an atmosphere that eliminates anxiety or tension. If you are relaxed, it helps the employee to relax. The appropriate atmosphere gives the impression that you are really caring, interested, and willing to exchange ideas. Genuine interest in a person makes the evaluation interview more pleasant and more productive.

Give your undivided attention to the interview, and you get the respect and attention of the employee. Just because you are face-to-face with a person does not assure you of his or her attention. Your manner can indicate that you expect attention and help you make the employee feel important and accepted. This manner may take the form of paying a genuine compliment for a job well done or of asking a question that shows you value the employee's opinion.

At the start of the interview make sure that the staff member understands the purpose of the evaluation. Even though you are having an annual evaluation interview, it is advisable to state the purpose of the session. Your ultimate goal is employee improvement, and saying so to persons shows that you and the organization are interested in them and in their professional growth. By your words and actions, indicate that you value their contributions to the health care agency and that you care about their level of job satisfaction.

Allow employees to read the evaluation, and give them time to think about what they have read. Never give the impression that you are rushed. If you must indicate a weakness to staff members, make sure you include a method for improvement, or at least allow time to discuss the possible ways to improve.

After employees have read the evaluation form and you have made any necessary comments, give them time to talk. Be sure to listen carefully and open-mindedly to anything they have to say. The goals of the evaluation interview are destroyed if you talk constantly. Doing so puts up a screen of words that makes any two-way communication impossible. Just the courtesy of attentive listening conveys to employees that what they have to say is important and that they are important.

Once the initial discussion has ended, try to arrive at a plan for further development and improvement. Here you must be specific. It is necessary to have concrete plans to help the improvement take place. Hopefully, employees will be able to assume some initiative in the planning stage, and you will only provide direction and guidance.

Prepare for follow-up to the interview. No evaluation session is finished until a specific time for follow-up has been established. At the close of the interview, make sure that employees feel good about the session and have expressed any feelings that they may have. Make sure that all areas have been covered and that the interview has been productive. If areas of improvement have been indicated, counsel employees carefully so that you are certain that mutual understanding has been reached.

Counseling

The evaluation interview serves many purposes, not the least of which is the opportunity for some real employee counseling. There are two types of counseling: (1) direct and (2) nondirective.

DIRECT COUNSELING   In this purposeful conversation, the supervisor attempts to help the employee grow by advising, telling, instructing, or suggesting. Direct counseling has been referred to as "advice-giving" and "fact-centered." It could also be called "supervisory-centered" because the supervisor gives the advice or facts. Another way of looking at this technique is to understand that administration relies on the supervisor's superior knowledge and judgment: knowledge of the job to be done and of the performance required to satisfactorily do the job, as well as the judgment to define any real problems and to recommend action. The supervisor's role is a decisive one in direct counseling.

Supervisors or head nurses may find it necessary to draw out information from the employee when engaged in direct counseling. This intent is most easily accomplished by direct questioning, but such questioning does not always get the results you expect. Encourage participation in the conversation on a factual or intellectual level, and attempt to minimize the emotional element as much as possible.

In direct counseling situations employees are often advised of decisions made for them. In this sense, the direct technique appears to be the least democratic of all possible approaches to evaluation.

Direct counseling deals with job performance, job behavior, and prescribed courses of action. You should begin every direct counseling situation with a distinct plan in mind. The goal for the session must be clearly defined, and there must be no question about attaining it. There is no room for vacillation and weakness when dealing with standards of job performance, job behavior, and indicated courses of action.

Use of the direct approach to counseling is indicated when:

1. employees have little or no insight into themselves in their work situation, or when there is little reason to hope that they ever will show much insight;
2. the employee has a rigid mind-set;
3. the employee is indecisive;
4. emergency situations arise; and
5. in most instances of significant disciplinary problems.

NONDIRECTIVE COUNSELING   The nondirective approach is geared to enhance employees' growth and development by helping them gain insight in terms of the job and in terms of self-direction. The psychologist, Carl Rogers, played a major part in the development of nondirective counseling techniques. Rogers felt that if you can provide a certain type of relationship, the other person discovers the capacity to use that relationship for growth and for a process of change. As a result, personal development occurs. "There can be no doubt about the effectiveness of such a relationship in producing personality change."[1]

Obviously, the emphasis is placed on relationships, for which there are three criteria:

1. *Be genuine.* The degree of helpfulness found in a counseling situation is directly proportionate to its genuine elements. The relationship should not allow a facade of one attitude or feeling to cover up another.
2. *Accept and like the individual.* Acceptance, as used here, means the "warm regard for him as a person of unconditional self-worth." Such acceptance promotes a feeling of being liked and therefore a feeling of safety. Feeling safe is vital to any helping relationship.
3. *Feel a continuing desire to understand.* Acceptance means little until understanding starts. To understand, you must rule out any moral and diagnostic evaluation, for these are always threatening.

The clinical, nondirective counseling technique of Rogers and other counselor–psychologists is not what we, as nurses, are prepared to use. The nondirective approach has been adequately modified, however, to allow for its effective use in evaluation interviews. The modifications permit us to employ a nondirective technique that is less deep than that practiced by the trained counselor–psychologist and not threatening or traumatic. For the nondirective technique to be used effectively, it is mandatory that you exercise keen judgment as to when and with whom it is used and that you are prepared to carry through with your technique. It is also essential that you have some knowledge and observance of your own limitations.

In nondirective counseling you deal with the picture that employees have of themselves. Nondirective counseling permits employees to express attitudes and feelings, and it allows supervisors to reflect upon and to clarify their employees' feelings. This sort of counseling permits all this only if you, as the supervisor, listen:

First, you listen to communicate that, "I care." Undivided attention tells employees that you are interested, that they have something of value to say, and that they are worthy of concern. Listening communicates "I care" by means other than silence: Facial expressions, gestures, eye contact, and posture are all part of your listening skills.

[1] C. R. Rogers, *Counselling and Psychotherapy* (Boston: Houghton-Mifflin Company, 1942).

Second, you listen to "stay on the beam." There is no other way to grasp what is being said and later to reflect and clarify what was said. There is no more effective way to disrupt the whole counseling situation than to respond with a comment or question that is completely inappropriate.

Third, you listen for what is not said, or for what is said only with great difficulty. Listening for what is not said may make the difference between successful and unsuccessful counseling. Attitudes and feelings that remain unexpressed by employees may still affect a decision they make. Any decision made on the basis of only a portion of one's feelings and attitudes is an unstable one, and it often goes unimplemented because it conflicts with unexpressed feelings and ideas. Further, the fact that something is difficult to discuss may mean it has an important and depth of meaning for the individual.

You may listen with a fourth purpose in mind: to glean something of what the employee is conveying by means other than words. In a sense, then, you listen with a third ear, which enables you to pick up such clues as a change in vocal pitch, undue emphasis on certain words, hesitation in speech, a shift in posture, a tensing of muscles, inappropriate gestures, the ability to make and/or hold eye contact, changes in color, and flights of ideas.

So when do you talk? In nondirective counseling, you talk or ask questions only:

1. when the employee seems to want to say something, but finds it very difficult to do so;
2. to direct the interview toward an omitted or imcompletely discussed topic; or
3. to clarify and to give approval. (Approval is not to be given indiscriminately, however. It is best given in recognition for insight, as this is developed by the employee.)

You should know how to use the pause, another difficult skill. Perhaps the very reason for the awkwardness of the pause is that it can represent growth taking place—and that process can be painful. During the pause, employees may be seeing an unpleasant picture of themselves, their deficiencies, and their need for improvement.

The use of the nondirective approach is indicated if you estimated that the employee has insight. More important, you must have the strength and capacity to take action based on insight. As a nurse/supervisor, you must estimate whether you, as a person, are capable of employing the nondirective technique in counseling. Much has been said about the importance of attitudes and their expression, but nowhere are attidues of greater significance than within supervisors or head nurses. Do you see each person as one of worth and significance?

Do you see each person as one of individual dignity? Does your attitude allow you to see within the other individual the capacity and right for self-direction? Or do you have such needs for domination that a non-directive approach is an impossibility for you? These are questions you must answer for yourself. Obviously, some supervisors cannot and should not attempt nondirective counseling.

A COMBINED COUNSELING APPROACH   Counseling is not strictly limited to either the direct or nondirective techniques. There is value in a combination of approaches. At no time should supervisors be inflexible in their choice of counseling methods, as long as they recognize certain fundamental principles underlying all counseling sessions:

1. *Counseling involves relationships between people, and emotional elements are therefore always present.* Because of the importance of this principle, recent writers on the counseling process stress the area of relationships rather than techniques; they stress the "climate" rather than rules of behavior.

2. *All evaluation has a therapeutic or helping aspect to it.* Any evaluation situation is far more than advice-giving, and it can be truly therapeutic. When it is, employees are helped to develop on the job. They become receptive to the supervisor's ideas and advice, to looking within themselves and their attitudes. Only as attitudes change can behavior on the job change, and you can "trigger" on-the-job behavior by helping to change or build attitudes. You also should recognize that the whole of any evaluation calls for as much honesty as possible.

3. *Each employee has different counseling needs.* With one employee, successful counseling may mean giving support, while another employee may need telling, advising, and defining. The exercise of judgment to determine which counseling approach to employ is as challenging and exacting as the counseling itself. Selecting the counseling approach means knowing the personnel for whom you are responsible. Such a selection can be predicated only on a supervisor's and head nurse's knowledge of "their" personnel.

Regardless of the approach, counseling takes skill, but its results can be extremely gratifying.

HANDLING A DIFFICULT EVALUATION INTERVIEW

What about when the shoe is on the other foot? How do you deal with disagreement over the evaluation? Giving constructive criticism is just as important as giving praise. Yet what happens if the employee disagrees with your evaluation? The best way to deal with this problem is to plan ahead for conflict. Thinking about how you would deal with certain problems helps you to avoid conflicts in evaluation interviews.

If employees think that your evaluation does not provide enough information or that the ratings are unfair, allow them to discuss the additions or corrections they think should be made. Discuss the changes with an open mind, and admit any errors or oversights you may have made. If the two of you still disagree, allow the employee to write a statement to that effect and file it with the evaluation.

If an area is extremely low, give specific examples to support that rating. If employees feel that they have done extremely well in certain area, don't hesitate to add it to the evaluation—if it is indeed true. The evaluation is a record of behavior; it is no place for modesty or error. Counsel employees in such a way that if they receive a low rating, they start working immediately to improve that rating.

Many staff members complain that the evaluation interview is unnecessary because, "Everyone knows what they are going to hear." This is exactly as it should be. If supervisors and staff are exchanging views, suggesting changes, and helping each other everyday, then the once-a-year formal evaluation won't surprise anyone. Evaluation interviews should be a time for complimenting performance, for reaffirming mutual goals, for arriving at a mutual pact to make things even better, and for setting the time for a follow-up conference, if necessary.

DISCUSSION QUESTIONS

1. What is the aim or purpose of employee evaluations?
2. What is meant by "measurable" items?
3. What factors must be taken into consideration when weighing an employee's performance rating?
4. What is job description evaluation? How can it be applied to your health care agency?
5. What is the role of the supervisor in evaluation?
6. Compare and contrast directive versus nondirective counseling.
7. Do you have a personal prejudice about a specific item or behavior?

APPLICATION: EVALUATING EVALUATION FORMS

1. Using the information you have read in this chapter, look at the sample evaluation forms in the appendix, and analyze them. Find examples of:
   a. nonmeasurable items,

    b. items that are merely personality traits and unnecessary on an evaluation form,

    c. "colored" rating words on the evaluation form, and

    d. grid pattern evaluation forms.

2. Select the form you feel most adequately meets the needs of employee evaluation at your health care agency.

    a. What are the best features of this form?

    b. How can the form be improved?

3. Using the best features from each example, design a new evaluation system for your health care agency. Use any evaluation system that you feel best meets your needs, and prepare a form.

APPLICATION: SUPERVISOR'S RATING SHEET FOR THE GROUP

Size Up Your Group

You will get an idea of their efficiency—whether they are producing as much as you have a right to expect.

Method of Scoring

Read the questions carefully, evaluate, then place your evaluation on the line to the right of the question. Score on this basis:

- Outstanding—5
- Above-Average—4
- Average—3
- Below Average—2
- Poor—1

Let's Go

1. Do your group members have plenty of enthusiasm?   ——

2. Do they keep busy at all times instead of loafing?   ——

3. Do they know the reason behind the work they do rather than just "grind it out"?   ——

4. Are they quick to understand your instructions?   ——

5. How is their teamwork? Do they work well together?   ——

6. Can you get results by asking them to do a job instead of commanding them?   ——

7. Does their work conform to standard practice?   ——

8. Does each one carry a full share of the load?   ——

9. Is their routine work kept in shape so that special jobs can be handled efficiently?   ——

10. Are they improving themselves by night school courses, lectures, outside reading? ___
11. Does the group make helpful suggestions? ___
12. Do they come to you for help? ___
13. Are they inclined to do their work without needless fretting and worry? ___
14. Are they accepting responsibility for assigned work rather than annoying you with every small detail? ___
15. Do they respond to constructive criticism and reprimands? ___
16. Do they get their work out on time? ___
17. Do they perform their job in a planned manner instead of hit-or-miss? ___
18. Is the quality of their work high? ___
19. Is the group vigilant in checking for errors? ___
20. Is your group careful in the proper use of materials and equipment? ___
Add 'em up: ===

It's Done

You have just rated your group. More important, you have rated your own ability as a supervisor, because the qualities of good leaders are reflected in the people they lead and the amount of quality production their personnel turn out.

If your total score is near 100, either you are an optimist or out of this world. If around or under 60, you need a good shot in the arm.

Self-improvement begins with an honest recognition of our weak points, then doing something about them.

TABLE 13–3
A supervisor's self-rating chart

EVIDENCES ON SUPERVISOR'S PART	EFFECTS ON SUBORDINATES	SUGGESTIONS FOR IMPROVING
Unfairness, partiality	Will lose respect of favored one; arouses resentment of others; slack work.	Give square deal; put yourself in others' shoes; treat everyone fairly; play no favorites.
Not practicing what you preach	Contagious; others will try to get away with it; disrupts discipline.	Watch your step; set only good example.

TABLE 13–3 (*cont.*)

EVIDENCES ON SUPERVISOR'S PART	EFFECTS ON SUBORDINATES	SUGGESTIONS FOR IMPROVING
Shirking responsibility, "passing the buck"	Loses respect of superiors and followers; others begin passing buck; active dissatisfaction; disrupts morale.	Shoulder own responsibilities; take blame if due; don't pass the buck.
Not interested in work	Lack of interest on part of staff; poor results.	Get interested or get out!
Overbearing, "high hat," unapproachable	Staff becomes "jumpy"; kills initiative; uneasiness and uncertainty, resentment.	Put yourself in others' shoes; be human and reasonable.
Quick-tempered, "going off half-cocked"	Same as for "overbearing."	Take time to cool off; look into various angles before making decision.
Lack of patience	Can't get results, discourages the staff; afraid to admit they don't understand.	Self-analysis; work on self-control; put yourself in others' place; take time to do job well.
Inconsistent	Staff uneasy and unsettled. Hesitate to go ahead; kills initiative.	Self-analysis; adopt a uniform policy and hold to it.
Leader ignorant of job, bluffing	No respect or confidence; staff won't follow lead; will short-circuit and go to higher-up for orders.	Apply yourself to learn what you don't know.
Continually finding fault, nagging.	Kills initiative; creates ill will.	Be fair; remember, everyone makes mistakes.
Leader failure as instructor	Staff not properly instructed; can't perform work properly; loss of production or property and even life.	Plan your work in advance; change your methods; study how to teach.
Unwilling to take suggestions, won't admit mistakes, bullheadedness, conceited	Kills initiative; loose benefit of valuable suggestions; kills cooperation.	Be open to suggestions at proper time and place; admit mistakes if occasion arises.

TABLE 13–3 (*cont.*)

EVIDENCES ON SUPERVISOR'S PART	EFFECTS ON SUBORDINATES	SUGGESTIONS FOR IMPROVING
Failure to give credit, grabbing credit where not due	Lack of credit; resentment; kills initiative; stops cooperation.	Put yourself in others' place; give credit when due.
Lack of consideration for, or interest in, staff	Staff will lie down on job whenever supervisor's back is turned.	Place yourself in others' place; be human.
Snooping	Loss of respect; creates suspicion; arouses resentment.	Don't do it; discourage in others.
Too familiar with staff	Loss of respect; loss of teamwork; loss of discipline.	Maintain a certain reserve befitting a position as leader.
Lax discipline	No teamwork; loss of respect.	Tighten up gradually but firmly and hold for results.
Staff lacks confidence	Won't follow supervisor's lead; will wait for orders from higher-up; no teamwork.	Self-analysis; under certain conditions do job yourself; actually lead group; make no promises you can't fill.
Dislike of group for leader	Staff will only carry out *direct orders*; no teamwork; unpleasant feeling.	Check up on self instead; lead instead of drive; put self in others' place; talk over on one-to-one basis; be courteous and human.

REFERENCES

FLESCH, RUDOLPH, *The ABC of Style: A Guide to Plain English*. New York: Harper & Row, Publishers Inc., 1964.

HAYAKAWA, S. I., *Language in Thought and Action*. New York: Harcourt, Brace and World, Inc., 1949.

PARRY, JOHN, *The Psychology of Communications*. London: University of London Press Ltd., 1967.

SAYLES, LEONARD, "On-the-Job Communications," *Supervisory Management* (August 1967).

APPENDIX: SAMPLE EVALUATION FORMS

Sample standardized evaluation forms are shown on pages 312 to 327.

EMPLOYEE DEVELOPMENT

Last Name	First Name	Middle Initial	Facility	Department	Position

Reason for Rendering Report (check one)	Date Last Salary Increase	Period Covered by this Evaluation
_____ Annual _____ End of Probationary Period _____ Termination _____ Change of duty _____ Other _____		From: To:

	Above Average	Average	Needs Improvement
ADAPTABILITY - Adjusts to new or changing situations and stresses; bears up under pressure			
APPEARANCE - Is neat and well groomed			
COOPERATION - Works in harmony with others as a team member			
DEPENDABILITY - Consistently accomplishes desired actions with minimum supervision			
INITIATIVE - Takes necessary and appropriate action on his/her own			
INTELLIGENCE - Acquires knowledge and grasps concepts readily; thinks logically and makes practical decisions			
SELF-DISCIPLINE - Conducts himself in accordance with accepted standards			
TACT - Says or does what is appropriate without giving unnecessary offense; is understanding of other's viewpoint			

STRENGTHS: In which areas does he/she perform particularly well?

IMPROVEMENTS: In which areas are improvements desirable?

JOB EFFECTIVENESS: In what ways has he/she become more effective during the last 12 months? (Including seminars, study, experience, and any other self development.)

DEVELOPMENT: What specific recommendations did you make that will contribute to further job-effectiveness of this employee.

Signature of Supervisor	Date	My review indicates no further action _____
Signature of Employee	Date	See comments on reverse _____
Signature of Department Head	Date	Signature of Administrator Date

Figure 13–2.

EMPLOYEE PERFORMANCE REVIEW   REVIEW DATE: / /

EMPLOYEE	CLASSIFICATION	COST CENTER	DATE
			/ /

I. ASSIGNMENTS SINCE LAST REVIEW:

II. PERFORMANCE ASSESSMENT
  A. PRODUCTIVITY (COMPARE VOLUME OF WORK OUTPUT TO STANDARDS OR REQUIREMENTS):

CONSISTENTLY EXCEEDS WORK GROUP STANDARDS/REQUIREMENTS ☐   MEETS WORK GROUP STANDARDS/REQUIREMENTS ☐
OFTEN EXCEEDS WORK GROUP STANDARDS/REQUIREMENTS ☐   DOES NOT MEET WORK GROUP STANDARDS/REQUIREMENTS ☐

  B. WORKMANSHIP (COMPARE QUALITY OF WORK TO REQUIREMENTS FOR THIS ASSIGNMENT. CONSIDER ACCURACY, NEATNESS, ERRORS, REJECTS, THOROUGHNESS, AND COMPLETENESS OF WORK PERFORMED):

CONSISTENTLY EXCEEDS WORK GROUP STANDARDS/REQUIREMENTS ☐   MEETS WORK GROUP STANDARDS/REQUIREMENTS ☐
OFTEN EXCEEDS WORK GROUP STANDARDS/REQUIREMENTS ☐   DOES NOT MEET WORK GROUP STANDARDS/REQUIREMENTS ☐

  C. PROFICIENCY (COMPARE JOB KNOWLEDGE TO REQUIREMENTS FOR THIS ASSIGNMENT. CONSIDER APPLICABLE METHODS, PROCESSES, AND PROCEDURES; PROPER USE OF EQUIPMENT; AND GENERAL ADEQUACY OF SKILLS):

CONSISTENTLY EXCEEDS WORK GROUP STANDARDS/REQUIREMENTS ☐   MEETS WORK GROUP STANDARDS/REQUIREMENTS ☐
OFTEN EXCEEDS WORK GROUP STANDARDS/REQUIREMENTS ☐   DOES NOT MEET WORK GROUP STANDARDS/REQUIREMENTS ☐

  D. SUMMARY APPRAISAL (CONSIDER THE PERFORMANCE FACTORS ABOVE (A THRU C) AND ANY OTHER JOB RELATED BEHAVIOR WHICH IMPACTS PERFORMANCE POSITIVELY OR NEGATIVELY):

OVERALL PERFORMANCE EVALUATION

CONSISTENTLY EXCEEDS WORK GROUP STANDARDS/REQUIREMENTS ☐   MEETS WORK GROUP STANDARDS/REQUIREMENTS ☐
OFTEN EXCEEDS WORK GROUP STANDARDS/REQUIREMENTS ☐   DOES NOT MEET WORK GROUP STANDARDS/REQUIREMENTS ☐

III. STRENGTH ASSESSMENT (DESCRIBE THE EMPLOYEE'S STRENGTHS; EMPHASIZE AREAS IN WHICH HE/SHE EXCELLS):

IV. PERFORMANCE IMPROVEMENT AND DEVELOPMENT NEEDS (SUPERVISOR AND EMPLOYEE PLAN FOR SPECIFIC TRAINING, EDUCATIONAL, AND/OR ON THE JOB EXPERIENCES NEEDED TO IMPROVE PERFORMANCE AND/OR CAREER GROWTH):

V. SUMMARY OF EMPLOYEE'S REACTIONS AND COMMENTS:

SUPERVISOR: _____ SIGNATURE _____ DATE _____ ORGANIZATION
APPROVED: _____ SIGNATURE _____ PERSONNEL: _____ SIGNATURE
I ACKNOWLEDGE RECEIPT OF THIS REVIEW. EMPLOYEE: _____ SIGNATURE

WHITE—PERSONNEL   GREEN—SUPERVISOR   YELLOW—EMPLOYEE

Figure 13–3.

INSTRUCTIONS TO REVIEWER:
Carefully analyze employee's performance. Study each factor and the description of each degree. Place an X in the square which most nearly fits the employee's performance. Where necessary, make comment below any factor to explain your evaluation. Read over each section of the form before indicating your rating. After completion, return the form to the Personnel Office The information recorded on this form is to be treated as **CONFIDENTIAL INFORMATION.** The purpose of this review is:

1. To encourage the employee toward a better performance.
2. To give the employee an evaluation of his present performance.
3. To be used as a reference for future promotions.
4. To recognize employee performance by basing salary increases on merit.

Avoid a negative reaction by placing emphasis on positive and objective encouragement within the capacity of the individual's ability.

PART I ABILITY AND APPLICATION

INITIATIVE Ability to exercise self-reliance & enterprise.	Grasps situation and goes to work without hesitation.	Works independently. Seldom waits for orders.	Usually waits for instructions. Follows others.	Does only what is specifically instructed to do.

COMMENTS:

QUALITY OF WORK Accuracy and effectiveness of work. Freedom from error.	Consistently good quality. Errors rare.	Usually good quality, few errors.	Passable work if closely supervised.	Frequent errors. Cannot be depended upon to be accurate.

COMMENTS:

QUANTITY OF WORK Output of work. Performance. Speed.	Works consistently and with excellent output.	Works consistently with above average output.	Maintains group average output.	Below average output. Slow.

COMMENTS:

KNOWLEDGE OF WORK Technical knowledge of job. Ability to apply it.	Knows job thoroughly. Rarely needs help.	Knows job well. Seldom needs help.	Knows job fairly well, requires instruction.	Little knowledge of job. Requires constant help.

COMMENTS:

ATTITUDE & COOPERATION Enthusiasm, cooperativeness, willingness.	Enthusiastic. Outstanding in cooperation. Tries new ideas.	Responsive. Cooperates well. Meets others more than half way.	Usually cooperates. Does not resist new ideas.	Uncooperative. Resents new ideas. Displays little interest.

COMMENTS:

Figure 13–4.

DEPENDABILITY	☐	☐	☐	☐
Willingness to accept responsibility, to follow through.	Outstanding ability to perform with little supervision.	Willing and able to accept responsibility. Little checking required.	Usually follows instructions, normal follow up.	Refuses or unable to carry responsibilities. Needs constant follow up.

COMMENTS:

ATTENDANCE	☐	☐	☐	☐
Reliability to be on the job.	Always can be relied upon to be at work absent only when real emergency.	Usually can be relied upon to be at work on time, explained absence occasionally.	Comes in late with reasonable excuses. Fairly frequent explained absences.	Frequent unexplained lateness and absences.

NUMBER OF DAYS ABSENT:
COMMENTS:

COURTESY	☐	☐	☐	☐
With the patients and fellow employees.	Always pleasant and courteous.	Usually pleasant and courteous.	Abrupt at times. Must be reminded occasionally to use tact and courtesy.	Requires constant reminder to display tact and courtesy.

COMMENTS:

PERSONAL APPEARANCE	☐	☐	☐	☐
Personal grooming, hair, nails, shoes, and general.	Always presents clean and tidy appearance.	Usually presents clean and tidy appearance.	Negligent of appearance at times.	Presents a poor appearance too often.

COMMENTS:

LEADERSHIP	☐	☐	☐	☐
If applicable. Ability to lead others.	Others naturally follow his example or direction.	Willingly assumes guidance of others. Is fairly well accepted in this role.	Is accepted reluctantly by his group as a guide or example.	Shows no aptitude or skill in leadership.

COMMENTS:

_____
(Employee's Signature)   Employee's Comment:_____

Figure 13–4 (*cont.*)

PART 2
CAPACITY AND AMBITION FOR ADVANCEMENT

A. Check (✓) applicable sections.

REGRESSING	NOT SUITED TO JOB	NOT LIKELY TO ADVANCE	PROGRESSING	SATIS-FACTORY	MAXIMUM PERFORMANCE ON JOB	READY FOR PROMOTION
☐	☐	☐	☐	☐	☐	☐

B. Review your ratings and comments, then briefly outline what actions you will take or suggest to maintain, to improve, or to correct the behavior and/or output of this employee.

_____

_____

_____

Time set for necessary improvement to take place_____

C. Employee reaction to review and suggestions was:

APPRECIATION ☐   INTEREST ☐   DISINTEREST ☐   RESENTMENT ☐
(Completely willing   (Will try to follow   (Satisfied with   (Feels review
to strive for   suggestions.)   present status.)   is imposition.)
improvement.)

Other: (explain) _____

D. Conclusion drawn from interview: _____

_____

_____

_____

DATE _____   SIGNATURE _____
                                              (Reviewer)

Figure 13–4 (*cont.*)

APPRAISAL OF SUPERVISORY EMPLOYEES

IMPORTANT! Consider only one characteristic at a time, regardless of how good or poor he may be in the others.

A. Fails to meet requirements
B. Needs some improvement
C. Meets requirements
D. Exceeds requirements
E. Not observed by appraiser

NAME OF EMPLOYEE _____ DATE _____

PRESENT POSITION _____ DEPARTMENT _____

	A	B	C	D	E	COMMENTS
1. Judges employees objectively and fairly on their ability, and situations on the facts and circumstances.						
2. Maintains poise and adjusts to change, work pressure, or difficult situations without undue stress.						
3. Considers new ideas, the views of others, or divergent points of view.						
4. Exhibits confidence, positive attitude, and firmness of position with an indication of flexibility.						
5. Establishes rapport, gains respect and cooperation, inspires and motivates, and works effectively with subordinates who have a variety of backgrounds and training.						
6. Accomplishes the quality and quantity of work expected, with adequate controls and within set limits of cost and time.						
7. Plans and organizes work, defines assignments, and carries out assignments effectively.						

APPRAISAL OF SUPERVISORY EMPLOYEES (*cont.*)

	A	B	C	D	E	COMMENTS
8. Coordinates the work with that of other related activities.						
9. Demonstrates skill in developing improvements in work methods or designing new procedures.						
10. Establishes rapport, gains respect and cooperation, inspires and motivates, and deals effectively with individuals or groups.						
11. Adjusts work operations to meet emergent or changing requirements within available resources, maintaining proper control, and minimizing sacrifice in quantity or quality.						
12. Establishes work objectives and standards, programs to accomplish objectives, and assesses progress.						
13. Coordinates and integrates the work activities of several organizational segments or several different projects.						
14. Absorbs new concepts, analyzes organizational and operational problems and issues, and develops timely and economical solutions.						
15. Communicates with others effectively both orally and in writing on matters related to work.						
16. Understands and applies the principles required to further management's goals in relation to normal work operations.						
17. Represents the activity both within and outside the organization or agency, and gains support for the agency's program goals.						
18. Accepts responsibility, exercises practical judgments, and makes sound and effective decisions.						
19. Gives clear directions to subordinates and delegates authority appropriate to program needs and the capacity of individuals.						
20. Maintains discipline, supports subordinates, and provides the basis for good morale without loss of effectiveness.						

APPRAISAL OF SUPERVISORY EMPLOYEES (*cont.*)

	A	B	C	D	E	COMMENTS
21. Resolves work-related employee problems and counsels employees.						
22. Understands and applies the theories and techniques of sound personnel management in dealing with employees and special interest matters.						
23. Instructs, guides, and reviews the work of others, and provides necessary training.						
24. Makes maximum utilization of employee skills, capabilities, and training.						

Summary and Recommendations (must be filled in)

SIGNATURE AND TITLE OF APPRAISER	DATE
SIGNATURE OF EMPLOYEE (to be signed after review and discussion)	DATE OF APPRAISAL

PERFORMANCE EVALUATION GUIDELINES

I. *Quality of Performance:*
   1. Friendliness, cooperation, and respect can promote good relationships with patients, medical staff, and hospital personnel.
   2. Management can promote the overall objective of quality patient care with minimum cost by a positive attitude toward the established goals.
   3. Management applies and interprets hospital policies and goals with the department by sharing information through scheduled department meetings, individual counseling, and in-service training.
   4. Evaluations are discussed in detail; goals are set for future individual attainment; and personnel are encouraged to better performance.

II. *Managerial Efficiency:*
   1. *Scheduling:* Is consistent in granting vacations, weekends, and holidays off, leaves of absence, and the like.
   2. *Sick leave, overtime, and turnover:* Encourages high morale by treating each staff member in a fair and consistent manner. Provides immediate consideration for problems of subordinate personnel. Encourages staff to be innovative and creative.
   3. *Turnover:* Differentiate from employee dissatisfaction and female resignations due to husband transfer, maternity leaves, illness, or family problems when the employee needs to stay home.

HEAD NURSE/CHARGE NURSE
MANAGEMENT EVALUATION

DATE: _____

NAME: _____ TITLE: _____

DEPARTMENT: _____ SHIFT: _____

EVALUATION: 90-day ☐   6-month ☐   Annual ☐   Other _____

Demonstrates management skills by planning, leading, organizing, and controlling management work in a manner that accomplishes the department goals and objectives.

PLANNING:
   1. Anticipates needs of department and develops a realistic supply and equipment budget.

COMMENTS _____

_____

FUTURE OBJECTIVES _____

2. Assesses the patient nursing care needs on a daily basis, and assigns and delegates the nursing care activities to staff members based on this forecast.

   COMMENTS _____

   _____

   FUTURE OBJECTIVES _____

   _____

3. Develops or has developed, with assistance of staff members, a written patient care plan for each patient.

   COMMENTS _____

   _____

   FUTURE OBJECTIVES _____

   _____

LEADING

1. Promotes good relationships among subordinates, patients, medical staff, and hospital personnel.

   COMMENTS _____

   _____

   FUTURE OBJECTIVES _____

   _____

2. Recognize overall nursing department goals by sharing staff when able and alerting supervisor in ability to do so.

   COMMENTS _____

   _____

   FUTURE OBJECTIVES _____

   _____

3. Head nurse assumes 24-hour patient care responsibility through delegation to charge nurses, P.M. and nights.

   COMMENTS _____

   _____

   FUTURE OBJECTIVES _____

   _____

4. Head nurse/charge nurse usually attends monthly Joint Administrative Nurses meeting.

    COMMENTS _____

    _____

    FUTURE OBJECTIVES _____

    _____

5. Evaluates staff on the basis of performance as specified in the job description.

    COMMENTS _____

    _____

    FUTURE OBJECTIVES _____

    _____

6. Interprets, applies and enforces hospital policies and goals within department consistent with intent of management.

    COMMENTS _____

    _____

    FUTURE OBJECTIVES _____

    _____

ORGANIZING

1. Efficiently directs and coordinates the patient care activities with ancillary departments.

    COMMENTS _____

    _____

    FUTURE OBJECTIVES _____

    _____

2. Has developed a systematic and efficient "desk" routine.

    COMMENTS _____

    _____

    FUTURE OBJECTIVES _____

    _____

3. Follows an established routine regarding patient rounds and shift reports.

COMMENTS _____

_____

FUTURE OBJECTIVES _____

_____

4. Maintains or causes to be maintained an orderly and up-to-date filing system of memos, policies, and procedures on his or her unit.

COMMENTS _____

_____

FUTURE OBJECTIVES _____

_____

5. Adjusts staffing "organizational" structure during low census period.

COMMENTS _____

_____

FUTURE OBJECTIVES _____

_____

CONTROL

1. Exercises judicial cost control in the use of supplies.

COMMENTS _____

_____

FUTURE OBJECTIVES _____

_____

2. Conducts periodic review and/or exercises of Code 99 procedure, fire drill, disaster procedures, and patient and employee safety measures.

COMMENTS _____

_____

FUTURE OBJECTIVES _____

_____

3. Recognizes abuse of sick leave and excessive or unauthorized overtime and institutes corrective measures.

   COMMENTS _____

   _____

   FUTURE OBJECTIVES _____

   _____

4. Recognizes the causes of turnover, and takes appropriate measures to reduce the percentage of turnover.

   COMMENTS _____

   _____

   FUTURE OBJECTIVES _____

   _____

5. Conducts monthly in-service unit conferences on patient care needs or unit and personnel needs.

   COMMENTS _____

   _____

   FUTURE OBJECTIVES _____

   _____

Additional Comments

Comment on professional and technical skills, economy in use of supplies, staff utilization, sick leave, and so on.

_____

_____

_____

_____

_____

_____

_____

_____

EMPLOYEE COMMENTS: _____

_____

_____

_____

_____

_____

RATED BY: _____

TITLE: _____

A copy of this report has been shown and discussed with me.

_____
(Employee's Signature)

_____
(Date)

PRESENT SALARY STEP: _____
ACTION TO BE TAKEN:

Merit Increase ( )   Probation ( )   Freeze Salary ( )

PERFORMANCE REVIEW
FOUNTAIN VALLEY COMMUNITY HOSPITAL

SECTION 1 IDENTIFICATION DATA

Name _____ Dept. _____ Classification _____

Present Pay Rate $ _____ Shift _____ Hrs. Per Week (Avg.) _____

SECTION II DUTIES

SECTION III RATING FACTORS

Knowledge of Duties

_____ Serious gaps in knowledge of fundamentals of the job.
_____ Satisfactory knowledge of routine phases of the job.
_____ Well informed on most phases of the job.
_____ Excellent knowledge of all phases of the job.

Performance of Duties

_____ Quantity or quality of work fails to meet job requirements.
_____ Performance meets only minimum job requirements.

Evaluation

_____ Quantity and quality of work are very satisfactory.
_____ Produces very high quantity and quality of work—always timely.

Initiative

_____ Often weak—fails to show initiative or accept responsibility.
_____ Initiative and acceptance of responsibility adequate in most situations.
_____ Satisfactorily demonstrates initiative and acceptance of responsibility.
_____ Demonstrates a high degree of initiative and acceptance of responsibility.

Judgment

_____ Decisions and recommendations often wrong and ineffective.
_____ Judgment is usually sound but makes occasional errors.
_____ Shows good judgment resulting from sound evaluation of factors.
_____ Sound logical thinker—considers all factors to make accurate decisions.

Adaptability

_____ Unable to perform adequately in any but simple, routine situations.
_____ Performance declines under stress or other than normal situations.
_____ Performs well under stress or in unusual situations.
_____ Performance excellent even under stress and unusual conditions.

Learning Ability

_____ Unsatisfactory for the job—fails to grasp simple instructions.
_____ Able to assimilate simple instructions if repeated several times.
_____ Learns at a steady rate to accomplish all phases of the job.
_____ Very quick learner—fully grasps abstract ideas and concepts.

Effectiveness in Working with Others

_____ Ineffective in working with others—does not cooperate.
_____ Sometimes has difficulty in getting along with others.
_____ Gets along well with most people under normal circumstances.
_____ Works in harmony with others—very good team worker.

Dependability

_____ Cannot be depended upon.
_____ Is of doubtful dependability.
_____ Usually reliable.
_____ Very dependable—wins confidence of all.

Punctuality

_____ Usually late.
_____ Frequently late.
_____ Usually always on time.
_____ Above average punctuality.

Personal Appearance

_____ Sloppy appearance—below acceptable hospital standards.
_____ Careless appearance detracts from effectiveness.
_____ Appearance creates an acceptable impression.
_____ Exceptionally well groomed at all times—creates favorable impression.

SECTION IV OVERALL EVALUATION
    —— Unsatisfactory.
    —— Below average.
    —— Effective and competent.
    —— Exceptional.

SECTION V COMMENTS: (By Rating Supervisor)

Position ———————— Date ————————

SECTION VI COMMENTS BY PERSON BEING RATED: This report has been discussed with me by the rating supervisor and I have no comment: ————
the following comment: ————

Signature ———————————————— Position ———————— Date ————————

SECTION VII REVIEW BY ENDORSING SUPERVISOR:

Signature ———————————————— Position ———————— Date ————————

SECTION VIII REVIEW BY PERSONNEL DEPARTMENT:

Signature ———————————————— Position ———————— Date ————————

14

Morale and discipline

THE NEED FOR
WELL-ADJUSTED EMPLOYEES

The nursing supervisor recognizes that in the health care agency, emphasis must be placed on the psychological adjustment and morale of employees if they are to perform the health care function effectively. While some supervisors are inclined to feel that the personal adjustment of subordinates is not their responsibility, they should realize that good mental health is essential not only to the individual, but also to the organization and to the public that it serves. Whether or not health care managers and supervisors are aware of the crucial importance of employee adjustment and morale, the employees themselves, as well as the associations that represent them, are well aware that employment conditions that are detrimental to adjustment and morale need not be tolerated. Neither do such conditions benefit the agency in the long run.

Many psychological studies have indicated that one of the leading factors in high employee turnover rates is poor morale. When we consider the cost of training a new staff member, it immediately becomes apparent that low morale is too expensive a luxury for a health care agency to allow.

It is therefore highly desirable that the individual members of an organization find satisfaction in what they are doing and that they be able to maintain good emotional adjustment. Attaining these goals is a management responsibility, but the individual members of the organization also have some responsibility for reaching these objectives for themselves as well as for their colleagues. The attitudes and feelings of each member of the group influence the behavior of other group members and affect the degree to which the goals and standards of the organization are met.

Since morale is closely associated with discipline, you, as a supervisor, must concern yourself with the quality of conduct or discipline of your subordinates. You do so by establishing reasonable standards of conduct, by informing your staff of these standards, and by enforcing them wisely. Such conditions are conducive to good morale, and the group itself will tend to enforce the standards by applying social pressure to members who tend to "get out of line." A basic managerial responsibility is to have an established procedure for handling employees who fail to conform to these standards of performance and conduct. There must also be a procedure for employees to express their complaints and grievances to management with the assurance that they will be given careful consideration.

MORALE

Problems of Employee Adjustment

Any reference to human wants and needs must include needs such as love, self-respect, social approval, or any need other than physiological origin. We become quite aware of our physiological needs if our lunch hour is postponed or if we can't get to a drinking fountain when we are thirsty. On the other hand, our other needs are not so easily defined, but they are nonetheless a part of our psychological makeup and require satisfaction. Hence we need to refer once again to the classification of human needs as developed by Maslow:

1. *The Physiological Needs* In this group are the needs for food, water, air, rest, and the like that are required for maintaining proper body equilibrium.

2. *The Safety Needs* This group includes the need for safety and security in both a physical and psychological sense, that is, the need to protect ourselves from external dangers to our bodies and to our personalities. For example, most employees want to work at jobs that provide a reasonable degree of freedom from physical and psychological hazards as well as providing a reasonable degree of job security.

3. *The Belongingness and Love Needs* The need for attention and social activity are the major needs in this category. Individuals want affectionate relationships with people and desire respected places in their groups.

4. *The Esteem Needs* Included in this group are the desires for self-respect, strength, achievement, adequacy, mastery, competence, confidence in the face of the world, independence, and freedom. This group also includes the desire for reputation, prestige, respect, and esteem from other people.

5. *The Need for Self-Actualization or Realization.* This need refers to individuals' desires for self-fulfillment, their dreams of fulfilling their potential and achieving all that they are capable of achieving.

In looking at the problems of human motivation, you cannot focus attention on any one need to the exclusion of the others. Since almost all behavior is multimotivated, several needs usually demand satisfaction at the same time. However, different needs may differ in their relative importance to the individual. Supervisors must recognize that the need pattern of each individual is different. They must be able to recognize these differences and utilize knowledge of them so as to provide satisfaction to individuals as they work toward the accomplishment of organizational goals.

How to Satisfy Human Needs

Ordinarily, only an incentive that is important to the individual may serve as a satisfier. Normally, positive incentives, such as pay and praise, are used because they bring pleasure and satisfaction to the individual, as well as achieving organizational goals. However, at times it is necessary to utilize negative incentives, such as fear and punishment. The positive incentives can be tangible or intangible, depending on the needs of the group. Some common incentives in health care are money, security, praise, competition, or knowledge of results and participation.

MONEY   In our society money is the incentive used most frequently to stimulate people to produce more. Ironically when employees are asked to state what they would most like to receive from their jobs, pay is seldom at the top of the list. As nurses, we choose to believe that salary is not at the head of our motivations list, but everyone needs enough money for food and shelter. Few of us are able to work for free.

SECURITY   Most people want to feel secure in their jobs. They want to feel that they have protection against the loss of their jobs and earnings, whether it be because of accident, illness, arbitrary firing, or other reasons. They are also concerned about security in their old age following retirement. Thus security becomes a positive incentive to work. The reasonable security provided by good employee protection systems in progressive health care agencies allows employees to enjoy a freedom that can stimulate them to work more wholeheartedly on the job. They are able to direct their energies toward the job rather than toward the achievement of personal goals.

PRAISE AND RECOGNITION   It is important to people that they be recognized and praised for a job well done.

COMPETITION   Employees may compete with themselves, other employees, or members of a group competing with other groups. When persons compete with themselves, as when nurses try to improve their own care records, they may obtain satisfaction, and no one loses face by not being the winner. Competition between individuals or groups may be useful in stimulating safety or increasing work output, and so on. The use of progress charts, such as those showing nursing care activities in relation to patient satisfaction, may also stimulate competition between departments to improve their delivery of nursing care.

The development of a personal interest in and enthusiasm for the attainment of high performance standards required the practice of good human relations in supervision and careful communication to the employee of the level of performance desired. It is not inconsistent with good human relations to establish standards and promote wholesome competition to meet those standards.

KNOWLEDGE OF RESULTS   Knowing the results of activities serves as an incentive to better performance and facilitates the learning of the job. For example, what happened to that patient when she was discharged to the rehabilitation center?

PARTICIPATION   This factor is recognized as one of the best incentives for stimulating employee productivity and providing job satisfaction. Subordinates may participate in meetings and conferences, on committees, or through a suggestion system. You may also encourage employee participation in decision making about the job itself and about the conditions under which it is to be done within the work group. Because the staff has a personal stake in the success of a change in procedures, their participation in the making of decisions about such changes minimizes resistance to the changes you wish to initiate. Where practicable, wise supervisors consult their staffs and heed their counsel in advance of any proposed changes in operation or procedures. Allowing the group to establish its own patient care delivery system is a good example.

Negative incentives most commonly used are:

- reprimand—either verbal or written and made a part of the person's permanent personnel record;
- imposition of overtime duty without compensation;

- suspension without pay;
- loss of some part of weekly or annual leave;
- demotion to a lower staff position or pay classification;
- separation from the department; or
- nonpunitive action—including all efforts short of punishment made by a superior to correct a weakness in a subordinate. When proper use is made of nonpunitive forms of discipline, it is seldom necessary to apply punitive measures.

Human Adjustment

People are continuously accommodating a broad variety of situations in an effort to satisfy their needs and to maintain an emotional equilibrium that might be defined as "adjustment." They are not so much concerned at the conscious level with the satisfaction of physiological and safety needs as with the satisfaction of the needs for belongingness, esteem, and self-realization. The frustration of these latter needs causes most maladjustment; and, since the satisfaction of these needs is dependent largely on other persons—particularly persons in authority (supervisors)—you must attempt to understand something about the nature of adjustment and maladjustment. One source considers as mentally healthy all persons who meet the following three criteria:

1. *They feel comfortable about themselves.* They are not bowled over by their own emotions—by their fears, anger, love, jealousy, guilt, or worries. They take life's disappointments in stride and have a tolerant, easy-going attitude towards themselves and others; they can laugh at themselves. They neither overestimate nor underestimate their abilities and accept their own shortcomings. They have self-respect and feel able to deal with most situations that arise. They get satisfactions from the simple everyday pleasures.

2. *They feel right about other people.* They are able to give love and consider the interests of others. Their personal relationships are satisfying and lasting. They expect to like and trust most other people and expect that others will like and trust them. They respect the differences between people, and they do not push people around; nor do they allow themselves to be pushed around. They can feel that they are part of a group and feel a sense of responsibility toward other persons.

3. *They are able to meet the demands of life and do something about problems as they arise.* They accept responsibility and welcome new experiences and ideas. They shape their environment whenever possible and adjust to it when necessary. They plan ahead without fear of the future. They make use of their natural capacities and set realistic goals for themselves. They think for themselves and make their own decisions. They put their best effort into what they do and obtain satisfaction from doing it.

"Adjustment" does not imply that individuals are free of all life's problems, but rather it implies an emotionally mature orientation toward life that enables persons to solve their problems in a constructive manner and to weather storms as they encounter them. No one is free of problems. However, some people are better equipped than others to handle them.

Problem employees are likely to be employees with problems. At least in part, emotional disturbance may play a major role in such problems as chronic absenteeism, accidents, high turnover rates, grievances, alcoholism, dishonesty, and other problems, including the many different forms of job dissatisfaction commonly found in employment situations. The crank, the bully, the chronic complainer, the gossip, and other types of problem employees, who demand so much of your time, are usually people who are having trouble in adjusting to the world about them. They are usually problems to themselves as well, and they often feel uncomfortable about their own behavior. However, you should never allow yourself to fall into the trap of labeling as "maladjusted" anyone who merely happens to hold a point of view different from your own.

From the time persons are hired until the day they leave, a large part of their lives is influenced by the personnel policies and procedures of the administration, the supervisor they work under, and their relationships with fellow staff members. It has been said that being a good nurse is not just a job, but a way of life. All these influences, together with all life experiences, determine how people adjust to their jobs as well as to other areas of their daily lives.

By setting up policies and procedures that tend to facilitate employee adjustment, the organization not only contributes to the mental health of the staff but also finds itself benefiting from the standpoint of efficiency, public relations, and lack of employee turnover. Good supervisors are able to recognize the symptoms of emotional problems in staff members and take steps to either handle them personally, if they are of a minor nature, or refer them to someone else who is equipped to handle them, if they are of a serious nature.

THE RELATIONSHIP OF MORALE TO DISCIPLINE

It should be obvious that merely teaching people the skills necessary to be good nurses and providing them with uniforms and equipment are not enough. Such qualities as enthusiasm, personal satisfaction, and a willingness to work as part of a team (which may be considered components of morale) are also essential for the continued success of the organization's operations. Only if all department members are interested in and satisfied with their jobs will there be the over-all, wholehearted, and cheerful cooperation that is essential to the functioning of the organization.

When morale is high in a department, there is likely to be less absenteeism and turnover than when morale is low: the higher the morale in an agency, the less discipline problems you encounter. People who are interested in their jobs and find their working relationships with supervisors and with fellow nurses pleasant are less likely to stay away from work or quit the agency than people who work under less desirable circumstances. As a result, at any given time there is more manpower available for patient duties and lower costs to the organization in terms of orientation budgets.

The attitude of staff members toward the health care agency soon becomes common knowledge in the community. As they associate with friends, neighbors, and the public at large, they cannot help revealing their attitudes, both favorable and unfavorable. Criticism expressed by a small minority of nurses can spread through the community and offset the best efforts to build good public relations for the agency. Low morale is also likely to affect recruitment. Well-qualified nurses will not make application to an agency when they feel that they would be unhappy working there.

Factors in Morale

Morale is not something that can be dictated by management or built overnight. It is developed over a long period as a result of sound personnel policies and procedures, good supervisory practices, and other factors. These influencing factors should receive careful attention from health care management, and a continuous, positive effort should be made to build good morale. While it is important to correct undesirable conditions, it is even more important to place emphasis on positive action to develop the type of work environment that contributes to high morale.

WANTS AND NEEDS   Developing high morale depends on taking proper action to satisfy as many of the employee's *needs*, both conscious and unconscious, as consistent with the goals of the organization. Much motivation is at the subconscious level, and for this reason individuals may not be clearly aware of their own needs. On the other hand, *wants* are individuals' conscious desires for those things or conditions that they feel will give them satisfaction. While the individual's wants go far beyond employment, their nature, as far as the job is concerned, is of vital interest to management in the development of high morale.

Which needs are most important to people? Psychologists have done many surveys to determine which satisfactions people want from their jobs, and a host of factors—the type of job a person holds, the economic and social conditions at the time of the survey, the length of time on the job, and so on—all appear to have had some effect on the results of the survey. Because of the differences that develop in survey results, making any completely conclusive statements about the priority or ranking of wants for employees is not really possible. However, it has been noted that in all cases where supervisors have been asked to rate what they feel are the wants of their subordinates, the rankings of the supervisors vary, often considerably, from the rankings applied to the same factors by subordinate employees. (Table 14–1 contains a fairly typical set of results in ranking ten job conditions.) The differences between the supervisors' and the workers' points of views are important in that they should indicate to alert supervisors that they must study subordinates and avoid making an assumption that the wants of subordinates are the same as their own.

DISCIPLINE

Discipline, a function of supervision, must be exercised in order to develop a group amenable to direction and control. Unfortunately, the term "discipline" has taken on a disagreeable and negative meaning. There is a tendency to think of discipline entirely in its most limited sense—an action taken against employees who are guilty of some violation of good behavior. This version is sometimes referred to as "corrective discipline." While this is one use of the term, there is a broader and more positive meaning. Discipline is not an entirely negative force. A form of training, it is an extremely important and constructive tool of leadership for eliminating weaknesses and for preventing their development. We speak of employees as being "well disciplined" or "poorly disciplined." The conduct of well disciplined employees con-

TABLE 14–1
Comparison of supervisors' and workers' need ratings

JOB CONDITIONS	WORKER RATING	SUPERVISOR RATING
Full appreciation of work done	1	8
Feeling "in" on things	2	10
Sympathetic help on personal problems	3	9
Job security	4	2
Good wages	5	1
"Work that keeps you interested"	6	5
Promotion and growth in company	7	3
Personal loyalty to workers	8	6
Good working conditions	9	4
Tactful disciplining	10	7

335

forms to recognized standards of behavior; poorly disciplined employees do not conduct themselves in this manner.

The word "discipline" has its roots in the Latin word *disciplina*, which means "instruction, teaching, or training." Discipline should therefore be thought of in terms of instruction and training rather than in terms of punishment and penalties. An undisciplined group is one that is incompletely trained, not due to a failure of the formal training program, but because supervisory personnel have not required that subordinates conform to organizational rules and procedures. The best disciplined groups are the best trained and, for this reason, the least punished. The conduct of well disciplined employees is therefore the result of training that has caused them to accept and live according to certain behavior patterns.

In this type of situation, employees voluntarily, and often without conscious thought or effort, act in accordance with established standards of conduct. This conduct, which may be either self- or group discipline, results when proper working habits are established and maintained over a long period. Proper working habits gradually become the regular behavior of every member of the group. A high morale and *esprit de corps* develop within such a group, and a self-administering group discipline results. In addition to preventing situations from developing that demand corrective disciplinary action, such a group feeling creates within individual employees a desire and determination to reach their work objective regardless of the obstacles encountered.

However, punitive action must be applied when rules and regulations are violated. When recommending punishment, you must make important judgments about the motive and intent of the offender. You must decide whether the violation came as a result of deliberate defiance of rules and regulations or inadvertently, from ignorance or carelessness. If ignorance or carelessness is the cause, punishment should be aimed at retraining the nurse and assisting in improving his or her value to the organization. However, if the act was one of defiance, immorality, or dishonesty, punishment should be severe.

The consequences of poor discipline are many, and you must be aware of these results. A few of the more common signals of a lack of discipline are:

1. lack of *esprit de corps* and low morale;
2. lackadaisical attitude toward the job, superiors, the organization, and the public;
3. lack of direction or objectives;
4. inattention to duty;
5. violations of rules and regulations; and
6. disregard for the rights of the client, with attendant loss of public confidence and trust.

The problem of discipline is not restricted to health care, of course, but due to the critical nature of the health care organization, it assumes a role of somewhat greater importance than in other agencies of government or industry. The special requirements of trust imposed by the mission of providing health care to the public make the problem of discipline especially important. Employees who have difficulty abiding by the regulations are of doubtful value in caring for others and in administering their health care needs.

Supervisory Responsibility in Discipline

You, as the supervisor, are responsible for developing and maintaining good working relationships with your subordinates. You are also responsible for developing and maintaining the highest level of efficiency among your staff. The effectiveness of the organization depends largely on how well you and the other supervisors measure up to this responsibility. One of your principal values to the organization is the extent to which you create and maintain working relationships, thus enabling subordinates as individuals and as a group to voluntarily put forth their best efforts. Each person represents a large financial investment by the organization. To protect this investment the organization, through its supervisors, must make every effort to help each person become and remain an efficient, productive, and satisfied worker. This necessity places on you the responsibility of seeing that your subordinates know:

- the objectives of their jobs and of the units in which they work;
- the tasks they are to perform;
- the accepted methods of doing these tasks;
- how well they are expected to do these tasks, that is, the standards of performance for the jobs;
- how well they meet these standards of performance;
- how they can improve their work and develop their capabilities;
- the policies and regulations that govern their work, and
- what is considered proper conduct or good discipline in the work group.

Securing Proper Discipline

The following suggestions help you develop and maintain proper discipline in your staff. These suggestions are based on the belief that creating and maintaining conditions that make corrective discipline unnecessary are far more important than developing successful techniques of handling corrective disciplinary cases. In other words, the emphasis should be placed on preventive, not corrective, action.

337

PUT ACCEPTED STANDARDS OF CONDUCT IN WRITING   In cooperation with other supervisors in the department, write out the standards of conduct that are expected of the people in the department, and see that each new employee receives a copy of them. Every person wants to know and is entitled to know what is considered good behavior or conduct, the "rules of the game." Here, as in other supervisory contacts, it is well to follow the admonition, "Do not overestimate employees' knowledge or underestimate their intelligence." Establishing such standards and having employees understand them are two measures that go a long way toward preventing many instances of misconduct. People have a natural sense of fairness that causes them to abide by the rules of the game—providing they know the rules.

When these standards of conduct have been followed long enough to become automatic, less and less of your time will be occupied by corrective disciplinary actions. You will have more time to spend in developing job enthusiasm and satisfactions that are so essential to high morale.

SET REASONABLE WORK OBJECTIVES FOR YOUR STAFF   There is considerable truth in the statement that supervisors can forget about corrective disciplinary actions if they set reasonable work objectives for their employees and keep them vitally interested in reaching these objectives.

CREATE A FAVORABLE WORKING ATMOSPHERE   Create a working situation that encourages subordinates to want to do their best work. A good working situation involves not only physical conditions, but also personal and other intangible relationships. Remember that a word of commendation and support for a job well done is just as essential to the maintenance of proper discipline as is the correction of a person who has been guilty of some act of misconduct.

The staff should feel free to bring you suggestions for improvement, as well as grievances, when and if they arise. The existence of grievances is not necessarily a reflection of your skill as a supervisor. What is important is the willingness of subordinates to come to you with grievances, knowing that you will be fair and open-minded in handling the problem. Be alert constantly to anticipate and eliminate any conditions that might lead to an employee grievance. At all times you must be ready to listen as quickly as possible to grievances when they arise. Adjust the situation, if it calls for an adjustment, and you are in a position to take action. Refer the case to a higher authority if it cannot be satisfactorily disposed of at your level. No employees should be denied the right to discuss a problem with a higher supervisor if they care to do so, and if they follow the established lines of authority.

SET A GOOD EXAMPLE   Good conduct starts with you, the supervisor. Your subordinates watch you, and you set the pattern of acceptable conduct for your staff in what you do and don't do. Unless you set an example of good conduct for your staff, it is useless to expect good conduct from them. There is a certain amount of truth in the old adage, "What you do speaks so loudly, I cannot hear what you say."

MAINTAIN FIRM, IMPARTIAL CONTROL   Firm and impartial control creates respect and lessens the disciplinary problem. Correct in private all infractions of the standards of conduct as soon as possible after they occur. In reprimanding or correcting a subordinate, remember that they need to maintain self-respect. Do not humiliate them. Avoid general criticism. Be specific and objective. Be fair, and don't jump to conclusions.

Infractions should not be allowed to go uncorrected. If they are not corrected, employees come to regard them as accepted practice. Also, do not allow uncorrected infractions to accumulate and become so aggravated that, as the first corrective act, you recommend separation from the organization. Call instances of misconduct or lack of self-discipline to the person's attention and record the instances when they occur. These records are helpful in the preparation and discussion of performance reports, and they can be referred to if formal corrective disciplinary action becomes necessary. In a health care agency with a union, this documentation is essential.

FIND AND ELIMINATE CAUSES FOR MISCONDUCT   This is sometimes referred to as the "clinical approach." The procedure is based on the premise that a cause prompts every action. If the action is undesirable, an attempt should be made to find out what this cause is and then eliminate it. If all your attention is devoted to the employee's unacceptable behavior, you are treating the symptoms rather than the disease. Causes must be eliminated in order to prevent a recurrence of the unacceptable action.

When subordinates have apparently done something that is contrary to the accepted standards of conduct, discuss the matter with them in private. In such discussions, start with a question that permits employees to tell their own story. Good listening on your part is essential if you are to acquire a real understanding of what actually happened, as employees see it, and if you are going to find out why the employees did what they did. You must try to maintain a free exchange of ideas with employees, since this atmosphere is the most conducive to reaching a mutual understanding.

The vast majority of the people in any organization are competent, conscientious, and efficient. However, any organization, large or small, occasionally hires one or more persons who willfully, thoughtlessly, or unwittingly violate the accepted standards of good behavior or who do not turn out a fair day's work. The actions of such individuals reflect unfavorably on the entire organization and on every person in it.

If such circumstances are allowed to go without reprimand or correction, they undermine the morale of other employees in the agency and lower the confidence of the public in all health care personnel. It is to your advantage to see that inefficient or uncooperative employees mend their ways or are separated from the service. This should be viewed not as punishment but rather as a device for eliminating the nonproductive from the organization in order to provide better care.

Supervisors are charged with the duty of taking prompt disciplinary action (when they have the authority) against subordinates, or of promptly calling such instances to the attention of the proper authority. The administration of prompt, fair, and effective corrective disciplinary action is essential to effective operations and good employee relations. If you take steps to correct workers who break the rules of good behavior, or take steps to rid the department of uncooperative, incompetent, or dishonest employees, you increase the respect of your subordinates. You also raise the prestige of all employees by proving that merit is necessary for continued employment in the health care field.

Proper discipline cannot be maintained, and appropriate corrective disciplinary actions cannot be taken, if you shirk your responsibilities or refuse to attempt discipline because of the time and effort necessary to work through the "red tape." Employees expect and want uniform adherence to recognized standards of conduct, and they respect the superior who maintains these standards. When corrective disciplinary action seems necessary, take action even if you feel that nothing will be accomplished. It is not a quick, easy process, and you do not always get the desired results, but you must continue to try. If you give up, so will your staff. Act as soon as you can, so the employee's action and your corrective action come close together. This advice does not mean that you should act before you have gathered and weighed the facts. It does mean that you should act as soon as possible after you have all the facts (including the employee's side of the story), have weighed the evidence, and have decided what to do on the basis of the facts. When you delay the corrective action too long, it seems unjustified and unfair to the employee and to fellow staff members.

In deciding on the corrective disciplinary action to take (or to recommend), consider the following:

- all the circumstances surrounding the situation;
- the seriousness of the person's misconduct in relation to the individual's particular job and record with the organization;
- what the agency has done to help prevent this type of behavior;
- the corrective disciplinary actions suggested in the organizational manual for the type of offense involved;

- any contemplated corrective action in light of its training value, rather than strictly as a punishment or reprisal for the offense;
- what corrective disciplinary actions the agency has taken in similar instances;
- the staff member's previous conduct record in the department;
- the probable cause for the behavior;
- what corrective action will most likely eliminate the cause and prevent a recurrence;
- the person's probable reaction to the corrective action; and
- the possible reactions of the other staff members to the corrective action. (Take action that will not violate the group's sense of fair play, if possible.)

Above all else, be fair and impartial in arriving at the corrective action you decide to take. Nothing does more to undermine the morale of your staff and their confidence in you than the feeling that you are being arbitrary or unfair in your treatment of them or any of their group. Resist any temptation to postpone action in the hope that it may not be needed. When a subordinate repeats a mistake after you have ignored the first one, the most recent mistake is the fault of you, the supervisor.

DISCUSSION QUESTIONS

1. What are the five basic types of human needs? Explain each.
2. What is the relationship of morale to discipline?
3. What are the commonly used incentives for satisfaction of needs? How are they used by health care agencies?
4. What are the negative incentives or punitive disciplinary actions most frequently used in health care agencies? In what circumstances might each be used?
5. What are the criteria that are met by mentally healthy persons?
6. What are some of the problems likely to be caused by emotional disturbance? How do they affect the worker on the job?
7. What role does the supervisor play in developing high morale?
8. Discuss the positive and negative connotations of discipline. How is it related to training?
9. What are the results of poor discipline? Good discipline?
10. What is the role of supervisors in relation to discipline? How should they discharge their responsibilities?
11. What are the points to remember when contemplating corrective disciplinary action?
12. Formulate a list of nonpunitive and punitive corrective actions that could be employed in your agency. Start with the least severe and move to the most severe punishment.

APPLICATION: A CASE STUDY
OF VICTORIA WARREN, A STUDY
OF MANAGERIAL JUDGMENT

Objectives

To practice various ways of dealing with a situation.
To see the possible results of your action.

Directions

This exercise presents a new way of thinking about the way you act as a manager. There is no right answer and no wrong answer. Each step that you take—each decision that you make—leads you in a different direction. The following pages contain numbered boxes (1, 2, 3. . .), which we will refer to as "pages." "Page" (box) 1 in this case contains the statement of a problem that you, the supervisor, are having with one of your staff. Then you are called upon to make a decision from a number of choices. The choice you make determines which page (box) you go to next. Do *not* read the entire case sequentially—"page" 1, 2, 3, and so on.

As you can see, there is no "right path" to take. The paths you take depend on your attitudes and actions at each decision point.

As you proceed through each point, record your choices on the Path Record Chart (Figure 14–1). Then, when you have completed the exercise, go through it again, this time selecting all the opposite choices to those you chose the first time.

We think you will find this exercise interesting and rewarding.
Now turn to page (box) one and begin.

You are a supervisor in a 330-bed community hospital. You are staffed with 20 head nurses for the 7–3 shift.

Vicki Warren is one of your head nurses who has been in this position for three and a half months. (She has been with the hospital for two years.)

Vicki is absent today (Monday). You know she has been absent quite a bit, but, when you note today's absence in your log, you are surprised to see that she has been absent for three Mondays out of the past four.

This absenteeism has no doubt interfered with staffing and has been part of the cause of your understaffed departments. You have had to call in part-time per diem help for the last two months to try to fill out the staff. You note that, on occasion, Vicki has been asked to work overtime because of the load in her area.

You feel that some action must be taken about Vicki Warren.

Which of the four steps listed below would you take first? Select the first step you would take from those below and turn to only the page number indicated for the one you select.

a. Call Vicki aside on her return and have a talk with her.   Turn to page 9
b. Ask some of the women on her floor if they know what her problem might be.   Turn to page 4
c. Ask the head nurse on her previous floor what her record was there.   Turn to page 7
d. Discuss the matter with the other supervisors.   Turn to page 11
e. Transfer her at the next opportunity.   Turn to page 34

Reasons for your choice:

Page 2

> *You are not following instructions:* Nowhere are you instructed to turn to this page.
>
> *Remember*—we said this would not be like any regular book where you follow the pages in sequence. Instead, you will skip around, depending on the action you decide to take.
>
> Now turn back to page one and select the number of the page you should be on.

Page 3

> You asked the employees who laughed to tell you what they saw. The women are embarrassed, but one of the more outspoken says:
>
> > We were just laughing at a joke Sue told at lunch time. It didn't have anything to do with you or Vicki.
>
> What would you do now?   Turn to page 24 and select another answer.

Page 4

> You decide to ask others on the staff if they know what Vicki's problem might be. You wonder if she has a drinking problem, a family problem, real illness, or what.
>
> You talk to three of the women talking at lunch time. They seem hesitant to talk, but one finally admits that an evening shift nurse reported seeing Vicki and a man speeding in a car early this morning. It looked like they were heading for the beach. She reported that Vicki:
>
> > . . .could have been drunk—anyway the girl who saw it said she looked like it.
>
> What would be your approach to Vicki now?   Turn to page 1

You decide to keep calling Vicki's home at regular intervals during the day. Late that afternoon, the phone is answered. The same man, still sounding peculiar, says that Vicki is not there. When you ask where Vicki is, he says nothing. After a few minutes of silence Vicki comes on the phone and asks who it is. When you tell her, she says,

I can't talk to you now, goodbye. [Hangs up.]

Tuesday morning when Vicki comes to work, what would be your approach to her? Turn to page 9

You have asked Vicki if she has really been ill. Vicki says:

Now look, I know the rules! They say either your illness or that of someone in your immediate family is allowable as sick leave. And it's been one of the two, I can assure you.

What would your general approach to Vicki be?

a. Explain to Vicki that her annual sick leave has long since been used up. Even though she's not now being paid when she is absent, you've got a job to do—that you are in charge and she should respect that fact. Turn to page 13

b. Tell her that her personal problems are her business, but that staffing is your business. Tell her to "shape up or ship out." Turn to page 24

c. Say, "I didn't mean it that way, Vicki, and I'm sorry you have been having so much trouble. But I'm concerned about how your absences have been affecting your work." Turn to page 28

d. Tell Vicki she is fired. Turn to page 25

e. Transfer Vicki at the first opportunity. Turn to page 34

Reasons for your choice:

Page 7

You have decided to ask the head nurse in Vicki's previous department what her experience with Vicki was. She says:

> Vicki Warren? Why I know Vicki very well. I think a lot of her, too. She was one of my best nurses, and I was sorry to see her go. If it hadn't been a promotion for her, I would have really tried to keep her.
> How is Vicki doing, anyway? I hear she married a widower with two teenaged kids. Boy, that's really getting a ready-made family.

Turn back to page 1, and decide on your next step.

Page 8

You have decided to call Vicki over to a more private place and ask her what is on her mind. She is reluctant to discuss it at first, then she blurts out:

> You know very well what's wrong. Everything seems to be screwed up! At first it was just at home, but now you're picking on me, too. It's enough to drive a person to drink!
> The least you could do would be to get off my back and keep off!

What general response would you make to Vicki following that rather blunt outburst?

a. Remind her you are the one in charge of this floor and of her, that you are just doing your duty, and that she should have more respect for this fact.   Turn to page 13

b. Suggest that she go back to work and cool off, and you will talk later.   Turn to page 19

c. Warn her that if there are any more comments from her like that, you will see that she is severely dealt with.   Turn to page 20

d. Tell her you think it might help if you discussed it. You don't wish to intrude, but you are concerned over her absences.   Turn to page 28

e. Tell Vicki she is fired.   Turn to page 25

f. Transfer Vicki at the first opportunity.   Turn to page 34

Reasons for your choice:

In discussing her absences with Vicki, which of the following general approaches would you take?

    a. Explain to her the importance of good attendance to the patient care of the hospital. Point out to her what would happen if everyone was absent on Monday. Urge her to try to do better.   Turn to page 10

    b. Tell her that her personal problems are her business, but that staffing is your business. Tell her to "shape up or ship out."   Turn to page 24

    c. Wait until Vicki brings the matter of her absences up so as not to embarrass her.   Turn to page 16

    d. Ask her what difficulty she is having.   Turn to page 12

    e. Be friendly, but tell her that you are going to place a warning letter in her personnel folder that states she must improve the following month.   Turn to page 17

    f. Tell her she is fired.   Turn to page 25

Reasons for your choice:

Vicki says, "I'll try to do better." However, the following Monday she is absent again and someone who says he is her husband phones in to say that she is ill. He sounds queer—as if he has been drinking. What would you do then?

    a. Telephone her home to verify her illness.   Turn to page 14

    b. Send some inexpensive flowers to her home with a "Get Well Soon" card?   Turn to page 27

    c. Ask others in the staff if they know what Vicki's problem might be (if you have not done so before).   Turn to page 4

    d. Wait until her return to deal with Vicki.   Turn to page 26

    e. Contact another supervisor to get some help on the problem.   Turn to page 40

Reasons for your choice:

Page 11

You have decided to discuss the problem with the personnel manager before taking any other action. He says:

> No, I don't know Vicki Warren, but I do know how understaffed that floor is. We just had a staff meeting on it, and, brother, I don't want to go through another meeting like that one! It was embarrassing. So for Pete's sake, get back down there and shape things up. I don't want per diem brought in unless it is absolutely necessary. Go to it and give it everything you've got!

Turn back to page 1, and decide on your next step.

Page 12

You have asked Vicki what difficulty she is having. She says:

> Well, it's rather personal and I would rather not talk about if it you don't mind.

What general approach would you follow now?

a. Tell her she is fired. Turn to page 25

b. Ask Vicki if she has really been ill for the last three Mondays. Turn to page 6

c. Tell her that her personal problems are her business, but that staffing is your business. Tell her "shape up or ship out." Turn to page 24

d. Be friendly, but explain that you are going to place a warning letter in her personnel folder that states she must improve the following month. Turn to page 17

e. Say something like: "Vicki, I don't want to butt in where I'm not wanted, but at the same time you must see how your Monday absences are affecting your work. I'm concerned about this and I know you are too." Turn to page 28

Page 13

You have told Vicki that you are in charge and that she should have respect for this fact. Vicki says:

> Well, one thing I have respect for is myself. Too much respect to keep on with this dumb hospital. *I quit!*

Vicki then leaves. How do you feel at this point?

a. That you might have handled yourself differently somewhere along the line? Would you like a chance to retrace your steps to see what could be done differently?   Turn to page 9

b. That you did what any supervisor would do to correct the staff and keep them in line and make sure they know who is the boss.   The exercise is over for you.

Page 14

You telephone Vicki's home to verify her illness. There is no answer. Now what would you do?

a. Keep calling at regular intervals during the day.   Turn to page 5

b. Ask your department clerk to keep calling.   Turn to page 21

c. Wait to handle it when Vicki returns.   Turn to page 26

Reasons for your choice:

Page 15

You have responded to Vicki, "You have talked about it with your husband?" Vicki says:

> Yes, but he is so wrapped up in his two kids that he won't listen. I knew I would have problems when I married a widower, but I didn't expect this.

Which general approach would you follow then?

    a. Say, "I'm glad you realize the serious-
    ness of this, and I hope you can make
    him see it, too. I hope you will try to do
    better. Turn to page 10
    b. Say, "It's pretty tough being married to
    a widower with kids, I guess. Turn to page 33
    c. Say nothing, but continue to listen. Turn to page 18

Reasons for your choice:

Page 16

You have decided to wait until Vicki brings up the matter of her absence. She does not. However, she was present each day for the next two weeks and then misses Monday and Tuesday of the next week and is absent today (Monday). When (and if) she comes in tomorrow, what approach will you take with her?

Turn to page 9

You have placed a warning letter in Vicki's personnel folder telling her that she must improve during the following month. Vicki is absent the first two Mondays in the next month. At this point what would you do?

a. Warn Vicki what will happen if she is absent again on either of the next two Mondays?   Turn to page 35

b. Wait to see if Vicki is absent the remainder of the month?   Turn to page 37

c. Transfer her at the first opportunity.   Turn to page 34

d. Tell Vicki you don't wish to intrude on her personal problems, but you are concerned over how her absences continue to affect patient care.   Turn to page 28

e. Express to Vicki your hope that she will be able to improve this month. Then wait to see if she is absent the remainder of the month.   Turn to page 37

Reasons for your choice:

You have decided to say nothing but to continue listening. Vicki continues:

> Bill, my husband, has a teenage daughter who has been married, but it is breaking up, I guess. Also, his boy who is two years younger is supposed to be living with us, but he has run away twice in the past two months. Everything seems to happen on weekends!
>
> First the daughter comes home mad at her husband, then the husband follows and they have a scene. Sometimes they make up and go back to their house and sometimes not.
>
> Then the boy takes off and the police phone me to come and get him. Sunday night at midnight I had to drive to the next state to get him out of jail. I didn't get back till eight last night.
>
> All these things happening on weekends are very upsetting to Bill. I think he is drinking too much. He cannot help in any way. I have been afraid to leave him. But I know it is causing you problems in the hospital. I hope I can get it worked out soon.

What would your general approach be?

Page 18
(Cont.)

a. Explain to Vicki that you understand what she is dealing with and tell her that you suggest you wait two weeks to see how things look then.

Turn to page 22

b. Tell her that her personal problems are her business but that staffing is your business. Tell her to "shape up or ship out."

Turn to page 24

c. Suggest that Vicki take her problem to her family doctor or minister.

Turn to page 41

d. Explain that you are going to place a warning letter in her personnel folder that states she must improve the following month.

Turn to page 17

Reasons for your choice:

Page 19

After the situation involving Vicki and the staff, things seem calm for the next several days except for some loud laughter in her department when you are nearby. You must schedule a special assignment, for extra pay, for two-thirds of the staff on next Saturday and Sunday. Would you?

a. Exclude Vicki from special work but say nothing about it to her.

Turn to page 30

b. Exclude Vicki but tell her if she "shapes up" she will be included in the future.

Turn to page 32

c. Tell Vicki that you are scheduling her for the special assignment, but ask her to pitch in and be on your team to help with staffing. Stress the importance of everyone doing her part.

Turn to page 10

d. Call Vicki in and explain that you have wondered what to do to help her improve her attendance because it is affecting her work and you don't want to schedule her for extra work if this will complicate the problem.

Turn to page 28

Page 19 (*Cont.*)

Reasons for your choice:

Page 20

You have warned her that any more comments will be severely dealt with. Vicki says:

> That's what I mean by everybody being on my back. Well, I don't have to take it from you! *I quit!*

Vicki then heads for the exit with tears in her eyes. At this point, how do you feel?

a. That you might have handled yourself differently somewhere along the line? Would you like a chance to retrace your steps to see what could be done differently?

Turn to page 9

b. That you did what any supervisor would do to correct the staff, keep them in line, and make sure they know who is the boss?

The lesson is over for you.

Page 21

You have asked the department clerk to keep calling Vicki's home. At three P.M., he calls to say there has been no answer. When Vicki returns on Tuesday morning, what will be your approach?

Turn to page 9

Page 22

Now that Vicki has spelled out some of the main problems causing her Monday absences, let's talk about them.

There is no clear-cut "ending" to the problems given here—nor do we find one, usually, in real life. First-line supervisors are constantly dealing with people on the crew, fellow supervisors, the public, and themselves in problems such as these. Their attitudes and approach to taking action often determine "how they come out."

Vicki's problem raises some interesting questions that we might discuss:

1. Now that you know some of Vicki's problems, is it easier or more difficult to "handle" Vicki's absences?
2. Do you feel the hospital should be understanding and give Vicki time to work out her problem?
3. Would just telling you about her problem help Vicki?
4. Are you familiar with where in the hospital or community Vicki might be referred for help?

Jot down any thoughts on the above questions.

Page 23

The staff committeeperson says:

Well, Vicki's story sounded pretty wild to me. Why don't you talk it over with her and let's see how it comes out. I see no reason to be there.

Turn to page 8

Page 24

After your comment to Vicki, she doesn't say anything at the time but goes to work. That afternoon, one of the women tells you that Vicki has been telling all the staff how dirty you have treated her. Later the same afternoon as you pass Vicki, you catch a glimpse of a gesture she makes behind your back. Three other women on your staff laugh. When you turn around, Vicki is back at work. What would you do?

a. Do nothing, continue on your rounds, but keep an eye on Vicki. Turn to page 19
b. Ask the employees who laughed to tell you what they say. Turn to page 3

c. Warn Vicki that she better stick to work and forget about making comments about you and gestures toward you. Then continue walking.

Turn to page 19

d. Call Vicki over to a more private place and ask her what is on her mind.

Turn to page 8

e. Tell Vicki she is fired.

Turn to page 25

Page 24
(Cont.)

Reasons for your choice:

Page 25

You have fired Vicki. Do you feel that—without previous warning—you could make this stick? My guess is that you couldn't. At any rate, here are some questions for you:

1. Would your action cause any problems with others on the staff?
2. Were you responding to her feelings with your feelings?
3. Were you admitting to Vicki that you didn't know what else to do with her?
4. Is there nothing more to know about Vicki?

If you have answered yes to any of these questions, you may be admitting you have something to learn about the managing of people. If so, turn to the previous page and take another choice.

If you have answered no to all four, there is evidently no doubt in your mind that how you operated is the correct way.

This exercise can teach you no more.

Page 26

You have decided to wait until her return to deal with Vicki.

Turn to page 9

Page 27

> You decide to send some inexpensive flowers to her home with a "Get Well Soon" card. Tuesday, when Vicki returns, she does not mention the flowers. What would be your approach to Vicki now?
>
> Turn to page 9

Page 28

> You have told Vicki you didn't want to intrude but expressed your concern over how her absences were affecting her work. Vicki says:
>
> > I know you are concerned and I have been, too. I'm sorry it's happening but I just can't help it. I've told my husband that I might lose my job if it keeps up.
>
> What general approach would you follow then?
>
> **a.** Say, "I'm glad you realize the seriousness of this and hope you can make him see it too. Vicki, I hope you will try to do better."   Turn to page 10
>
> **b.** Say, "You have talked about it to your husband?"   Turn to page 15
>
> **c.** Say nothing, but continue to listen.   Turn to page 18
>
> **d.** Impress Vicki with the seriousness of this in a business situation, and warn her that she must improve or take the consequences.   Turn to page 35
>
> *Reasons for your choice:*

Page 29

> You have removed the warning letter from her file and told her you hoped she would keep up the good record she has started. Vicki may or may not be absent on future Mondays. If she is, then that is another problem. Did you ever wonder just what Vicki's problem was? Other paths led to her telling you, and perhaps you would like to hear her describe it also. If so. . .
>
> Turn to page 18
>
> Then turn to page 22, and let's discuss the questions there.

Page 30

You decide to exclude Vicki from special assignments. You say nothing to her directly, but inform the other staff people of your decision.

Turn to page 36

Page 31

After Vicki was present each Monday for the remainder of the month, you told her to "keep up the good work." Vicky says, "I'm certainly trying." Vicki is in attendance for the next three weeks, including the special assignment. At the end of this time, what would you do?

    a. Nothing?   Turn to page 39
    b. Tell Vicki that you were removing the letter from her file, and express the hope that she is able to keep up the good record she has started.   Turn to page 29

Reasons for your choice:

Page 32

You decide to exclude Vicki from the special assignment, but you tell her if she "shapes up," she will be included in the future. Vicki says nothing but goes back to work.

Turn to page 36

Page 33

You remarked to Vicki how tough it must be to be married to a widower with kids. Vicki says, "Boy, I'll say." She then clams up. What general approach would you use then?

    a. Say, "I'm glad you realize the seriousness of this, and I hope you can make him see it too. Vicki, I hope you will try to do better."   Turn to page 10
    b. Say nothing, but continue to listen.   Turn to page 18

Reasons for your choice:

Page 34

You have transferred Vicki at the first opportunity. That got rid of your problem nicely, didn't it? Yet what about the hospital, of which you are part of the first-line management? Did you really fulfill your responsibility as a supervisor?

Return to your previous page, and make another decision.

Page 35

You have reminded Vicki what will happen if she is absent again on Monday. Vicki is there the next Monday.

On the following Monday, you notice Vicki at lunch time sitting by herself looking flushed and ill. When you ask her what the trouble is, Vicki says she feels quite sick. You send her to the emergency room, and they send her home. You receive word that Vicki had a fever of 103° and was dangerously ill.

Vicki was reported to have told the nurse that she was afraid you would have her fired if she stayed home ill. Vicki is absent for six days.

When she returns, what will be your approach to her?

a. Tell her that, despite her illness, she is still under the warning letter because of her Monday absences and that she must improve.   Turn to page 24

b. Tell her that you are "wiping the slate" and hope she has no more trouble in the future.   Turn to page 10

c. Say that you are sorry she was ill—that you don't want to intrude, but ask her if the difficulty she was having with the Monday absences looks cleared up.   Turn to page 28

d. Say nothing to Vicki.   Turn to page 36

Page 36

That afternoon, the hospital grievance committeeperson tells you that Vicki has brought a grievance against you, and she charges you with persecuting her. Would you?

a. Tell the committeeperson the charges are ridiculous and dare him to put them in writing and into arbitration.   Turn to page 38

Page 36
(*Cont.*)

b. Tell the committeeperson the situation
and say that you wish to talk to Vicki
about it, and he also can be present if
he and Vicki wish.   Turn to page 23

Reasons for your choice:

Page 37

You have waited to see if Vicki is absent the remainder of the month.
She is not. At this point, what action would you take?

a. You would do nothing.   Turn to page 39
b. You would tell Vicki to keep up the
good work.   Turn to page 31
c. You would tell Vicki that you were removing the letter from her file and express the hope that she is able to keep
up the good record she has started.   Turn to page 29

Reasons for your choice:

Page 38

You have dared the committeeperson to put the charges into writing.
The next day he comes in with a lengthy statement of charges con-
taining not only Vicki's remarks, but testimony from quite a few others
on your staff. After a few minutes, it is apparent there is nothing to be
gained by discussing it; so you sign it and kick it upstairs.

So there it is. You may win the final arbitration on this basis of Vicki's
absenteeism, but it will be a long road between here and there. And
it certainly won't help your relations with your staff—and there is still
Vicki to deal with. At this point, how do you feel?

a. That you did what any supervisor would
do to correct the staff, keep them in
line, and make sure they know who is
the boss.   The lesson is over
for you.

Page 38
(*Cont.*)

b. That you might have handled yourself differently along the line? Would you like a chance to retrace your steps to see what could be done differently?

Go back to page 9

Page 39

You would do nothing after Vicki was not absent the remainder of the month. Why not? Vicki seems to be trying to do what you wish her to. One principle of teaching desired behavior is to reward it when it happens.

Turn back to your previous page and reward Vicki.

Page 40

You have contacted the personnel counselor to get some help on your problem. The counselor is unable to help since you are unable to say what Vicki's problem is. You then decide to discuss it with Vicki.

Turn to page 9

Page 41

You have suggested that Vicki take her problem to her family doctor or minister. Vicki says:

Well, we are not really churchgoers, and we don't have a regular doctor.

Turn to page 18

Page 42

No place in this book were you instructed to turn to this page! Return to your previous page, and get back on the track.

APPLICATION: SUPERVISORY ROLE PLAYING

Objectives

Nursing supervisors can use the techniques of role playing to teach and to enforce proper actions to their staffs. It is very helpful to use role playing in your staff meetings to assist the group in improving their dealings with others. The nonthreatening atmosphere and actual

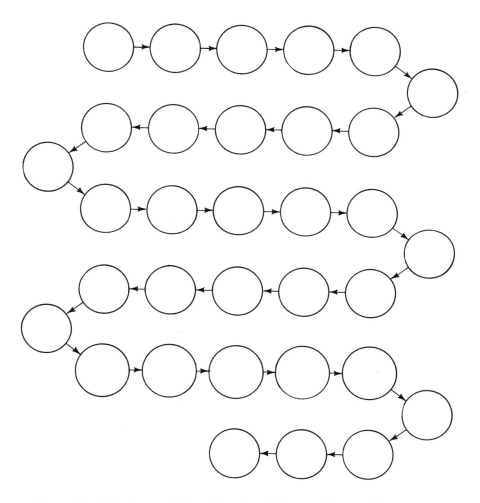

Figure 14–1. Path record chart. Starting with page #1, record in sequence the pages to which you turn in solving this personnel problem. As mentioned in the case booklet, there is no one way of solving this problem. Your answers, however, can provide insight on your particular managerial style.

fun of acting out parts give you valuable insight into the feelings and actions of your subordinates and your fellow supervisors. This type of situation creates a very favorable learning experience for you and for everyone involved.

It takes no special training to set up a role-playing situation. The only requirements are that you and your group are willing to commit yourselves to the task and that you are willing to use the experience for a learning tool. The interpretation of the situations becomes easily apparent as the role playing progresses. It is very easy to see errors in judgment and to correct them. Practicing the interpersonal relationships necessary to deal with others gives you an opportunity to hear how words and actions hear and feel, and you can take steps to eliminate any problems in the future.

As a supervisor, you should become familiar with this technique and use it often to help develop the leadership skills of your staff. Role playing also serves to give you feedback on how your subordinates would like to be treated, if you allow them to play the leadership role and display how they would handle a given situation.

Henry C. Smith, in his *Psychology of Industrial Behavior,* outlines a format for a role-playing session in leadership training. Role playing can be extremely effective in practicing disciplinary actions. The chance to practice techniques in a classroom setting is helpful to avoid errors when the real situations occur.

Directions

1. Begin with a short discussion of the general area of the problems to be discussed.
2. Select two of the trainees, and send them out of the room.
3. Describe to the group the problem that will be acted out.
4. Select a member of the group still in the room to play the role of the subordinate.
5. With the help of the class, decide the various methods by which the "supervisor" should be able to solve the problem. Instruct the group to look for these factors while the play is in progress so that they may be discussed in a critique later.
6. Set the stage. Use as many props as possible to make the situation realistic.
7. Call in one of the two trainees waiting outside. Instruct him or her as to the role as the "supervisor" in the play and present the problem. Have the trainee take a place and proceed.
8. End the play when you have decided it has gone on long enough.
9. Recap the play, and outline the action and solutions to the problems—if any—that were accomplished during the play. Use a blackboard or flip chart to record the impressions. The evaluation should include a discussion of the following questions:
   a. How well did the actors fit the roles they were playing?
   b. How well and how often did the "actor" playing the part of the supervisor alter his or her behavior to fit the reactions of the partner in the play?
   c. How much and in what ways did the actors change their behavior to fit their roles?
   d. What method(s) was (were) used to solve the problem?
   e. How could the play have been "performed" better?

10. Cover the board or chart so that it is not visible during the next session.
11. Call in the second trainee, and go through the routine again, using the same actor to play the part of subordinate.
12. After the second play, recap the action as in the first. Compare the two.
13. Ask the three players to critique their own actions. This allows them to save face in front of the group by pointing out their own errors.
14. Using the blackboard or flip chart again, work out with the players and the other trainees a third solution to the problem, based upon the experiences gained during the plays and the consensus of the group.
15. Select another member of the group who has not yet played a part and have him or her play the part of the supervisor as outlined by the group (the third solution). Instruct the group to watch carefully for any flaws in what they have set up as "preferred" behavior.

HYPOTHETICAL ROLE-PLAY PROBLEMS

Role-Playing Situation #1 (Self-test)

Assume for the moment that you are a 21-year-old RN, a vision in white, working at last on a real ward of a real hospital. You've been there only a few weeks when you're made a team leader and assigned an aide you've never worked with before. She is 47 years old. She has worked at the hospital for 15 years, and she does not respond to your eager smile as you divide the work. Oh yes, you are white, and she is black.

It's midmorning now, and you note that the aide has done only two of her five patients. You find her visiting with two other aides, and you tell her, with a smile, "Miss Johnson, you'll have to hurry to do your other patients before the lunch trays get here." Miss Johnson's expression does not change. She eyes you silently for a moment and then says, "Well, if you're in such a hurry, maybe you'd better take care of them yourself."

Which of the following do you say?

a. Nothing. You leave as gracefully as possible; then, after lunch, you do the patients.
b. "Now look, we have to get the work done. And it's a lot easier if everyone cooperates."

363

c. "Would it help if we did them together?"

d. "I have my own work to do. I expect you to finish with them by 12:00 o'clock.

e. "Are you refusing to do your work?"

If you chose a or c, you have a lot of company:

1. What else is there to do but do it yourself?

2. I just try to avoid friction. It means that I must do the aide's work sometimes, but that is what I do. I know I should be able to handle it better, but I sure don't know how.

3. Aides think that desk work is loafing.

4. The problem is that the aides cannot be disciplined, and they know it.

If you chose b, you will be as frustrated as those who picked a and c:

1. Trying to develop a team spirit along with team nursing.

2. Patient care meetings, allowing the aides to contribute, handling everything democratically—it still seems that they do as little as possible.

3. Trying to get along on a social level—okay unless they do not accept.

If you chose d:

1. If you really mean it, that response may work. Too often this is an empty threat.

2. All the nurse has to do is let that aide know she means it, and that's the end of the problem. Yet you'd be surprised how many experienced nurses still haven't learned that.

If you chose response e:

1. The key to this answer is "letting them know."

2. We tell our nurses to stand their ground—not to hassle, not to give in, not to apologize. Most of the time, the aide intends to do the work all along. Saying no is just a challenge some of them need, especially if they have an audience.

3. Ask them if they are refusing. If they are, that is insubordination, and disciplinary steps will be taken.

4. The aide knew she was wrong all along, and as soon as she finds out the RN is not going to take that answer, the chances of her trying it again with that RN are greatly reduced, especially if she does have an audience. She may show personal hostility for a while, but the RN has an effective person working for her.

5. But what about the union?
  a. Do not be afraid. The union works for the nurse.
    1. Spells out the aide's job.
    2. The union contract spells out the meaning of insubordination.
6. What about nonunion places?
  a. Everything may be centralized. No decisions in the patient care area.
  b. Head nurses had full responsibility for the personnel, but no authority over them.
  c. Get 24-hour-a-day supervisors with full authority to hire and fire aides and ward clerks. With authority, discipline improves and morale is higher.

The aide's point of view:

1. Every year they are confronted with new graduates who dictate to them, even though they may have more experience.
2. Some new girls like to prove that they are running the show.
3. Aides don't know what they are expected to do.
4. Nurses worry more about the functioning of the floor, whether everything is getting done on time, than they do about patient care.

Role-Playing Situation #2

PARTICIPANTS Supervisor—Mrs. Know-it-all
Staff Nurse—Miss Easy-go
Staff Physician—Dr. Freelove

SITUATION You are the day supervisor in a small hospital in a community where everyone knows everyone else.

Nurse Easy-go is 25 years old, single, and very pretty. You have heard rumors that she is too friendly with one of the more prominent married doctors on staff, Dr. Freelove. This situation has been brought to your attention many times, by many people. The reports indicate that their behavior is obvious to other staff members and to patients. It has even been said that they are carrying on a blatant affair in the hospital. You have never personally witnessed any behavior that would indicate the truth to these rumors, but you feel that you should talk to Miss Easy-go about the situation.

DIRECTIONS FOR THE SUPERVISOR You are calling Miss Easy-go into your office to talk to her. Handle the situation in any way you wish.

DIRECTIONS FOR MISS EASY-GO You have been called into the supervisor's office. You do not know why you have been called in, but you have a sneaking suspicion that it might concern your relationship with Dr. Freelove, and you are very anxious.

Allow the play to continue until it no longer accomplishes work, and then allow a lengthy period of time to discuss the actions and how they could be improved.

Additional Role-Playing Situations

1. A supervisor finds a nurse missing from the hospital and finds her sleeping in her car.
2. A nurse, arriving late at report, creates a disturbance by her raucous behavior in the back of the room.
3. A nurse is reported to have been punching in and out for her friends.
4. A nurse is observed going through a patient's drawer; later the patient's family reports missing money and jewelry.
5. A nurse is consistently arriving for work in dirty uniforms.
6. A nurse gives her supervisor two tickets to the Laguna Art Festival and then, a week later, asks for a special day off that she is not actually entitled to.
7. A nurse is habitually 10 to 15 minutes late to report, but she is likewise habitually working late a half hour to 45 minutes at the end of the day.
8. A new graduate, obviously a misfit who somehow passed her boards, asks a stupid question in front of about six of her fellow nurses. She has asked this same question and received a detailed answer to the question at least 47 times already.

REFERENCES

NEWMAN, WILLIAM, H., *Administrative Action*, 2nd ed. Englewood Cliffs, N.J.: Prentice-Hall, Inc., 1963.

NIGRO, FELIX, A., *Modern Public Administration*. New York: Harper & Row, Publishers, 1965.

15

Collective bargaining in nursing

Nursing associations have been in existence for over fifty years. Just recently these associations and many outside labor unions have sought a voice in labor negotiations with management. These associations seek to be the voice of nurses in expressing their grievances with health care management.

The social change within our society has created a new militancy within the ranks of nurses. Nurses look at themselves differently today. They see no reason why, in an affluent society, they should be discriminated against and expected to accept, without complaint, salaries and working conditions worse than those of employees in business or industry. Nurses have the same desire as any other worker to participate in management decisions and to be treated with dignity. In a period of social upheaval, as one group succeeds in making gains, other groups are bound to try to improve their status also, imitating the tactics used by the private business sector to accomplish these goals.

To a large extent, the union movement in health care is a revolt of professional workers who are redefining their roles and remaking their self-images. Nurses are seeking greater control over decisions affecting patient care. The major issues facing nurses today involve this lack of control. Some of these issues are:

1. *A Voice in Nursing Assignments:* Traditionally, the assignment of patient care has been the sole privilege of management. Nurses are expressing fears that managements, in the interest of greater profits, are sending unprepared nurses into specialized units and that they are reducing the nurse-patient ratio to dangerous levels

2. *The Use of Paraprofessionals:* One of the concerns frequently raised by nurses is to seek curbs on replacing registered nurses with personnel not qualified to give professional nursing care.

3. *Relief from Non-Nursing Duties:* Nursing organizations are making efforts to relieve registered nurses from clerical and housekeeping chores.

4. *Continuing Education:* Nurses want time off and financial assistance to obtain continuing education. They want the health care agency to provide quality programs during working hours on all shifts.

5. *Salary Increases:* Along with pay boosts, nurses seek increased finge benefits; hospitalization, longer vacations, more days off, less frequent weekend and holiday assignments, and extra pay for overtime.

These are only a few of the problems confronting nurses today, but they seem to be the major issues expressed by the majority of nurses. For these reasons, some nurses feel the only solution is to unite in the form of collective bargaining to accomplish their goals. This movement does not mean that nurses want a revolution. Actually, they are very willing to work cooperatively with management, as long as they are assured that some change will occur. How quickly these changes occur depends on several variables:

1. The degree of the nurses' determination in an individual health care agency.
2. The attitude of nurses toward a union.
3. The activity of state and other associations.
4. The impact of non-nursing unions.
5. The geographic location of the health care agency. Urban areas seek change more aggressively than rural areas.

Why do so many nurses want to see changes made? Many nurses have the feeling that they are being left behind in the economy and also in their own health care agency. Nurses feel that they are no longer the doctor's handmaidens but defenders of patients' rights. Nurses are getting more aggressive in protecting patients' interests. One of the most direct new ways is by setting up private nursing practices to offset impersonal medical care.

Other nurses are fighting for patients within traditional hospital channels. The impact of the women's movement has done much to raise the level of consciousness in some nurses. Nurses are thinking in terms of their rights as women and of their rights as employees. The first stage of the militants' approach is therefore to assert their equality with doctors. When doctors walked into a hospital room years ago, the nurse automatically stood up to give them a seat. Today nurses sit tight. The subordinate relationship of the nurse to the doctor has sometimes interfered with the nurse's ability to give good care. Many nurses are hesitant to make suggestions to the doctor because they feel they would be stepping out of their role.

Another target of the nurses' militancy is the hospital administration. One of the main complaints voiced by nurses is that poor hospital organization prevents them from treating patients as human beings. The organization's quest for profit seems to detract from quality patient care.

Will nurses take all the trappings of collective bargaining and continue to strike? Most nurses feel that this is not necessary. Nurses who were dissatisfied in the past had only one alternative, to leave their jobs. Now, with the assistance of collective bargaining units, there is a channel for bargaining and negotiation. Union leaders state that the flare-up of strikes seen in the past was just a reaction of those few nurses who felt that all necessary change should be accomplished "yesterday." All unions agree that the "strike" is a poor alternative, and that it should not be used unless absolutely necessary.

The question of whether or not to allow unions to enter nursing is no longer pertinent. The unions *are* in nursing, and they will remain. The situation for the nursing supervisor is to understand the labor union and to be able to work cooperatively with its representatives.

HOW ORGANIZING WORKS

Assume that a health care agency does not have a collective bargaining unit at the present time. The nurses in this hospital may feel that their interest would be best served by the negotiations of a bargaining agent. The usual first step is to seek help from a professional group, such as a state nursing association. This is done because the state nursing associations are usually well aware of the problems facing nursing. The feeling of may nurses is that uniting with an outside agency such as the Teamsters Union would swallow up nursing and cause the profession to lose its identity. In some cases, the union takes the initiative and contacts the nurses in an agency to see if there is any interest in joining a labor union.

If the nurses in the agency decide that they do indeed wish to use a collective bargaining association, the next step is to get support signatures from 30-percent of the nurses in the agency. Without this 30-percent support, the association is not allowed to make approaches to the staff. After the petition with the 30-percent of signatures is obtained, the bargaining agency files the petition with the National Labor Relations Board. This indicates to the Labor Relations Board that the agency is interested in representing the nurses and that the nurses have shown the required desire. If the National Labor Relations Board agrees that the petitioning union has the right to represent the nurses, the union goes back to the health care institution to enlist membership. For a bargaining agency to work in a health care agency, a secret ballot election must be held.

All nurses in the agency are asked whether or not they wish to have the union represent their interests. The vote must pass a 50-per-cent-plus-one-vote majority of all the nurses who took part in the election. Notice, this is 50-percent-plus-one of the nurses *participating* in the election, not of all the nurses in the institution. If the vote passes, the union is the official representative of the nursing staff with management.

What if the vote passes by a razor thin majority? Do all nurses have to join the union and participate in its decisions? This subject is open to negotiation between the union representatives and the health care agency management. The nurses may or may not be forced to participate. The question of paying dues is also an issue for negotiation. In many cases, all nurses in an agency that has collective bargaining are required to pay dues to the union, whether or not they voted for its approval. The only exception to this is a nurse who is not permitted to join a collective bargaining agency on religious grounds. In one important court case, though, a nurse who declined to pay dues on religious grounds was forced to donate the amount of her dues to that religious agency.

Once the vote has passed, the union then gets together with the management of the health care agency to work out a contract proposal. When the contract proposal has been written, the nurses are asked again to vote on the issue: whether or not to accept the proposal. These negotiations take many months, even years, to develop.

THE STRIKE QUESTION

When the subject of collective bargaining is discussed, the first thought in everyone's mind is always the question of striking. In a critical industry such as nursing the power of a strike is a real threat. Although most collective bargaining agencies try to avoid strikes, they do occur if arbitration between labor and management cannot be reached. Because of the necessity of providing health care needs to the community, the National Labor Relations Board has set strict requirements for the strike process.

If a union is proposing a strike, they must give the health care agency thirty days written notice of the intent to strike. Once the notice has been served, a Federal Mediation and Conciliation Service is called in to try and prevent the strike by settling the dispute. If no agreement can be reached, then the organization must give ten days written notice to the health care agency so that emergency procedures can be set up.

WHO CAN JOIN A LABOR UNION?

In the question of collective bargaining, the position of the nurse/leaders must be taken into consideration. The guidelines set up by the Labor Relations Board for industry do not fit into nursing. The basic rule of union membership is that a person in a supervisory capacity is not allowed to join a labor union. The industrial definition of supervisory capacity is "any person who functions using independent judgment and action." In nursing, that definition fits every nurse who works in any type of patient care function. It means that no one in nursing could participate in collective bargaining. Although each state requirement is different, the basic criterion for who is management and who is not centers around the degree of professional responsibility the nurse possesses. Nurses are not considered supervisors if their professional responsibility is solely related to patient care. The ability to hire and fire or to work with time schedules is one factor that automatically places a nurse in the "management" category.

There is much disagreement on whether or not supervisors should be allowed to enter negotiations. Some health care agencies want their supervisors to participate so that they have a voice in the proceedings. Other agencies want head nurses and above excluded so that the staff is not too powerful in the arbitration. Most supervisors do not wish to participate in labor unions because they feel that it causes a conflict of interest and reduces their effectiveness in their positions.

The decision as to whether or not to participate in labor unions is an individual decision, which nurses must consider carefully. One study of labor unions showed that if there is a labor union working in a health care agency, their representatives are at times inclined to oppose, on principle alone, any change suggested by management. You must realize that the union was not hired to cooperate with management, but to change it. The role of the union is to protect the interests of each individual member. Management tends to be the "big bad wolf." The employee is usually more comfortable with a fighting union representative than with one who cooperates fully with the organizational management. When you consider the function of the representative, you can understand that the members figure the representatives are doing a good job only if they are constantly battling.

Unions are always met with some resistance, even in cases where the health care agency leaders recognize that the proposed changes are good both for the union members and for the health care facility. The whole question of collective bargaining brings a multitude of emotions into play. You, as a supervisor, must deal with these feelings and learn to work within the framework set by the union.

Using the union as an excuse for not accomplishing the work of supervision is not acceptable. Granted, the grievance procedures of the labor unions make it difficult to initiate discipline. Difficult, but not impossible. Follow the established procedures and follow through on all grievance procedures, and your diligence will eventually be rewarded. No one promises that it will be easy, but working *with* unions reaps more benefits that fighting the system or giving up.

WHERE IS IT ALL GOING?

What will hospitals be like when nurses get more power? One example is a New York hospital established for recuperative periods for clients. Although physicians check up on their patients and order medications, nurses are in charge of the hospital. The nurses have abolished rigid rules and routines. Patients eat when they are hungry and sleep when they are tired. No longer are patients tied to the organizational clock. Most agencies are seeking to meet the total needs of each patient by allowing registered nurses the freedom to meet the emotional and physical needs of patients. Nurses use primary care and are able to plan, direct, and coordinate the care of patients. Licensed practical nurses are given only routine patient care duties or housekeeping duties.

Other health care agencies are trying new and creative ways to keep the professional nurses functioning in a nursing role. The idea of flexible scheduling is one way to keep inactive nurses in the health care setting by allowing them the freedom to pursue their professional responsibilities as well as their home commitments.

One California hospital is using a vastly different approach to administer patient care. In this institution, all staff members are paid a minimum wage, no matter what their position. The hospital has set stringent criteria for levels of expected behaviors, and each member of the staff is paid according to his or her own individual output. In the case of nursing service, a nurse given an assignment that should take eight nursing hours is paid for those hours. If she does less than that amount of work, she is paid less. In essence she is paid per patient. Admittedly, this is a very controversial plan, but it does illustrate quite vividly one agency's plan to revamp the image of nursing.

Other agencies are charging the patient for services rendered similar to a hotel setting. In other words, the patient pays a standard room rate for sleeping in the bed. If the patient requires 8 hours of nursing care in 24, he pays for that service on a standard scale. Lab, X-ray, linen, housekeeping, and the like are all additional charges. The food service is charged as it would be in a restaurant. The patients who are NPO pay nothing for food. For a liquid diet, they may pay $2.50

per meal. When patients progress to a regular diet, they are given a menu with prices listed. If they choose meatloaf, they pay for meatloaf; lobster has a much higher price tag. This particular hospital feels that this system answers the constant question, "Why is health care so expensive?"

Some health care agencies are taking the clerical duties away from the nursing staff by installing complex computer systems that eliminate the need for charting, requisitions, and any other paperwork. All patient care needs are ordered and recorded by a computer. The nursing staff uses the computer to punch in and out, to record care, to read patient charts, and to plan the patient care loads.

There have been some encouraging developments for nurses outside the hospital, too. Some nurses are setting up private practices to fill the gap left by the medical community. These nurses feel that doctors do not spend enough time talking over their patients' problems. These nurses are on call 24 hours a day and make home visits to meet the needs of patients. They also offer free counseling on the phone and charge a modest fee for home visits.

Although nurses cannot diagnose disease or prescribe medication except under standard orders, they can independently take steps to prevent illness and make nursing interventions. The important thing to remember is that today's nurses have options. They are not tied to the traditional role unless they choose to be. Nurses can assist patients in obtaining objective facts about their medical care and in learning to make their own decisions concerning medical care.

The trend, as most nurses see it, is toward a newly aggressive nurse. We can anticipate a new era in health care, when the nurse is a partisan for patients, instead of a mere handmaiden blindly following orders. The nurse/supervisor or nurse/leader will be a contributing member of the team, not a slave to the medical bureaucracy.

NURSING ASSOCIATIONS (UNIONS)

Definitions

Agreement   A written contract between an employer and an employee organization, usually for a definite term, defining conditions of employment (wages, hours, vacations, holidays, overtime payments, working conditions, and so on) and procedures to be followed in settling disputes or handling issues that arise during the life of the agreement.

Arbitration   A method of settling disputes through recourse to an impartial third party. The primary use of arbitration involves the interpretation of the terms of an existing contract. Arbitration involving the interpretation of the terms of an existing contract is usually final and binding, which means the award is enforceable in court.

Collective Bargaining A process by which an employee organization negotiates with an employer in good faith with a view toward reaching agreement on wages, hours, and conditions of employment. The process does not require either party to agree to any particular proposal, nor does it require the making of a concession.

Injunction A court order restraining individuals, groups, or employee organizations from committing unlawful acts or acts which, in the court's opinion, will cause irreparable harm or endanger public health, safety, or welfare.

Strike Temporary stoppage of work by a group of employees (not necessarily union members) to express a grievance, to enforce a demand for changes in the conditions of employment, to obtain recognition, or to resolve a dispute with management. *Wildcat strike* is a strike that is not sanctioned by the union and that violates a collective agreement. *Quickie strike* is a spontaneous or unannounced strike. *Showdown* is a deliberate reduction of output without an actual strike in order to force concessions from an employer. *Sympathy strike* is a strike of employees not directly involved in a dispute, but who wish to demonstrate employee solidarity or bring additional pressure upon employer. *Sitdown strike* is a strike during which employees remain in the workplace, but they refuse to work or allow others to do so. *General strike* is a strike involving all organized employees in a community or country. *Walkout* is the same as a strike.

Employee Any person employed by a public or private agency except elected officers.

Employee Organization An organization that includes employees of the public or private agency and that has as one of its primary purposes representing such employees in their relations with such agencies.

Employee Relations The employer/employee relationship between the agency and its employees and their legally constituted employee organizations.

Fact Finding The investigation of an impasse by an impartial third party for the purpose of describing the issues in dispute, stating the positions of the parties, making findings of fact on the issues in dispute, making advisory recommendations for settlement of the dispute.

Management Employee Includes both administrative management employees and supervisory employees.

Mediation The efforts of an impartial third party functioning as an intermediary, to assist the parties in reaching a voluntary resolution of an impasse through interpretation, suggestion, and advice.

APPLICATION: A CASE STUDY
IN HEALTH CARE LABOR RELATIONS
AND MANAGEMENT

Statement of the Problem

Whether to officially recognize the State Nurse's Association as a legally constituted and exclusive bargaining agent, dealing with all employee grievances and labor-relations problems, or to accept an outside labor union, nationally recognized (A.F. of L.–C.I.O.) as the new bargaining agent in all health care employee/labor-relations negotiations.

Relevant Facts
Concerning the Situation

This problem takes place in a large metropolitan city in the Eastern part of the United States. The city has been a major focal point of massive changes over the past twenty years. With a large commercial airport and one of the nation's largest seaports, it is a year-round tourist attraction.

The hospital in question is a large publicly financed institution, having at its head an administrator and a governing board. Within the organization is a nursing association that has been in existence for over fifty years. It has been the nurses' exclusive bargaining agent for the past ten years, although it has not been recognized as an official bargaining agent by the administration or the board. The nursing association has intervened in a number of labor relations and employee grievance problems, essentially in an arbitration capacity. Recently the association has become a rather powerful political organization, having a strong lobby within its framework, and has tended to become a more militant foe in contractual negotiations. Important, however, is the fact that under its leadership, the association has opposed unions and strikes.

In the recent past, relations between the administration and the staff have been fragmented. Serious problems have arisen dealing with specific questions such as the principle of salary standardization ("equal pay for equal work"), promotion, nursing care ratios, merit determinations, disciplinary problems, requirements for promotional advancement, uniform allowance, and others.

The most critical problem facing the administration is the association's demand for a contractual guarantee that the nursing units would be staffed with a realistic ratio of patients to staff. The association was worried that the hospital might return to the practice of assigning only

375

minimum staff to each unit and of using on-call, float, or registry help to fill in the gaps. The administration refused to bargain this question, on the grounds that it was management's responsibility, not the employees, to decide how to carry out the nursing function. As a result of this decision, fragmentation has grown to monstrous proportions. There have been massive work slowdowns, "sick-ins," and other actions. The A.F. of L.–C.I.O. has been working in close harmony with the nursing association as it is currently seeking the implementation of a full-scale nursing union as a collective bargaining agent for the nursing association. If implementation occurs, there is no doubt that the administration will lose a great deal of power in all aspects of labor relations and grievance questions.

Possible Decisions

After evaluating the various possibilities and a number of alternatives, a final reduction of possible decisions was presented to the administration for their selection and ratification:

1. Continue to recognize the nurses' association as an exclusive bargaining agent.
2. Accept the A.F. of L.–C.I.O.'s organization of an independent nursing union to represent the employees in all labor–management disputes.
3. Utilize a hospital commission "ad hoc" committee comprised of equal representation from the nursing staff and the management.
4. Allow the use of a previously tried method of administrator's "open-door" policy, which permits any and all nursing leaders to make an appointment, whenever the occasion arises, and meet with the administration on an informal basis to discuss any grievances. This approach had the approval of the nursing association.
5. Establish the use of both the formal and informal communications channels to deal with the administration using a liaison person (a nurse) assigned as a facilitator for all collective bargaining sessions.
6. Adopt the use of the city Labor Commission as a labor–management body to engage in all grievance matters requiring arbitration.
7. Establish a new Employees Relations Division to provide liaison between the management of this hospital and those of legitimate organizations to which employees of the hospital presently belong.
8. Reorganize the present Personnel Division so as to include an equally represented (employee–management) Collective Bar-

gaining Unit, to handle all personnel and labor relations grievance problems.

9. Establish a twelve-person Personnel Grievance Board to look into, evaluate, and make recommendations regarding labor–management disputes.

10. Establish a neutral Labor Relations Office outside the hospital structure, which would be responsive to all employees and management personnel. It would have major labor relations responsibilities, including preparation for contract negotiations as well as monitoring of contract interpretations.

What Would You Do?

FINAL DECISION   The decision was made to institute new Personnel and Labor Relations Units, to deal more effectively with management–employee relations.

DECISION IMPLEMENTATION   This solution was implemented by establishing an Employee Relations Section within the Personnel Department. The administrator placed the personnel officers within the management unit, while the Employee Relations Section (ERS) was a staff unit. As a staff unit, the Employee Relations Section engages in programs to carry out management's obligations, to discover potential grievances so that they can be brought to the attention of the line and administrative units concerned for resolution.

The ERS's function includes advising supervisors concerning management–employee problems, as well as procedures and assistance in identifying and resolving frictions.

EVALUATION AND COMMENTS   The Employee Relations Section was staffed by a nursing supervisor, several head nurses, and from nine to twelve staff nurses.

Organizationally situated in the Personnel Bureau, ERS, in fact, is the Administration Unit, reporting directly to the Bureau and to no one else. Such is the ERS leader's role, that she does not go through her nominal superior, the Director of Personnel, and she does not attend the staff meetings of the Personnel Bureau. This special relationship has meant that ERS recommendations concerning individual labor–relations and grievances problems carry very special weight in the hospital.

Recently there has been a period of refinement for the hospital's labor and personnel relations. For the first time, an outside expert has become the Director of Labor Relations and, after a review, has reorganized the nursing care delivery systems.

Finally there have been some very important changes that have brought a closer relationship with the nursing association.

APPLICATION: LIFE/CAREER
PLANNING EXERCISE

> Man has to live with the body and soul which have fallen to him by chance. And the first thing he has to do is to decide what he is going to be.
>
> *Jose Ortega Y Gasset*

Life Inventory

Imagine that you will die ten years from now. Write a letter from one of your best friends, to another good friend, telling him or her about you and your life. What do you *want* that letter writer to be able to say about you?

- What do I do well?
- What do I dislike doing that I must do in my present circumstances?
- What do I want (or need) to do better?
- What dreams do I have (that is wishes that I have not turned into plans)?

Career Inventory

Now prepare a "Career Inventory" (as a subset to "Life Inventory") that answers the following questions:

- Which kinds of work experiences give the greatest satisfaction?
- Which of my skills and talents are most highly valued by the organization?
- What are my "flat sides" in the work environment in terms of interpersonal competence, technical competence, managerial competence, and so on?
- What do I dislike in my present situation?
- Which rewards mean the most to me: status, money, power, recognition, achievement, sense of growth, sense of challenge, risk-taking, winning, close team relations, doing my own thing, and so on?
- What new career areas would I like to explore?
- What new skills do I want to develop?

Finally, write down goals, steps to be taken to reach them, and target dates.

REFERENCES

DIEKELMANN, NANCY L. AND MARTIN M. BROADWELL, *The New Hospital Supervisor*. Reading, Mass.: Addison-Wesley Publishing Company, 1977.

DOUGLASS, LAURA MAE AND EM OLIVIA BEVIS, *Nursing Leadership in Action*. St. Louis: The C.V. Mosby Company, 1974.

MAHLER, WALTER R. *Diagnostic Studies*. Reading, Mass.: Addison-Wesley Publishing Company, 1974.

RUBIN, IRWIN M., RONALD E. FRY, AND MARK S. PLOVNICK, *Managing Resources in Health Care Organizations*. Reston, Va: Reston Publishing Co., 1978.

Index

Index